Effective Techniques for Managing Trigeminal Neuralgia

Steven Chang
Stanford University, USA

Allen Ho
Stanford University, USA

A volume in the Advances in Medical Diagnosis, Treatment, and Care (AMDTC) Book Series

IGI Global
DISSEMINATOR OF KNOWLEDGE

Published in the United States of America by
IGI Global
Medical Information Science Reference (an imprint of IGI Global)
701 E. Chocolate Avenue
Hershey PA, USA 17033
Tel: 717-533-8845
Fax: 717-533-8661
E-mail: cust@igi-global.com
Web site: http://www.igi-global.com

Library of Congress Cataloging-in-Publication Data

Names: Chang, Steven D., editor. | Ho, Allen, 1987- editor.
Title: Effective techniques for managing trigeminal neuralgia / Steven Chang and Allen Ho, editors.
Description: Hershey PA : Medical Information Science Reference, [2018]
Identifiers: LCCN 2017040554| ISBN 9781522553496 (hardcover) | ISBN 9781522553502 (ebook)
Subjects: | MESH: Trigeminal Neuralgia--therapy
Classification: LCC RC346 | NLM WL 544 | DDC 616.8--dc23 LC record available at https://lccn.loc.gov/2017040554

This book is published in the IGI Global book series Advances in Medical Diagnosis, Treatment, and Care (AMDTC) (ISSN: 2475-6628; eISSN: 2475-6636)

British Cataloguing in Publication Data
A Cataloguing in Publication record for this book is available from the British Library.

Advances in Medical Diagnosis, Treatment, and Care (AMDTC) Book Series

ISSN:2475-6628
EISSN:2475-6636

MISSION

Advancements in medicine have prolonged the life expectancy of individuals all over the world. Once life-threatening conditions have become significantly easier to treat and even cure in many cases. Continued research in the medical field will further improve the quality of life, longevity, and wellbeing of individuals.

The **Advances in Medical Diagnosis, Treatment, and Care (AMDTC)** book series seeks to highlight publications on innovative treatment methodologies, diagnosis tools and techniques, and best practices for patient care. Comprised of comprehensive resources aimed to assist professionals in the medical field apply the latest innovations in the identification and management of medical conditions as well as patient care and interaction, the books within the AMDTC series are relevant to the research and practical needs of medical practitioners, researchers, students, and hospital administrators.

COVERAGE

- Cancer Treatment
- Internal Medicine
- Patient Interaction
- Disease Prevention
- Patient-Centered Care
- Medical Testing
- Chronic Conditions
- Disease Management
- Medical Procedures
- Diagnostic Medicine

IGI Global is currently accepting manuscripts for publication within this series. To submit a proposal for a volume in this series, please contact our Acquisition Editors at Acquisitions@igi-global.com or visit: http://www.igi-global.com/publish/.

The Advances in Medical Diagnosis, Treatment, and Care (AMDTC) Book Series (ISSN 2475-6628) is published by IGI Global, 701 E. Chocolate Avenue, Hershey, PA 17033-1240, USA, www.igi-global.com. This series is composed of titles available for purchase individually; each title is edited to be contextually exclusive from any other title within the series. For pricing and ordering information please visit http://www.igi-global.com/book-series/advances-medical-diagnosis-treatment-care/129618. Postmaster: Send all address changes to above address.

Titles in this Series

For a list of additional titles in this series, please visit:
https://www.igi-global.com/book-series/advances-medical-diagnosis-treatment-care/129618

Complementary and Alternative Medicine and Kidney Health
Mayuree Tangkiatkumjai (Srinakharinwirot University, Thailand) Annalisa Casarin (The NIHR Research Design Service East of England, UK) Li-Chia Chen (University of Manchester, UK) and Dawn-Marie Walker (University of Southamptn, UK)
Medical Information Science Reference • ©2018 • 308pp • H/C (ISBN: 9781522528821) • US $265.00

Research-Based Perspectives on the Psychophysiology of Yoga
Shirley Telles (Patanjali Research Foundation, India) and Nilkamal Singh (Patanjali Research Foundation,India)
Medical Information Science Reference • ©2018 • 456pp • H/C (ISBN: 9781522527886) • US $225.00

Sustainable Health and Long-Term Care Solutions for an Aging Population
Ben Fong (The Hong Kong Polytechnic University, Hong Kong) Artie Ng (The Hong Kong Polytechnic University, Hong Kong) and Peter Yuen (The Hong Kong Polytechnic University, Hong Kong)
Medical Information Science Reference • ©2018 • 441pp • H/C (ISBN: 9781522526339) • US $225.00

Emerging Applications, Perspectives, and Discoveries in Cardiovascular Research
Ashim Malhotra (Pacific University, USA) and Shivani Soni (California State University, Fullerton, USA & Chapman University, USA & Alabama State University, USA)
Medical Information Science Reference • ©2017 • 439pp • H/C (ISBN: 9781522520924) • US $225.00

Healthcare Community Synergism between Patients, Practitioners, and Researchers
Valerie C. Bryan (Florida Atlantic University, USA) and Jennifer Lynne Bird (Florida Atlantic University, USA)
Medical Information Science Reference • ©2017 • 348pp • H/C (ISBN: 9781522506409) • US $210.00

For an entire list of titles in this series, please visit:
https://www.igi-global.com/book-series/advances-medical-diagnosis-treatment-care/129618

IGI Global
DISSEMINATOR OF KNOWLEDGE

701 East Chocolate Avenue, Hershey, PA 17033, USA
Tel: 717-533-8845 x100 • Fax: 717-533-8661
E-Mail: cust@igi-global.com • www.igi-global.com

Table of Contents

Detailed Table of Contents

Trigeminal neuralgia (TN) is a debilitating facial pain disorder with a rich history dating back over a thousand years. From early records of cases with suggestive features, to better descriptions of its symptomatology, to today's well-established diagnostic criteria, TN has evolved from a largely enigmatic condition to a now manageable disease. Paralleling our understanding of its pathophysiology, various therapeutic approaches have been developed, ranging from early medicines alleviating pain, to destructive procedures targeting the trigeminal nerve, to restorative surgery treating the source. As the pathology of TN becomes better understood, more effective strategies can be used to manage this condition. This chapter provides an overview demonstrating the parallel between understanding of the pathophysiology and the corresponding treatments that were developed over the years.

Trigeminal neuralgia is a rare syndrome classically described as brief paroxysms of severe, lancinating facial pain along a unilateral trigeminal nerve distribution. Numerous clinical presentations of trigeminal neuralgia exist, with various distinct etiologies. Several classification schemes have been designed for clinical and research purposes. However, varying terminology and inconsistent utilization of these systems can lead to diagnostic confusion and ungeneralizable research findings. Similarly, multiple pain scales have been used for trigeminal neuralgia with differing degrees of granularity, validity, and reliability. This chapter provides an overview of the commonly used classification systems and pain scales in the context of their evolution and utilization. Furthermore, the authors provide recommendations for application of these systems to clinical and research practice.

The first-line treatment of trigeminal neuralgia can be very effective, but side effects are often difficult for patients to tolerate. This chapter is a guide to the broad selection of medical therapies currently available for the treatment of trigeminal neuralgia which includes oral therapies and other non-surgical methods of treatment such as IV medications, nasal sprays, topical ointments, and injections. The discussion of each treatment includes discussion of its evidence in current literature, its proposed mechanism of action, its dosing and appropriate setting for clinical use, and its side effect profile.

Microvascular decompression (MVD) is a neurosurgical procedure used to treat various neuralgias of the cranial nerves. The clinical presentation, natural history, pathophysiology, and medical management of trigeminal neuralgia, hemifacial spasm, glossopharyngeal neuralgia, and nervus intermedius neuralgia is reviewed. A thorough discussion on the retrosigmoid approach for decompression of cranial nerves is presented, along with newer techniques and controversies on adjuvant therapies and neuromonitoring. The surgical outcomes of MVD are discussed, along with alternative techniques to open MVD.

Microvascular decompression (MVD) is a highly effective surgical treatment for patients with trigeminal neuralgia (TN) caused by arterial compression. In cases of TN without arterial compression of the nerve, however, a variety of other surgical treatments can be effective for pain relief including neurolysis, nerve section, and placement of a tentorial sling. In this chapter, the authors discuss the nuances of surgical interventions for TN outside of standard MVDs. They also explore recent innovations in MVD surgery for TN.

In this chapter, the authors discuss the use of glycerol rhizotomy (GR) as a treatment modality for trigeminal neuralgia. GR was first described by Håkanson and has been used for more than 40 years as a minimally invasive, safe option for the management of facial pain. Here, the authors discuss the history behind the discovery of GR, relevant biochemical mechanisms of neurolysis, indications, a step-by-step procedural outline for GR and intraoperative cisternography, potential side effects, efficacy of treatment, and new applications for the imaging technique. GR has stood the test of time in neurosurgery, and this chapter demonstrates its utility in patients who are poor surgical candidates for microvascular decompression and for whom medical treatment has failed to manage their intractable pain.

No single surgical procedure can achieve lasting pain relief in all patients with trigeminal neuralgia. Percutaneous balloon compression trigeminal rhizotomy is an alternative outpatient procedure for patients in whom open operation or other percutaneous procedures are infeasible or have failed. The instrumentation required and a stepwise description of the procedure are given. Limited information on results is available, but suggest that approximately 95% of patients will get immediate relief of their pain with a median duration of pain estimated between 20 and 28 months. As many as 20% of patients may remain pain free and off medication at 5 years. Serious complications are rare but include meningitis, hemorrhage, extensive facial dysesthesia or analgesia and cranial nerve dysfunction.

Trigeminal neuralgia is a debilitating neuropathic condition characterized by recurrent paroxysms of shock-like pain across the distribution of the trigeminal nerve, often

population. Despite the unclear understanding, the psychiatric comorbidities should be addressed as a part of comprehensive, multi-modal approach. Anticonvulsants or serotonin and norepineprhine reuptake inhibitors are viable pharmacological options that can supplement the currently used carbamazepine therapy. For medically refractory cases, surgical interventions are being suggested as effective alternatives in managing both the pain and the psychiatric complaints of TN. Examples include microvascular decompression, stereotactic radiosurgery, and repetitive transcranial magnetic stimulation. Continued research to understand TN should take into account the psychiatric burden in this population in order to promote a holistic treatment approach.

Preface

Trigeminal neuralgia is a surgeon's disease. Traditionally thought of as having a strong anatomic etiology, trigeminal neuralgia has fallen to the neurosurgeon for definitive treatment of patients with this affliction where medicines had failed. Successful treatment has relieved many patients of the debilitating pain and suffering that trigeminal neuralgia inflicts, but we need to continue to review our results in order to refine out outcomes. At Stanford we are fortunate to have access to the full complement of multi-modal approaches to the disease and can reap the benefits of what a comprehensive, multidisciplinary strategy can bring to patients. In this text, we have assimilated this ethos, and drawn from the experience of the experts in the field, not just in medical and open surgical management of trigeminal neuralgia, but of all relevant and novel approaches to treat the disease. In addition to reviewing the existing treatment options for trigeminal neuralgia, this text illustrates the emerging advances in the field including endoscopic approaches to surgery, interventional radiology-guided procedures, radiosurgery, neuromodulation, and other noninvasive options along with a cogent analysis of the evidence and efficacy of each approach. This book will be suitable first and foremost for advanced providers who care for trigeminal neuralgia patients on a daily basis, as well as trainees, and motivated patients and family members who seek to learn more about their disease. In this way, we provide a comprehensive resource for treatment of trigeminal neuralgia in a concise text that we know will be of lasting benefit to both providers and patients alike.

THE DISEASE

Trigeminal neuralgia is a devastating neurological condition characterized by episodes of unilateral sharp, stabbing, electrical shock-like pain in one or more branches of the trigeminal nerve. Painful episodes can either occur spontaneously or after triggers such as cold air, fine touch, and facial movements (e.g., talking, eating, etc.). The recurrent nature of the disease and anticipation of the next attack frequently cause functional impairment and debilitation.

Initial treatments were largely medicinal and aimed at masking the symptoms. As the source of the pain was determined to be nerves, destructive procedures gained attention. These procedures were further refined after identifying the trigeminal nerve as the culprit of the disease. Various processes including chemoneurolysis, nerve transection, ganglionectomy, and balloon compression were used to damage the trigeminal nerve in effort to provide symptomatic relief.

More recently, vascular compression of the trigeminal nerve was discovered to underlie the painful symptoms. Therefore, decompressive surgery became the mainstay therapeutic approach for TN. However, for those who are refractory to surgical decompression or are poor surgical candidates, destructive procedures remain a feasible option. Furthermore, novel approaches such as stereotactic radiation have also emerged as potential alternatives.

ORGANIZATION OF THE BOOK

The book is organized into 12 chapters. A brief description of each of the chapters follows:

Chapter 1 discusses the history of trigeminal neuralgia and describes how an increasing understanding of the pathophysiology underlying the disease has guided the evolution of treatment.

Chapter 2 discusses the classification system for trigeminal neuralgia and facial pain so that disease characteristics and severity can be standardized across patients and providers.

Chapter 3 discusses medical management strategies for trigeminal neuralgia that remain the first-line treatment modality for this disease.

Chapter 4 discusses general techniques for open microvascular decompression which remains the most definitive treatment available for severe medically refractory trigeminal neuralgia.

Chapter 5 discusses nuances and different microsurgical strategies for open microvascular decompression for trigeminal neuralgia, important techniques for the surgeon to have in their armamentarium.

Chapter 6 discusses novel techniques for treatment of trigeminal neuralgia beyond open microvascular decompression with varying degrees of invasiveness.

Chapter 7 discusses endoscope-assisted microvascular decompression and how use of the endoscope can increase operative efficiency, increase microscopic visibility, and decrease invasiveness.

Chapter 8 discusses glycerol rhizotomy as a treatment for trigeminal neuralgia, including patient selection, techniques, outcomes, and complication avoidance.

Chapter 9 discusses balloon rhizotomy as a treatment for trigeminal neuralgia, including patient selection, techniques, outcomes, and complication avoidance.

Chapter 10 discusses the evidence behind radiosurgery for trigeminal neuralgia as well as reviewing radiosurgical treatment planning and strategies.

Chapter 11 discusses V2 rhizotomy as a treatment for trigeminal neuralgia, including patient selection, techniques, outcomes, and complication avoidance.

Chapter 12 discusses the psychiatry of pain with respect to trigeminal neuralgia and critical mental health considerations for both providers and patients battling this disease.

Allen Ho
Stanford University, USA

Steven Chang
Stanford University, USA

Acknowledgment

We would like to sincerely thank Lily Kim. The conceptualization of this book would not have been possible without her valuable and highly professional collaboration as the Managing Editor for this publication.

Chapter 1
History of Trigeminal Neuralgia:
A Discussion of How the Understanding of Pathophysiology Guided Treatment

Alice L. Hung
Johns Hopkins University, USA

Michael Lim
Johns Hopkins University, USA

ABSTRACT

Trigeminal neuralgia (TN) is a debilitating facial pain disorder with a rich history dating back over a thousand years. From early records of cases with suggestive features, to better descriptions of its symptomatology, to today's well-established diagnostic criteria, TN has evolved from a largely enigmatic condition to a now manageable disease. Paralleling our understanding of its pathophysiology, various therapeutic approaches have been developed, ranging from early medicines alleviating pain, to destructive procedures targeting the trigeminal nerve, to restorative surgery treating the source. As the pathology of TN becomes better understood, more effective strategies can be used to manage this condition. This chapter provides an overview demonstrating the parallel between understanding of the pathophysiology and the corresponding treatments that were developed over the years.

DOI: 10.4018/978-1-5225-5349-6.ch001

INTRODUCTION

Trigeminal neuralgia, formerly known as tic douloureux and Fothergill's disease, is a devastating neurological condition characterized by episodes of unilateral sharp, stabbing, electrical shock-like pain in one or more branches of the trigeminal nerve. Painful episodes can either occur spontaneously or after triggers such as cold air, fine touch, and facial movements (e.g. talking, eating, etc.). The recurrent nature of the disease and anticipation of the next attack frequently cause functional impairment and debilitation.

Initial treatments were largely medicinal and aimed at masking the symptoms. Because the pathophysiology was poorly understood, many treatments were used to alter sensorium, thereby decreasing awareness of facial pain. As the source of the pain was determined to be nerves, destructive procedures gained attention. These procedures were further refined after identifying the trigeminal nerve as the culprit of the disease. Various processes including chemoneurolysis, nerve transection, ganglionectomy, and balloon compression were used to damage the trigeminal nerve in effort to provide symptomatic relief. Chemoneurolysis is the injection of a chemical substance into the trigeminal nerve to cause damage. Ganglionectomy is the resection of the associated ganglion to decrease neural signaling.

More recently, vascular compression of the trigeminal nerve was discovered to underlie the painful symptoms. Therefore, decompressive surgery became the mainstay therapeutic approach for TN. However, for those who are refractory to surgical decompression or are poor surgical candidates, destructive procedures remain a feasible option. Furthermore, novel approaches such as stereotactic radiation have also emerged as potential alternatives. Unfortunately, many patients still have pain that is refractory to current treatments. As more is learned about the pathophysiology, perhaps novel therapeutic options can be discovered for this group of patients.

EARLY MENTIONS OF TRIGEMINAL NEURALGIA

The very first accounts of TN are unclear. A few key figures have been identified by historians as the earliest people to encounter this mysterious disease. As shown by the selected passages from literature thought to be the earliest descriptions of TN, the unique characteristics of TN have been observed early in history. However, it wasn't until many years later was TN identified as a distinct disease.

Vague Historical References

The earliest writings about TN documented suggested symptoms without establishing it as a distinct clinical condition. As a result, there is no consensus on the very first record of TN. Some considered Aretaeus of Cappodocia, a prominent ancient Greek physician best known for his characterization of diabetes, to be the first person to identify the existence of TN in *Cephalaea* during the first century (Nurmikko & Eldridge, 2001; Rose, 1993; Stookey & Ransohoff, 1959).

But in certain cases, the parts on the right side, or those on the left solely, so far that a separate temple, or ear, or one eyebrow, or one eye, or the nose which divides the face into two equal parts; the pain does not pass this limit, but remains in the half of the head... For if at any time it sets in acutely, it occasions unseemly and dreadful symptoms; spasm and distortion of the countenance take place (Aretaeus, 1856, pp. 294-295).

However, this description was fairly non-specific, without convincing qualities suggestive of TN. The unilateral features and temporal distribution, while consistent with TN, could also be indicative of other conditions such as migraine and cluster headaches. Furthermore, *Cephalaea* was a chapter on headaches, supporting the notion that the description likely pertained to headache-type pain. There was no mention of facial pain per se to suggest otherwise. Aretaeus made the first mention of "spasm and distortion" of the face, which continued to appear throughout historical texts about TN. Although involuntary muscle spasms are not qualities of TN, it is possible that these descriptions referred to voluntary facial grimaces secondary to severe pain.

Others recognized Avicenna, a Persian physician, as the first person to document symptoms of TN close to a millennium later. Avicenna reported on a facial disorder, termed *Leqvet,* with paralytic and spasmodic variants. Historians have argued that while the paralytic type was unmistakably facial palsy, description of the spasmodic type might be consistent with TN (Ameli, 1965; Bretschneider, 1847; Krause, 1896).

Leqvet is a type of organic disease affecting the face, and it causes abnormal changes on one side of the face, including lips and eyelids. The cause of this affection is either paralysis or spasm... Know the signs of spasmodic Leqvet is that there is not much change in power and sensation. The skin of the forehead is pulled, and the muscles of the face are hard, and the part of the face affected is pulled down towards the neck. There is a diminution of saliva and moisture of the mouth. It is difficult to pull the face to its normal position. The other sign of the disease is pain in the face. The skin is dry and there are convulsions on that side of the face (Ameli, 1965, pp. 105-106).

The lack of weakness or changes in sensation, coupled with the associated pain and unilateral distribution, were suggestive of TN. However, these symptoms could also be consistent with other facial pain syndromes, such as shingles and post-infectious neuritis. Again, facial "convulsions" were less supportive of TN, unless they were in reference to expressions of pain. Coupled with the changes in muscle tone, drooling, and inability to "pull the face to its normal position" (p. 106), this description seemed more reflective of involuntary facial movements, which are not a feature of TN. While more convincing than Aretaeus's writing, this was still weakly descriptive of TN.

Non-written footprints in history have also left signs suggestive of early sufferers of TN. Between the 13th and 19th century in Wells, pilgrims with toothaches used to visit Bishop Button's tomb under the belief that his blessing would provide a cure. Carvings suggestive of people with severe toothaches have been found in the area. However, examination of the buried remains revealed a paucity of dental decay. This was thought to be early records of trigeminal neuralgia (Pearce, 2003; Stookey & Ransohoff, 1959). Again, there was no definite evidence in favor of TN. Despite the lack of concrete proof, these pieces of puzzle left traces in history that are valuable towards our speculation about the origins of this fascinating disease.

Discrete Case Portrayals

It wasn't until 1677 in a series of letters between John Locke and Thomas Syndeham, both famous English physicians, and their patient, did a detailed depiction of TN finally establish itself as a distinct clinical entity:

[The Lady was] found in a fit of such violent and exquisite torment… which extended all over the right side of her face and mouth. When the fit came, there was, to use My Lady's own expression of it, as it were a flash of fire all of a suddaine shot into all those parts, and at every one of those twitches which made her shreeke out… These violent fits terminated on a suddaine, and then My Lady seemed to be perfectly well, excepting only a dull pain which ordinarily remained in her teeth on that side, and an uneasienesse in that side of her tongue which she phansied to be swollen on that side, which yet when I looked on it, as I often did, had not the least alteration in it in colour, bignesse, or any other way (Dewhurst, 1957, pp. 24-25).

The distribution, quality, and episodic nature of the facial pain accurately reflected the features of TN. Furthermore, the lack of visible changes to the affected area suggested that it was unlikely to be secondary to an inflammatory or infectious etiology. This was a more convincing account universally agreed to reflect TN. At the time, Locke consulted several physicians, and it was thought that the pain was because of "weakness of the nerves traversing to the left side of the face," or "some pungent vapor which affects the nerve" (Dewhurst, 1957, pp. 28-30). The source of the pain was correctly localized to the nerves, but no further consideration was given towards this occurrence as a distinct medical condition.

A few years later in 1688, Johannes Michael Fehr also published a description indicative of TN in the eulogy of Johannes Laurentius Bausch. Even though the eulogy was published later, Bausch's symptoms predated those of Locke's patient, occurring in the early 1660s. Reproduced by Eadie, M. (2012), the excerpt powerfully portrayed Bausch's four years of struggle with "a harassing, sharp, shooting pain in his right maxilla [that] varied in intensity. It was less at times; at other times, it retreated deep into the tissues or even completely disappeared" (p. 245). The affliction led to speech limitations and reduced oral intake, illustrating the severity of symptoms and gravity of the situation (Eadie, 2012). Even with these pathognomonic qualities of TN, this case did not allude to the possibility of it as a distinct disorder.

Recognition as Clinical Disease

Despite the unique features of TN, it wasn't established as an official disease until 1756, when it was named "tic douloureux" in Nicholaus André's *Observations pratiques sur les maladies de l'urèthre et sur plusiers faits convulsifs* (André, 1756). In this report, as analyzed by Brown J.A. et al (1999), André uses five examples to emphasize the symptoms characteristic of TN, including its intermittent timing, "lancinating pain," and functional impairment (Brown, Coursaget, Preul, & Sangvai, 1999).

John Fothergill independently described TN in 1773 based on cases he had encountered and treated in his practice. He recognized it as its own disease, different from any other established disorder. Fothergill not only delineated its symptoms, but also accurately described the patient population:

This affection seems to be peculiar to persons advancing in years, and to women more than to men... From imperceptible beginnings, a pain attacks some part or other of the face, or the side of the head: sometimes about the orbit of the eye, sometimes the ossa malarum, sometimes the temporal bones, are the parts complained of. The pain comes suddenly, and is excruciating; it lasts but a short time, perhaps a quarter or half a minute, and then goes off; it returns at irregular intervals, sometimes in half an hour, sometimes there are two or three repetitions in a few minutes... Speaking, or chewing, or even slight touching the skin of the side affected with the softest handkerchief, would immediately excite the pain, which, after continuing perhaps a quarter or half a minute, gradually went off, till it was again awakened by some fresh motion (Fothergill, 1773, pp. 101-104).

Fothergill further distinguished it from toothaches, citing that some patients with this pain were of old age and had few remaining teeth. He wrote in extensive detail about the patient population, associated features, and theories about the underlying cause. Because of his contribution to the recognition of TN as a distinct entity, this disease is also called Fothergill's disease.

Although André and Fothergill were credited as the founders of TN, Eboli et al (2009) have recently acknowledged the efforts of John Hunter, a British anatomist, in his interpretation of the disease. In 1778, when theories about the cause of TN were greatly debated, Hunter accurately hypothesized that the pain likely came from the nerves. Furthermore, he correctly portrayed the idea that nerve compression led to pain distal to the site of compression (Eboli, Stone, Aydin, & Slavin, 2009). Unfortunately, his ideas were largely unvisited, dwarfing their potential contribution to the early understanding of this disease.

EARLY THEORIES AND TREATMENTS

From the initial identification of TN, both surgical and conservative therapies have prevailed. Although both types of treatment have drastically changed over time, it is interesting to note that the divergence occurred early in history. Furthermore, the two strategies originated from the two people the disease was named after: André and Fothergill.

Initial Attempts at Pain Relief

During the beginnings of appreciation for TN as a clinical entity, its pathophysiology was poorly understood. As a result, treatment approaches were mostly arbitrary. John Locke's patient, for example, was advised to try "mixtures of vapours" and opiates to calm the pain (Dewhurst, 1957, p. 26). Others, suspecting that the pain is dental in etiology, attempted tooth extractions without success (Stookey & Ransohoff, 1959). Additional treatments that have been used include bed rest, alcohol, bleeding, purging, and a variety of anesthetics (Wilkins, 2002). Many of these therapies resulted in decreased or altered consciousness, thereby reducing the sensation of pain.

Origins of Two Approaches

André and Fothergill, the two credited as founding fathers of TN, interestingly had vastly different theories and treatment methods. These led down two different paths of therapeutic strategies still used today. André's surgical approach aimed at destroying and "decompressing" the nerve was strangely similar to modern day destructive and decompressive procedures, despite different reasons. Fothergill, on the other hand, resorted to a more conservative methodology using oral medicines, much like modern day drugs used for TN.

André believed that TN resulted from the fluid obstruction of nerves, which he thought were hollow, causing irritation and disease of the nerve. Therefore, his goals were to surgically destroy adhesions of the nerve using mercury water and to allow drainage of the fluid to "decompress" the rest of the nerve. He left wounds open and created fistulas to allow continued drainage of fluid and prevention of scar formation, which would obstruct the nerve again, causing pain to return (Brown et al., 1999). Although André's technique is no longer used, his ideas of nerve destruction and decompression remarkably continue to underlie modern surgical procedures used to treat TN.

Unlike André, Fothergill persisted with medicinal treatments aimed at reducing pain. He prescribed opium and hemlock for his patients with TN pain (Fothergill, 1773). Hemlock, a poisonous plant, has been shown to have anti-nociceptive properties (Radulović et al., 2012). Fothergill's treatment selection was largely aimed at symptomatic relief without targeting the pathologic cause. However, the adverse effects of the medications rendered them as impractical long term solutions. Regarding the pathophysiology of TN, Fothergill had his suspicions in a cancerous source. He recounted prior experience with patients who had cancer and noted the inexplicable bodily pains without an obvious cause. Based on this theory, he proposed treatments such as repeated bleedings, laxatives, and hemlock (Fothergill, 1773). Fothergill's theory and drugs of choice have been disproven. Nonetheless, the conservative medicinal management of TN remains a feasible option today.

PROGRESSION OF MEDICAL MANAGEMENT

Conservative treatment of TN perhaps has the longest history out of all the therapies. However, the method by which drugs were selected has changed. Earliest drugs were chosen based on solely on previously observed effects, while later ones were selected for their mechanism of action and relation to the pathophysiology of the disease. Through these efforts, carbamazepine, an anti-convulsant medication, was finally found to be one of the most effective drugs used to treat TN.

Old Remedies for TN

Various medicines have been used in the treatment of TN. Most were randomly selected for their ability to reduce facial pain, without much consideration for the underlying mechanism of action. Therefore, drug classes and types were highly variable, and countless remedies have been tried. Unfortunately, most had severe side effects limiting their tolerability. This section covers a few representative examples demonstrating these features.

Since the acknowledgment of TN as a disorder by André and Fothergill, various mineral and herbal medicines were attempted. Because the pathophysiology of TN wasn't understood, there were no consistent thought processes guiding treatment. In 1822, Huchinson published a pamphlet, *Cases of Neuralgia Spasmodica, Commonly Termed Tic Douloureux Successfully Treated*, summarizing the successes and failures of treatments used up until his time. He wrote,

The curative capabilities of the conium maculatum of stramonium, of opium, of the different preparations of copper, of lead, and of silver, of the belladonna, of electricity, magnetism, the actual cautery, of the external applications of lyttae, the tar trite of antimony, and of tar, have been appreciated with sufficient accuracy and discrimination, by many distinguished members of our profession... in some few instances a little good has been produced... and in an unfortunately large majority of suffering patients, not the least relief has been afforded (Hutchinson, 1822, pp. 51-52).

As told by Hutchinson, medicinal efforts provided little relief during the early treatments of TN. Later in the pamphlet, Hutchinson further detailed what he thought was an effective remedy, involving a mixture of iron and carbonated soda. Hutchinson (1822) presented a few successful cases he had treated and concluded that he has discovered "the existence of a very considerable palliative, if not of a perfect cure, for the generality of cases of one of the most painful maladies to which human nature is subject" (p. 63). He thought that the iron improves the functions of the blood, thereby serving as a cure not only for TN, but potentially also for other illnesses (Hutchinson, 1822).

This drug was tested about a century later by Davidhoff, who determined that despite initial pain relief, most patients had recurrence of pain (Davidoff, 1950). This was not surprising considering our current understanding that iron content and blood are irrelevant in the pathogenesis of TN. It is unclear why many of the patients using ferrous carbonate experienced brief periods of effect. Given the intermittent nature of TN, it is conceivable that the periods of relief were spontaneous remissions that happened to coincide with the drug intake (Cosnett, 1990).

Trial and error of various medicines continued throughout much of the early 1900s. Many drugs were selected for their ability to cause numbness of the face (Antoni & Johnson, 1958; Cavanagh & Buxton, 1989; Woodhall & Odom, 1956). The mechanisms were rarely questioned. Thus, the drugs at best provided temporary symptomatic relief without long-term effects. Some, such as trichloroethylene and stilbamidine, were later shown to have severe toxicity, including immediate nausea, dizziness, and blurry vision, and long-term renal and hepatic damage (Chiu et al., 2012; Seager & Castelnuovo, 1947). Nonetheless, patients were still willing to take these drugs for brief alleviations of pain. The progression in conservative management of TN remained largely stagnant until the use of hydantoins.

Discovery of Anti-Convulsant Therapy

In 1853, Armand Trousseau was the first person to draw the connection between TN and epilepsy in that both were characterized by abnormal neural spasms (Sheinberg & Sagher, 2002; Watson, 2012). However, it wasn't until 1942 did Bergouignan present hydantoins, an anti-convulsant drug, as a treatment for TN. Usage of this drug was met with success. In 1958, Iannone, A. et al published a small case series of successfully treated patients and provided evidence explaining its efficacy. The authors cited the previous finding that Dilantin (phenytoin, a type of hydantoin) can decrease neural signaling in animal studies (Morrell, Bradley, & Ptashne, 1958), and further hypothesized that TN pain might be secondary to increased electrical firing. Therefore, Dilantin would reduce pain by decreasing neural firing. The results from the study were positive, supporting the use of anti-convulsant therapy (Iannone, Baker, & Morrell, 1958). This was also the first instance where a medical treatment was supported by empirical evidence.

Unfortunately, adverse effects of hydantoins limited their use at high doses, while low doses often did not provide symptomatic relief. In 1962, Blom discovered a new anti-convulsant drug, Geigy 32883 (currently known as carbamazepine), as a safer alternative (Blom, 1962). Follow-up study in 96 patients demonstrated long-term benefits in 68% of study population (Graham & Zilkha, 1966). Over the years, carbamazepine remain treatment of choice in conservative management of TN pain (Sindrup & Jensen, 2002; Wiffen, McQuay, & Moore, 2005; Zakrzewska & Linskey, 2014). For those with pain refractory to carbamazepine or are unable to tolerate the side effects, other drug options include lamotrigine, gabapentin, and baclofen (Fromm, Terrence, & Chattha, 1984; Shaikh, Yaacob, & Abd Rahman, 2011; Wiffen, McQuay, Edwards, & Moore, 2005).

EVOLUTION OF DESTRUCTIVE THERAPIES

The idea that nerve damage can reduce TN pain is one of the oldest theories in the management of TN. However, while the concept remained the same, the way it was achieved has changed drastically both in target and methodology. In the earliest examples, the peripheral nerve was transected via open surgery. As more was learned about the anatomy of the trigeminal nerve, the target became more proximal, involving the ganglion and root of the nerve. Furthermore, the approach has changed as well from open surgeries to percutaneous procedures. Given the efficacy in pain relief, it is not surprising that the idea persisted. Yet the approach has been continuously modified to reduce complications and maximize benefits.

Early Peripheral Neurotomy

While some physicians were experimenting with medical therapies, others believed that surgical destruction of the nerve was the most effective way to treat TN pain, which was thought to arise from diseased nerves. This practice dated back to Nicholaus André during the early 1700s. Early surgeries targeted the peripheral nerve. André did his trigeminal surgeries with Marechal, one of his colleagues and renowned surgeon at the time. They performed peripheral neurotomies of the infraorbital nerve and the maxillary nerve for two patients afflicted with TN. Although both surgeries were complicated by hemorrhage, the two patients reported short-term pain relief (Brown et al., 1999). This was the first known instance of temporary TN pain relief subsequent to the destruction of the trigeminal nerve. Remarkably, the trigeminal nerve and its associated anatomy had not been identified at the time.

Peripheral neurotomies continued as a treatment option for TN with considerable success. John Lizars, for example, described his experience in the early 1800s with a TN patient who achieved temporary pain relief after the procedure (Behrman, 1960). However, due to the lack of understanding of neural anatomy, transections of the facial nerve were not uncommon. This practice led to facial paralysis without much improvement in pain. Charles Bell, a notable Scottish physician, discussed the difference between the trigeminal nerve (cranial nerve V) and facial nerve (cranial nerve VII) in his publication, *The Nervous System of the Human Body*, in 1830 (Butler, 1962). His contribution was fundamental in the history of TN, marking the point at which the pathology of "trigeminal neuralgia" was correctly localized. After this discovery, surgical procedures have evolved to better target TN.

Development of Ganglionectomy

During the first half of the 19th century, great strides were made in the study of electrophysiology and neural conduction. Many studies suggested that electrical currents flowed through the body (McDonald, 2004). Therefore, it came as no surprise that Carnochan, surgeon and professor at New York Medical College, proposed the radical idea of Gasserian (ie. trigeminal ganglion) ganglionectomy as the surgical treatment for TN. In his paper from 1858, Carnochan wrote,

The ganglion of Meckel, being composed of gray matter, must play an important part as a generator of nervous power, of which, like a galvanic battery, it affords a continual supply; while branches of the ganglion, under influence of the diseased trunk, serve as conductors of the accumulated morbid nervous sensibility (Carnochan, 1858, p. 128).

Carnochan's usage of the terms "generator" and "galvanic battery" suggest that his ideas were likely influenced by the discoveries being made during that period. He accessed the Gasserian ganglion via the base of the skull, after making an incision through a V-shaped incision below the eye. Carnochan demonstrated the value of Gasserian ganglionectomy in his three case presentations, showing that all patients were healthy and pain free for up to 14 months post-resection (Carnochan, 1858). This breakthrough led the progression of TN surgery one step closer to the source of the pathology, away from simply targeting peripheral nerves.

Since the initial proposal, many surgeons have made headway in perfecting the Gasserian ganglionectomy via variations in the skull base approach (Fowler, 1886; W. Rose, 1890). Poor exposure, incomplete resection of the ganglion, blood loss, and infection remained major challenges. Mortality was as high as 18% (Murphy, 1896). In 1881, Horsley proposed an alternative intradural technique that accessed the ganglion via craniotomy (Horsley, 1891). However, proximity to the temporal lobe and risk of lacerating the brain generated hesitation in adopting this strategy. The following year, the Hartley-Krause procedure, which accessed the ganglion via a subtemporal craniotomy without penetrating the dura, was devised (Hartley, 1892). During the 1890s and early 1900s, significant effort was devoted to improving this technique (Cushing et al., 1983; Kellogg, Pendleton, Quinones-Hinojosa, & Cohen-Gadol, 2010).

There was no doubt that ganglionectomy provided symptomatic relief from TN pain. The complications and adverse effects, nevertheless, should not be overlooked. Injury to the middle meningeal artery was a major risk that accounted for a mortality rate greater than 20% (Kellogg et al., 2010). Apart from reported immediate post-operative complications such as hemorrhage and infections, long-term sequalae could also be devastating. For instance, transection of temporalis muscle and transection of the motor root could cause difficulty with chewing. Removal of the entire trigeminal ganglion would also eliminate corneal sensation, increasing the chance of ulcerations (W. Rose, 1890). Moreover, prolonged retraction of the brain during surgery could also affect cognitive functions (Hartley, 1892). With this in mind, it's not surprising that surgery was considered the treatment of last resort. Even as surgical methods were refined, alternative means continued being developed.

Percutaneous Nerve Injections

Nerve destruction can be achieved in multiple ways. Besides surgical transection, injection of corrosive substances was another option. Bartholow (1873) was one of the first physicians to propose injection of a chemical substance to burn the nerve. The needle was applied through the cheek until the tip reached the opening of the infraorbital foramen near the nerve. He advised the use of chloroform, but noted that alcohol was an acceptable substitute (Bartholow, 1876, 1873). Likewise, Neuber used the same approach in 1883 and injected osmic acid (Murphy, 1904). Both methods resulted in at least temporary improvement without local irritation, signs of necrosis, or other side effects. These were the first use of chemoneurolysis in the management of TN. The non-invasive nature and considerable success rendered it as an appealing alternative to high risk open surgeries during this period. This idea was well expressed by Ostwalt:

My aim has been to find a therapeutic method by which a serious surgical operation might be avoided, even in the very rebellious and chronic cases of tic douloureux, the uncertainty of the final result being too great to warrant such dangerous operations as those recommended in such cases (Ostwalk, 1906).

At the turn of the century, he proudly published about his experience with percutaneous chemoneurolysis using alcohol, which he had adapted from Schlösser. Moreover, Ostwalt had modified the technique to better reach the trigeminal ganglion. He had a 90% success rate in about 60 cases. Patients frequently required multiple injections to be completely pain free, and approximately a third of patients experienced a recurrence in pain, usually around 5 months later. The pain was typically milder and responsive to repeat injection. In addition, Ostwalt astutely suggested that the transient paralysis that followed was likely due to alcohol induced nerve damage. As the nerve recovered, its functions returned to normal (Ostwalt, 1906).

Ostwalt's reasoning was based on prior studies on the effect of alcohol on nerves. It was previously shown in guinea pigs that alcohol caused necrosis of peripheral nerves distal to the site of injury and subsequent loss of function (Culbertson,

1887). Unlike historical haphazard efforts in TN treatment, the usage of alcohol chemoneurolysis was a logical and systematic approach. From animal studies to clinical trial, followed by retrospective analysis of clinical results and explanations grounded in experimentally drawn conclusions, this was a representative example of how the approach towards TN treatment had changed over the years.

Numerous physicians continued to refine Oswalt's method, believing that direct injection into the ganglion would achieve better results than simply injecting near the nerves. Effort was taken to avoid injury of nearby structures and allow better targeting. Finally, in 1912, Härtel devised an extra-oral approach that penetrated the cheek near the second upper molar tooth, went through the muscles, and entered the foramen ovale, directly reaching the nerve before it exited, where the injection is performed. It was thought that Härtel's technique reduced risks of injury and was more precise. It became widely accepted in the treatment of TN and is still in use in current practice.

Härtel's technique improved the accuracy of percutaneous injections, but it still required considerable skill and finesse to accomplish. Localization was entirely dependent on minimal landmarks and prior experience. To further reduce risks and increase precision, Pollock et al. (1916) advocated for the use of radiographic-guided imaging to confirm adequate placement of the needle before injection. After its introduction, some embraced the novel tool (Putnam et al., 1936; Sweet et al., 1950). Others questioned its utility, suggesting that fluoroscopy unnecessarily complicated the procedure, and instead preferred to rely on anatomic knowledge (Cushing, 1920). Through the test of time, more surgeons adopted its use. Radiographic guidance prevailed as part of the standard protocol in modern day percutaneous injections for TN.

Minimizing Nerve Injury

Percutaneous procedures had lower risk with decent results, but not all patients were responsive. Moreover, it only provided a short-term solution. As chemoneurolysis was being developed, surgeons continued to modify open procedures to minimize complications while maintaining efficacy. The next breakthrough came in 1915 when Frazier first published his experience of what was called "subtotal division of the sensory root" on 25 patients (Frazier, 1928, p. 534). Subtotal division referred to partial transection of the trigeminal nerve with the goal of only cutting part of the sensory portion and sparing the ophthalmic and motor fibers. This idea was based on his and Spiller's prior observation in dogs showing that the trigeminal nerve was arranged in a consistent and orderly fashion (Frazier, 1928; Wilkins, 1963).

In a subsequent paper on over 500 cases, Frazier reported the tremendous success of the new technique. Saving the ophthalmic branch of the trigeminal prevented sensory loss of the eye, thereby reducing the incidence of corneal ulceration. Reduction in the areas of numbness also increased patient satisfaction (Frazier, 1928). Building on Frazier's development, Stookey (1928) further proposed "differential sectioning" of the nerve (p. 172). The idea was to selectively transect the maxillary or mandibular fibers within the trigeminal trunk, depending on the area of pain. The goal was to reduce post-operative numbness secondary to loss of trigeminal innervation (Stookey, 1928). The approach soon became widely popularized for TN treatment for the next few decades.

NERVE COMPRESSION THEORY

The notion that TN results from vascular compression of the trigeminal nerve is a widely accepted theory today. However, the idea wasn't well received when it was first proposed. Only after numerous reported observations of vessels contacting the nerve and many successful operations did the concept final gain acceptance.

Early Origins

The idea that TN might be due to compression of the trigeminal nerve dated back to André's initial theory on the built up of "nerve fluids." Since then, other surgeons had also alluded to the idea without much headway. In 1952, Taarnhøj 1952 discussed cases where instances of nerve compression were associated with TN pain. He cited two sources of compression: tumor and anatomic variant. It had been known that TN pain might be caused by tumors in the cerebellopontine angle (CPA). He treated a patient with a right CPA epidermoid who presented with facial pain. Intra-operative visualization showed tumor compression of the trigeminal nerve. After surgical resection, his TN pain was completely gone, suggesting that it was likely secondary to the mass. Taarnhøj further postulated that variations in anatomy might result in other forms of compression, leading to pain:

There is one site where it is possible to imagine that quite small changes in the tissue could give rise to a compression: that part of the root running from the ganglion posteriorly, through the narrow channel formed by the dura, to the sharp margin of the petrous bone. Small changes, either in the dura or adjacent tissues, perhaps vascular origin, could be assumed to narrow the channel so much that a compression takes place... It should be possible to treat patients with trigeminal neuralgia by dividing the dura over the root without trigeminotomy (Taarnhøj, 1952, pp. 288-289).

In a study of 10 patients, 100% had pain relief after surgery. Unfortunately, follow up duration was short, ranging between 1 and 8 months (Taarnhøj, 1952). In a later study, Taarnhøj reported that out of the 228 cases in which he operated using this approach, the rate of pain recurrence was 40% (Taarnhøj, 1982). Repeat studies by other surgeons revealed considerable success. More importantly, the reduction in side effects associated with nerve transections increased the appeal.

Revisit and Enhancement

While the subtemporal approach was commonly performed during this period, Dandy advocated for suboccipital access of the trigeminal root through the posterior fossa. He believed that this minimized cranial nerve injury and provided better exposure. Interestingly, despite Dandy being credited for this approach, it was actually first performed by Clairmont, a German surgeon. However, he did not have good results, and the technique was never publicized (Pinkus, 1984). As Dandy improved this approach, he also noticed vessels compressing the trigeminal nerve in a large number of patients, but did not further explore this observation (Jannetta, 1967).

Gardner took Dandy's findings one step forward. Using the suboccipital approach, he visualized arterial compression of the trigeminal root in many of his patients. Gardner proceeded to separate the vessel from the nerve using Gelfoam, performing the first vascular decompression. In addition, Gardner also hypothesized that prolonged contact between the vessel and the nerve resulted in chronic irritation and myelin loss, which predisposed the nerve to "short circuiting," thereby producing pain (Gardner, 1962, p. 956; Gardner et al., 1959; Rand, 1981). The demyelination theory was further supported by Kerr et al.'s (1966) description of degenerative changes in the myelin sheaths observed using electronic microscopy in trigeminal nerve samples of those with TN. These findings provided a pathophysiologic basis for this operation.

Gardner's technique piqued the interest of Jannetta in 1967. He further modified the decompression surgery to include usage of the operating microscope in assisting visualization of the nerve and vessel. In recognition of Jannetta's contributions, microvascular decompression became known as Jannetta's procedure (Jannetta, 1967). Vascular compression of the trigeminal nerve remains the current understanding of the pathogenesis of TN, and MVD is one of the first line treatments.

STANDARD SURGICAL THERAPIES TODAY

Modern management of TN can be grouped into three categories: open surgery, percutaneous nerve destruction, and radiation therapy. Open surgery refers to MVD, which is the only non-destructive option. It is preferred by younger patients and those in good health due to the non-destructive nature. Percutaneous procedures include radiofrequency ablation, glycerol rhizotomy, and balloon compression. These involve insertion of a needle or electrode to damage the nerve. Albeit minimally invasive, these methods have a higher risk of post-operative sensory abnormalities. Lastly, stereotactic radiosurgery is a novel approach using gamma beams to damage the nerve. However, long term outcomes are still lacking.

Microvascular Decompression

Since Jannetta's report, MVD became widely accepted as the preferred operation for TN. The reduced sensory loss relative to prior nerve sectioning and positive post-surgical results supported its popularity. Reported success rates had been 70-97% with 6.5-19% rate of recurrence over a period of 4 to 20 years (Barker, Jannetta, Bissonette, Larkins, & Jho, 1996; Bender et al., 2011; Ferguson, Brett, Peerless, Barr, & Girvin, 1981; Kolluri & Heros, 1984; Kondo, 2001; Rushworth & Smith, 1982; Sun, Saito, Nakai, & Ando, 1994; Wei et al., 2016). The most frequently encountered complications have been numbness, cerebrospinal fluid leak, and hearing loss due to the proximity of the eighth cranial nerve. Facial numbness was more likely in those who have undergone previous treatments (Theodros et al., 2016). Furthermore, the senior author has reported reduced CSF leak in patients who received calcium phosphate cement for bone reconstruction following MVD (Eseonu et al., 2015). In the late 1900s, numerous surgeons had recommended the usage of intraoperative brainstem auditory evoked responses (BAERs) to decrease the rate of hearing loss (Kuchta, Møller, Wedekind, & Jannetta, 1998; Møller & Møller, 1989; Nishihara et al., 1986; Sindou, Fob, Ciriano, & Fischer, 1992). Delays or reductions in BAERs suggested possible disruption of the eighth nerve signaling, alerting surgeons to take caution in preventing accidental injury. In a 2011 systematic review, the reported post-operative hearing loss was 1.9% in over 6,000 cases (Xia et al., 2014).

The goal of MVD is to decompress the vessel in contact with the trigeminal nerve to reduce demyelination. The most common offending vessels found are the superior cerebellar artery (SCA), anterior inferior cerebellar artery (AICA), and aberrant veins (Cutbush & Atkinson, 1994; Hardy & Rhoton, 1978; Xia et al., 2014). For these instances, the senior author has had positive experience with intraoperative glycerin injection into the trigeminal root. In a small study of 14 patients, this strategy was shown to result in a 100% improvement. Only one patient had a CSF leak post-operatively, and no patients had residual neurological deficits (Goodwin et al., 2013). These preliminary results suggested that for patients without a compressive etiology, an alternative effective treatment could be performed during the same session. However, the lack of vascular compression in some patients also suggest that the pathophysiology of TN remains incompletely understood. Additional causes of this challenging disease must be understood to formulate treatments for those who are refractory to the current therapies.

Radiofrequency Ablation

The role of electricity in managing TN pain did not gain much popularity until 1974 when Sweet and Wepsic published on radiofrequency coagulation of the trigeminal nerve. A few physicians had experimented with the idea earlier in history, but progress was slow because of poor control of electricity. The first major advance was made by Kirschner in 1931. He invented a headgear to direct the insertion of an electrode into the trigeminal ganglion via the foramen ovale, whereby he applied an electrical current to burn the nerve. After over 1,000 cases in the next 10 years, 95% of patients experienced an improvement in pain and 20% had a recurrence (Oddsson, 1944). Unfortunately, others who used this method had so many complications, including ulceration, blindness, facial palsy, hearing loss, and vascular injury, that the procedure was only infrequently used (Sweet & Wepsic, 1974).

Finally, Sweet and Wepsic modified the technique in several ways to increase the safety profile. In addition to radiographic confirmation of electrode placement, they also sought sensory feedback from the patient for reassurance. This was done by gentle stimulation once the electrode is placed, and patient reports of "humming, buzzing, vibrating, pressing, tingling or sense of something moving on or under the skin" in the affected distribution were indicative of adequate localization ((Sweet & Wepsic, 1974, p. 149). Once placement was established, the electrode was gradually heated to prevent excessive damage. These modifications yielded a 91% response rate and a 22% recurrence rate in the first cohort of patients (Sweet & Wepsic, 1974). The practice of radiofrequency ablation increased over the years and subsequent refinements were made to improve precision (Emril & Ho, 2010; Taha & Tew, 1996). Currently, it is one of the standard therapies used to treat TN, especially for patients with pain that is refractory to other modalities (Bender et al., 2013).

Glycerin Rhizotomy

The concept of using glycerol for TN treatment was only recently introduced in 1981 by Håkanson (Håkanson, 1981). Despite the efficacy of alcohol in reducing pain, the complications were challenging. Cases of local tissue necrosis have been reported, especially in patients requiring multiple injections. Other adverse effects included paresthesia, facial palsy, visual loss, and shingles outbreak in the treated area (Fardy & Patton, 1994). Håkanson proposed glycerol as an another option, presumably with fewer complications and good results. In his initial paper, he reported a 98.6% rate of patients who were pain free after the first injection out of a total of 74 patients. Over a 48-month follow-up period, 13 patients had pain recurrence. No adverse effects were reported for this cohort of patients (Håkanson, 1981). Later study demonstrated selective effect of glycerol on pain fibers, sparing other sensory fibers (Sweet, Poletti, & Macon, 1981). The targeted effects of glycerol may account for the decreased number of side effects.

Glycerol didn't gain immediate acceptance. Its viscous consistency made it challenging to administer, deterring some from using it (McLeod & Patton, 2007). Alcohol continued to be preferred by many physicians into the 1990s. At the turn of the century, numerous studies were published on the efficacy of the two. Approximately 90-99.6% of patients were pain free immediately after glycerol injection (Chen, Xu, & Zou, 2010; Erdem & Alkan, 2001; Sweet et al., 1981; Wilkinson, 1999; Xu-Hui et al., 2011), compared to 90% in those treated with alcohol (Han & Kim, 2010; McLeod & Patton, 2007; Ostwalt, 1906). Pain free interval ranged between 7-36 months post-glycerol administration (Erdem & Alkan, 2001), versus 6-24 months post-alcohol injection (McLeod & Patton, 2007). Overall, the results of the two were comparable. However, relative to alcohol, glycerol was less uncomfortable for patients upon initial injection (Fardy, Zakrzewska, & Patton, 1994). Alcohol was also thought to decrease in effectiveness after repeated use. In contrast, glycerol has been shown to maintain efficacy after repeated injections (Bender et al., 2012). Perhaps because of these reasons, glycerol rhizotomies have become the predominant percutaneous chemoneuroloysis procedure today.

Balloon Compression

Similar to glycerol rhizotomy and radiofrequency ablation, balloon compression is another destructive procedure that relieves TN pain by injuring the trigeminal nerve. This technique was devised by Mullan and Lichtor in 1983. It involved fluoroscopic guided insertion of a Fogarty catheter until it reached the foramen ovale, where the balloon became inflated, causing compression of the nerve (Mullan & Lichtor, 1983). Mullan and Lichtor drew their inspiration from Shelden et al (1955), who originally performed nerve compression via an open surgical approach. After exposure of the trigeminal root, a dental roll was used to create pressure on the nerve. This process produced good results in the initial cohort of 29 patients. The biggest drawback, however, was the high rate of dysesthesia (Shelden, Pudenz, Freshwater, & Crue, 1955).

There were 50 patients in the first cohort undergoing balloon decompression. Of these patients, 98% were pain free immediately post-compression. Recurrence occurred in 12% at 6-31 months of follow up. The biggest complication reported was sensory abnormalities (Mullan & Lichtor, 1983). Since its conception, those who attempted the technique have reported a 85-100% initial relief rate (J.-F. Chen, Tu, & Lee, 2012; Corrêa & Teixeira, 1998; Kouzounias, Lind, Schechtmann, Winter, & Linderoth, 2010; Lobato, Rivas, Sarabia, & Lamas, 1990; Trojnik & Ŝmigoc, 2012). Recurrence rate reported has been up to 50% by 21 months (Kouzounias et al., 2010). Physicians have continued to refine the technique in effort to produce better results (Asplund, Linderoth, & Bergenheim, 2010; Goerss, Atkinson, & Kallmes, 2009). It is considered one of the frontline treatments in today's management of TN.

Stereotactic Radiosurgery

Leksell's invention of stereotactic radiosurgery revolutionized the neurosurgical field, affecting the treatment of multiple diseases, including TN (Leksell, 1971; Rand, 1997). Gocht first started using radiation to treat TN in 1897 for those with pain refractory to other therapies. His efforts had considerable success in terms of pain relief, but radiation side effects (e.g. hair loss) were also inevitable (Artico, De Caro, Fraioli, & Giuffrè, 1997; Cole, Liu, & Apfelbaum, 2005). Leksell's Gamma Knife surgery further increased the efficacy of the original idea while reducing adverse effects.

Stereotactic radiosurgery uses a three-dimensional coordinate system to precisely focus radiation energy on the intended target using multiple low intensity beams from various directions. Because each beam only contains little energy, tissues in the path are minimally injured. Only when several beams converge on the target does the combined dose cause damage. Leksell used gamma rays with this technique, therefore resulting in the term "gamma knife surgery" (GKS).

Systematic review by Lopez et al (2004) assessed all available studies until 2003 and concluded that 75% of all patients became pain free after radiation, and rate of recurrence was up to 40% after two years. Unlike other modalities, it took between one week to 3 months to notice an effect after treatment. The most commonly experienced complication was numbness, which occurred in up to 54% of patients in those receiving 90 Gy. Interestingly, numbness was also associated with better outcomes (Lopez, Hamlyn, & Zakrzewska, 2004). A more recent prospective study of 497 patients treated between 1992 and 2010 showed an improvement. In this cohort, 91.75% of patients had some pain relief, and only 34.4% suffered a recurrence. Sensory abnormalities remained the most common complication at a rate of 21.1% (Régis et al., 2016). These findings show promise that stereotactic radiation as an effective treatment for TN. As a minimally invasive technique, it may be an attractive option for those intolerant of or refractory to other therapies.

CONCLUSION

Trigeminal neuralgia has been a mysterious and trying disease that remains incompletely understood even today. However, considerable progress has been made since its conception hundreds of years ago. Influenced by prevalent theories during each period in history, the understanding of its pathogenesis has evolved. Along with that, treatment strategies paralleled this knowledge. From initial probing of the peripheral nerves to identification of the trigeminal root, awareness of neuroanatomy allowed better localization of the disease. Between hemlock and carbamazepine, attention to the mechanistic actions and safety profiles of drugs gave rise to more effective medications. Countless surgeries and numerous innovative ideas amounted to today's microvascular decompression. Even though a substantial percentage of patients are still not responsive to current treatment options, the majority of patients are able to achieve pain relief. As more is understood about the pathogenesis, refinements of current therapies and invention of new ones are possible in the future.

REFERENCES

Ameli, N. O. (1965). Avicenna and trigeminal neuralgia. *Journal of the Neurological Sciences*, *2*(2), 105–107. doi:10.1016/0022-510X(65)90074-2 PMID:4862205

André, N. (1756). *Observations pratiques sur les maladies de l' urèthre et sur plusiers faits convulsifs, & la guérison de plusiers maladies chirurgicales, avec la décomposition d'un remède propre à réprimer la dissolution gangréneuse & cancéreuse, & à la réparer; avec des*. Paris: Delaguette.

Antoni, A. A., & Johnson, J. H. (1958). Treatment of tic douloureux with stilbamidine isethionate. *Journal of Oral Surgery*, *16*(3), 226–230. Retrieved from http://www.ncbi.nlm.nih.gov/pubmed/13526059 PMID:13526059

Aretaeus. (1856). *The extant works of Aretaeus, the Cappadocian* (F. Adams, Ed.). London: Sydenham Society.

Artico, M., De Caro, G. M., Fraioli, B., & Giuffrè, R. (1997). 1897--celebrating the centennial--Hermann Moritz Gocht and radiation therapy in the treatment of trigeminal neuralgia. *Acta Neurochirurgica*, *139*(8), 761–763. doi:10.1007/BF01420050 PMID:9309292

Asplund, P., Linderoth, B., & Bergenheim, A. T. (2010). The predictive power of balloon shape and change of sensory functions on outcome of percutaneous balloon compression for trigeminal neuralgia. *Journal of Neurosurgery, 113*(3), 498–507. doi:10.3171/2010.2.JNS091466 PMID:20345223

Barker, F. G., Jannetta, P. J., Bissonette, D. J., Larkins, M. V., & Jho, H. D. (1996). The Long-Term Outcome of Microvascular Decompression for Trigeminal Neuralgia. *The New England Journal of Medicine, 334*(17), 1077–1084. doi:10.1056/NEJM199604253341701 PMID:8598865

Bartholow, R. (1873). Therapeutics of the Nervous System and Mind. In The Chicago Journal of Nervous and Mental Disease (pp. 100–104). Chicago.

Bartholow, R. (1876). *A practical treatise on materia medica and therapeutics.* New York: D. Appleton and Company. Retrieved from https://archive.org/details/apracticaltreat03bartgoog

Behrman, S. (1960). John Lizars. Centenary of a forgotten pioneer of the surgery of trigeminal neuralgia. *British Medical Journal, 2*(5213), 1665–1666. Retrieved from http://www.ncbi.nlm.nih.gov/pubmed/13688719 PMID:13688719

Bender, M., Pradilla, G., Batra, S., See, A., Bhutiani, N., James, C., ... Lim, M. (2012). Effectiveness of Repeat Glycerol Rhizotomy in Treating Recurrent Trigeminal Neuralgia. *Neurosurgery, 70*(5), 1125–1134. doi:10.1227/NEU.0b013e31823f5eb6 PMID:22067421

Bender, M. T., Pradilla, G., Batra, S., See, A. P., James, C., Pardo, C. A., ... Lim, M. (2013). Glycerol rhizotomy and radiofrequency thermocoagulation for trigeminal neuralgia in multiple sclerosis. *Journal of Neurosurgery, 118*(2), 329–336. doi:10.3171/2012.9.JNS1226 PMID:23121430

Bender, M. T., Pradilla, G., James, C., Raza, S., Lim, M., & Carson, B. S. (2011). Surgical treatment of pediatric trigeminal neuralgia: Case series and review of the literature. *Child's Nervous System, 27*(12), 2123–2129. doi:10.100700381-011-1593-8 PMID:21965150

Blom, S. (1962). Trigeminal Neuralgia: Its Treatment with a New Anti-Convulsant Drug (G-32883). *Lancet, 279*(7234), 839–840. doi:10.1016/S0140-6736(62)91847-0 PMID:13870089

Bretschneider, H. (1847). *Versuch einer Begründung der Pathologie und Therapie der äusseren Neuralgieen.* Jena: Mauke.

Brown, J. A., Coursaget, C., Preul, M. C., & Sangvai, D. (1999). Mercury water and cauterizing stones: Nicolas André and tic douloureux. *Journal of Neurosurgery, 90*(5), 977–981. doi:10.3171/jns.1999.90.5.0977 PMID:10223470

Butler, R. (1962). Sir Charles Bell. *Resenha Médica, 3*(2), 56–62. doi:10.2218/resmedica.v3i2.389

Carnochan, J. M. (1858). Exsection of the Trunk of the Second Branch of the Fifth Pair of Nerves, beyond the Ganglion of Meckel, for Severe Neuralgia of the Face: With Three Cases. *The Southern Medical and Surgical Journal, 14*, 126–136. Retrieved from https://archive.org/stream/southern1858medi/southern1858medi_djvu.txt

Cavanagh, J. B., & Buxton, P. H. (1989). Trichloroethylene cranial neuropathy: Is it really a toxic neuropathy or does it activate latent herpes virus. *Journal of Neurology, Neurosurgery, and Psychiatry, 52*(3), 297–303. doi:10.1136/jnnp.52.3.297 PMID:2538571

Chen, J.-F., Tu, P.-H., & Lee, S.-T. (2012). Repeated Percutaneous Balloon Compression for Recurrent Trigeminal Neuralgia: A Long-Term Study. *World Neurosurgery, 77*(2), 352–356. doi:10.1016/j.wneu.2011.06.013 PMID:22120364

Chen, L., Xu, M., & Zou, Y. (2010). Treatment of Trigeminal Neuralgia with Percutaneous Glycerol Injection into Meckel's Cavity: Experience in 4012 Patients. *Cell Biochemistry and Biophysics, 58*(2), 85–89. doi:10.100712013-010-9094-z PMID:20717747

Chiu, W. A., Jinot, J., Scott, C. S., Makris, S. L., Cooper, G. S., Dzubow, R. C., ... Caldwell, J. C. (2012). Human Health Effects of Trichloroethylene: Key Findings and Scientific Issues. *Environmental Health Perspectives, 121*(3), 303–311. doi:10.1289/ehp.1205879 PMID:23249866

Cole, C. D., Liu, J. K., & Apfelbaum, R. I. (2005). Historical perspectives on the diagnosis and treatment of trigeminal neuralgia. *Neurosurgical Focus, 18*(5), E4. Retrieved from http://www.ncbi.nlm.nih.gov/pubmed/15913280. doi:10.3171/foc.2005.18.5.5 PMID:15913280

Corrêa, C. F., & Teixeira, M. J. (1998). Balloon compression of the Gasserian ganglion for the treatment of trigeminal neuralgia. *Stereotactic and Functional Neurosurgery, 71*(2), 83–89. doi:10.1159/000029651 PMID:10087472

Cosnett, J. E. (1990). Therapeutics in retrospect: Iron carbonate in chorea and tic douloureux. *Journal of the Royal Society of Medicine, 83*, 390–391. Retrieved from https://www.ncbi.nlm.nih.gov/pmc/articles/PMC1292693/pdf/jrsocmed00135-0060.pdf PMID:2199675

Culbertson, J. C. (1887). Artificial production of peripheral neuritis. *The Cincinnati Lancet, 58*. Retrieved from https://books.google.com/books?id=fktAAQAAMAAJ&pg=PA146&lpg=PA146&dq=Pitres+Vaillard+alcohol&source=bl&ots=18Qxur5Jbx&sig=a3wDF56ZUBkz-Lf7A16czA6mjWo&hl=en&sa=X&ved=0ahUKEwjSvLKFr5zRAhXDQSYKHStGCBMQ6AEIIjAD#v=onepage&q=PitresVaillardalcohol&f=false

Cushing, H. (1920). The role of deep alcohol injections in the treatment of trigeminal neuralgia. *Journal of the American Medical Association, 75*(7), 441. doi:10.1001/jama.1920.02620330001001

Cushing, H., & Keen, W. W. (1983). A Method of Total Extirpation of the Gasserian Ganglion for Trigeminal Neuralgia. *Journal of the American Medical Association, 250*(4), 519. doi:10.1001/jama.1983.03340040059035 PMID:6345823

Cutbush, K., & Atkinson, R. L. (1994). Treatment of trigeminal neuralgia by posterior fossa microvascular decompression. *The Australian and New Zealand Journal of Surgery, 64*(3), 173–176. doi:10.1111/j.1445-2197.1994.tb02171.x PMID:8117193

Davidoff, L. M. (1950). *Trifacial neuralgia. Oral Surgery, Oral Medicine, Oral Pathology* (Vol. 3). Mosby. 10.1016/0030-4220(50)90372-0

Dewhurst, K. (1957). A Symposium on Trigemonal Neuralgia With Contributions by Kocke, Sydenham, and other Eminent Seventeenth Century Physicians. *Journal of the History of Medicine and Allied Sciences, XII*(1), 21–36. doi:10.1093/jhmas/XII.1.21 PMID:13406256

Eadie, M. J. (2012). *Headaches: Through the Centuries*. Oxford University Press. doi:10.1093/med/9780199860975.001.0001

Eboli, P., Stone, J. L., Aydin, S., & Slavin, K. V. (2009). Historical characterization of trigeminal neuralgia. *Neurosurgery, 64*(6), 1183–1187. doi:10.1227/01.NEU.0000339412.44397.76 PMID:19487899

Emril, D. R., & Ho, K.-Y. (2010). Treatment of trigeminal neuralgia: Role of radiofrequency ablation. *Journal of Pain Research, 3*, 249–254. doi:10.2147/JPR.S14455 PMID:21311718

Erdem, E., & Alkan, A. (2001). Peripheral glycerol injections in the treatment of idiopathic trigeminal neuralgia: Retrospective analysis of 157 cases. *Journal of Oral and Maxillofacial Surgery, 59*(10), 1176–1179. doi:10.1053/joms.2001.26721 PMID:11573175

Eseonu, C. I., Goodwin, C. R., Zhou, X., Theodros, D., Bender, M. T., Mathios, D., ... Lim, M. (2015). Reduced CSF leak in complete calvarial reconstructions of microvascular decompression craniectomies using calcium phosphate cement. *Journal of Neurosurgery, 123*(6), 1476–1479. doi:10.3171/2015.1.JNS142102 PMID:26230465

Fardy, M. J., & Patton, D. W. (1994). Complications associated with peripheral alcohol injections in the management of trigeminal neuralgia. *British Journal of Oral & Maxillofacial Surgery, 32*(6), 387–391. doi:10.1016/0266-4356(94)90031-0 PMID:7849000

Fardy, M. J., Zakrzewska, J. M., & Patton, D. W. (1994). Peripheral surgical techniques for the management of trigeminal neuralgia?Alcohol and glycerol injections. *Acta Neurochirurgica, 129*(3–4), 181–184. doi:10.1007/BF01406500 PMID:7531385

Ferguson, G. G., Brett, D. C., Peerless, S. J., Barr, H. W., & Girvin, J. P. (1981). Trigeminal neuralgia: a comparison of the results of percutaneous rhizotomy and microvascular decompression. *The Canadian Journal of Neurological Sciences, 8*(3), 207–14. Retrieved from http://www.ncbi.nlm.nih.gov/pubmed/6169418

Fothergill, J. (1773). Of a painful affection of the face. *Medical Observations and Inquiries by a Society of Physicians, 5*, 129–142. Retrieved from https://archive.hshsl.umaryland.edu/bitstream/10713/3435/1/Fothergill1940.pdf

Fowler, G. R. (1886). I. The Operative Treatment of Facial Neuralgia. *Annals of Surgery, 3*(4), 269–320. doi:10.1097/00000658-188603000-00026 PMID:17856059

Frazier, C. H. (1928). Operation for the radical cure of trigeminal neuralgia: Analysis of five hundred cases. *Annals of Surgery, 88*(3), 534–547. doi:10.1097/00000658-192809000-00021 PMID:17865965

Fromm, G. H., Terrence, C. F., & Chattha, A. S. (1984). Baclofen in the treatment of trigeminal neuralgia: Double-blind study and long-term follow-up. *Annals of Neurology, 15*(3), 240–244. doi:10.1002/ana.410150306 PMID:6372646

Gardner, W. J. (1959). Response of trigeminal neuralgia to decompression of sensory root; discussion of cause of trigeminal neuralgia. *Journal of the American Medical Association, 170*(15), 1773. doi:10.1001/jama.1959.03010150017004 PMID:13672767

Gardner, W. J. (1962). Concerning the Mechanism of Trigeminal Neuralgia and Hemifacial Spasm. *Journal of Neurosurgery, 19*(11), 947–958. doi:10.3171/jns.1962.19.11.0947 PMID:13946557

Goerss, S. J., Atkinson, J. L. D., & Kallmes, D. F. (2009). Variable size percutaneous balloon compression of the gasserian ganglion for trigeminal neuralgia. *Surgical Neurology, 71*(3), 388–390. doi:10.1016/j.surneu.2007.09.040 PMID:18291447

Goodwin, C. R., Yang, J. X., Bettegowda, C., Hwang, B., James, C., Biser, A., ... Lim, M. (2013). Glycerol rhizotomy via a retrosigmoid approach as an alternative treatment for trigeminal neuralgia. *Clinical Neurology and Neurosurgery, 115*(12), 2454–2456. doi:10.1016/j.clineuro.2013.09.009 PMID:24161889

Graham, J. G., & Zilkha, K. J. (1966). Treatment of trigeminal neuralgia with carbamazepine: A follow-up study. *British Medical Journal, 1*(5481), 210–211. doi:10.1136/bmj.1.5481.210 PMID:5901730

Håkanson, S. (1981). Trigeminal neuralgia treated by the injection of glycerol into the trigeminal cistern. *Neurosurgery, 9*(6), 638–646. doi:10.1227/00006123-198112000-00005 PMID:7322329

Han, K. R., & Kim, C. (2010). The Long-Term Outcome of Mandibular Nerve Block with Alcohol for the Treatment of Trigeminal Neuralgia. *Anesthesia and Analgesia, 111*(2), 550–553. doi:10.1213/ANE.0b013e3181e4204c PMID:20584871

Hardy, D. G., & Rhoton, A. L. Jr. (1978). Microsurgical relationships of the superior cerebellar artery and the trigeminal nerve. *Journal of Neurosurgery, 49*(5), 669–678. doi:10.3171/jns.1978.49.5.0669 PMID:712389

Hartley, F. (1892). Intracranial Neurectomy of the Fifth Nerve. *Annals of Surgery, 17*, 511–526. doi:10.1097/00000658-189301000-00120 PMID:17859915

Horsley, V. (1891). Remarks on the Various Surgical Procedures Devised for the Relief or Cure of Trigeminal Neuralgia (Tic Douloureux). *British Medical Journal, 2*(1615), 1249–1252. doi:10.1136/bmj.2.1615.1249 PMID:20753459

Hutchinson, B. (1822). *Cases of Neuralgia Spasmodica, Commonly Termed Tic Douloureux Successfully Treated*. London: Second.

Iannone, A., Baker, A. B., & Morrell, F. (1958). Dilantin in the treatment of trigeminal neuralgia. *Neurology, 8*(2), 126–128. doi:10.1212/WNL.8.2.126 PMID:13504430

Jannetta, P. J. (1967). Arterial Compression of the Trigeminal Nerve at the Pons in Patients with Trigeminal Neuralgia. *Journal of Neurosurgery, 26*(1part2), 159–162. doi:10.3171/jns.1967.26.1part2.0159 PMID:6018932

Kellogg, R., Pendleton, C., Quinones-Hinojosa, A., & Cohen-Gadol, A. A. (2010). Surgical Treatment of Trigeminal Neuralgia: A History of Early Strides Toward Curing a "Cancerous Acrimony.". *Neurosurgery*, *67*(5), 1419–1425. doi:10.1227/NEU.0b013e3181f0ef13 PMID:20871443

Kerr, F. W. L., Miller, R. H., Bader, G., Coenen, H., Guarch, F. S., Lignac, G. O. E., ... Hager, W. (1966). The Pathology of Trigeminal Neuralgia. *Archives of Neurology*, *15*(3), 308. doi:10.1001/archneur.1966.00470150086014 PMID:5912011

Kolluri, S., & Heros, R. C. (1984). Microvascular decompression for trigeminal neuralgia. A five-year follow-up study. *Surgical Neurology*, *22*(3), 235–240. doi:10.1016/0090-3019(84)90005-3 PMID:6463831

Kondo, A. (2001). Microvascular decompression surgery for trigeminal neuralgia. *Stereotactic and Functional Neurosurgery*, *77*(1–4), 187–189. doi:10.1159/000064619 PMID:12378075

Kouzounias, K., Lind, G., Schechtmann, G., Winter, J., & Linderoth, B. (2010). Comparison of percutaneous balloon compression and glycerol rhizotomy for the treatment of trigeminal neuralgia. *Journal of Neurosurgery*, *113*(3), 486–492. doi:10.3171/2010.1.JNS091106 PMID:20187700

Krause, F. (1896). *Die Neuralgie des Trigeminus*. Leipzig: Vogel.

Kuchta, J., Møller, A. R., Wedekind, C., & Jannetta, P. J. (1998). Delayed hearing loss after microvascular decompression of the trigeminal nerve. *Acta Neurochirurgica*, *140*(1), 94–97. doi:10.1007007010050064 PMID:9522915

Leksell, L. (1971). Sterotaxic radiosurgery in trigeminal neuralgia. *Acta Chirurgica Scandinavica*, *137*(4), 311–314. Retrieved from http://www.ncbi.nlm.nih.gov/pubmed/4948331 PMID:4948331

Lobato, R. D., Rivas, J. J., Sarabia, R., & Lamas, E. (1990). Percutaneous microcompression of the gasserian ganglion for trigeminal neuralgia. *Journal of Neurosurgery*, *72*(4), 546–553. doi:10.3171/jns.1990.72.4.0546 PMID:2319312

Lopez, B. C., Hamlyn, P. J., & Zakrzewska, J. M. (2004). Stereotactic radiosurgery for primary trigeminal neuralgia: State of the evidence and recommendations for future reports. *Journal of Neurology, Neurosurgery, and Psychiatry*, *75*(7), 1019–1024. doi:10.1136/jnnp.2003.018564 PMID:15201363

McDonald, I. (2004). A History of Nerve Functions: From Animal Spirits to Molecular Mechanisms. *Brain*, *128*(1).

McLeod, N. M. H., & Patton, D. W. (2007). Peripheral alcohol injections in the management of trigeminal neuralgia. *Oral Surgery, Oral Medicine, Oral Pathology, Oral Radiology, and Endodontology*, *104*(1), 12–17. doi:10.1016/j.tripleo.2007.01.001 PMID:17428701

Møller, A. R., & Møller, M. B. (1989). Does intraoperative monitoring of auditory evoked potentials reduce incidence of hearing loss as a complication of microvascular decompression of cranial nerves? *Neurosurgery*, *24*(2), 257–263. doi:10.1227/00006123-198902000-00017 PMID:2918977

Morrell, F., Bradley, W., & Ptashne, M. (1958). Effect of Diphenylhydantion on Peripheral Nerve. *Neurology*, *8*(2), 140–144. doi:10.1212/WNL.8.2.140 PMID:13504433

Mullan, S., & Lichtor, T. (1983). Percutaneous microcompression of the trigeminal ganglion for trigeminal neuralgia. *Journal of Neurosurgery*, *59*(6), 1007–1012. doi:10.3171/jns.1983.59.6.1007 PMID:6631493

Murphy, J. B. (1896). Surgery of the Gasserian Ganglion with Demonstration and Report of Two Cases. In *Western Medical Review* (pp. 149–152). Western Medical Review Publishing Co.

Murphy, J. B. (1904). Osmic acid injections for relief of trifacial neuralgia. *Journal of the American Medical Association*, *43*(14), 947. doi:10.1001/jama.1904.92500140001f

Nishihara, K., Hanakita, J., Kinuta, Y., Kondo, A., Yamamoto, Y., & Nakatani, H. (1986). Importance of intraoperative monitoring of ABR and compound action potential of the eighth cranial nerve during microvascular decompression surgery. *No Shinkei Geka. Neurological Surgery*, *14*(4), 509–518. Retrieved from http://www.ncbi.nlm.nih.gov/pubmed/3713977 PMID:3713977

Nurmikko, T. J., & Eldridge, P. R. (2001). Trigeminal neuralgia--pathophysiology, diagnosis and current treatment. *British Journal of Anaesthesia*, *87*(1), 117–132. doi:10.1093/bja/87.1.117 PMID:11460800

Oddsson, B. (1944). Electrocoagulation of the Gasserian ganglion by the Kirschner method. *Acta Psychiatrica Scandinavica*, *19*(1–2), 293–299. doi:10.1111/j.1600-0447.1944.tb04571.x

Ostwalt, F. (1906). On deep alcohol injections in the facial and other neuralgias and in histrionic spasm. *Lancet*, *167*(4319), 1605–1607. doi:10.1016/S0140-6736(01)84034-4

Pearce, J. M. S. (2003). Trigeminal neuralgia (Fothergill's disease) in the 17th and 18th centuries. *Journal of Neurology, Neurosurgery, and Psychiatry*, *74*(12), 1688. doi:10.1136/jnnp.74.12.1688 PMID:14638891

Pinkus, R. L. (1984). Innovation in neurosurgery: Walter Dandy in his day. *Neurosurgery*, *14*(5), 623–631. doi:10.1227/00006123-198405000-00022 PMID:6374495

Pollock, L. J., Potter, H. E., Patrick, H. T., Patrick, H. T., Härtel, F., Grinker, J., & Maes, U. (1916). Experimental studies of injection of the Gasserian ganglion. *Journal of the American Medical Association*, *LXVII*(19), 1357. doi:10.1001/jama.1916.02590190019007

Putnam, T. J., Hampton, A. O., Harris, W., Härtel, F. F., Irger, I. M., Zander, P., ... Gama, C. (1936). A technic of injection into the Gasserian ganglion under roentgenographic control. *Archives of Neurology and Psychiatry*, *35*(1), 92. doi:10.1001/archneurpsyc.1936.02260010102007

Radulović, N., Đorđević, N., Denić, M., Pinheiro, M. M. G., Fernandes, P. D., & Boylan, F. (2012). A novel toxic alkaloid from poison hemlock (Conium maculatum L., Apiaceae): Identification, synthesis and antinociceptive activity. *Food and Chemical Toxicology*, *50*(2), 274–279. doi:10.1016/j.fct.2011.10.060 PMID:22063758

Rand, R. W. (1981). The Gardner neurovascular decompression operation for trigeminal neuralgia. *Acta Neurochirurgica*, *58*(3–4), 161–166. doi:10.1007/BF01407123 PMID:7315548

Rand, R. W. (1997). Leksell Gamma Knife treatment of tic douloureux. *Neurosurgery Clinics of North America*, *8*(1), 75–78. Retrieved from http://www.ncbi.nlm.nih.gov/pubmed/9018707 PMID:9018707

Régis, J., Tuleasca, C., Resseguier, N., Carron, R., Donnet, A., Gaudart, J., & Levivier, M. (2016). Long-term safety and efficacy of Gamma Knife surgery in classical trigeminal neuralgia: A 497-patient historical cohort study. *Journal of Neurosurgery*, *124*(4), 1079–1087. doi:10.3171/2015.2.JNS142144 PMID:26339857

Rose, F. C. (1993). European neurology from its beginnings until the 15th century: An overview. *Journal of the History of the Neurosciences*, *2*(1), 21–44. doi:10.1080/09647049309525550 PMID:11618442

Rose, W. (1890). Removal of the Gasserian Ganglion for Severe Neuralgia. *Lancet*, *136*(3505), 914–915. doi:10.1016/S0140-6736(01)78645-X

Rushworth, R. G., & Smith, S. F. (1982). Trigeminal neuralgia and hemifacial spasm: Treatment by microvascular decompression. *The Medical Journal of Australia*, *1*(10), 424–426. Retrieved from http://www.ncbi.nlm.nih.gov/pubmed/7099070 PMID:7099070

Seager, L. D., & Castelnuovo, G. (1947). Toxicity of stilbamidine; a study of the effects of chronic intoxication. *Archives of Pathology*, *44*(3), 287–296. Retrieved from http://www.ncbi.nlm.nih.gov/pubmed/20267695 PMID:20267695

Shaikh, S., Yaacob, H., & Abd Rahman, R. B. (2011). Lamotrigine for trigeminal neuralgia: Efficacy and safety in comparison with carbamazepine. *Journal of the Chinese Medical Association*, *74*(6), 243–249. doi:10.1016/j.jcma.2011.04.002 PMID:21621166

Sheinberg, M. A., & Sagher, O. (2002). Medical Management of Trigeminal Neuralgia. In K. J. Burchiel (Ed.), *Surgical Management of Pain*. Stuttgart: Georg Thieme Verlag; doi:10.1055/b-0034-45927

Shelden, C. H., Pudenz, R. H., Freshwater, D. B., & Crue, B. L. (1955). Compression Rather than Decompression for Trigeminal Neuralgia. *Journal of Neurosurgery*, *12*(2), 123–126. doi:10.3171/jns.1955.12.2.0123 PMID:14368343

Sindou, M., Fob, J.-L., Ciriano, D., & Fischer, C. (1992). Hearing Prognosis and Intraoperative Guidance of Brainstem Auditory Evoked Potential in Microvascular Decompression. *The Laryngoscope*, *102*(6), 678–682. doi:10.1288/00005537-199206000-00014 PMID:1602916

Sindrup, S. H., & Jensen, T. S. (2002). Pharmacotherapy of trigeminal neuralgia. *The Clinical Journal of Pain*, *18*(1), 22–27. doi:10.1097/00002508-200201000-00004 PMID:11803299

Stookey, B. (1928). Differential section of the trigeminal root in the surgical treatment of trigeminal neuralgia. *Annals of Surgery*, *87*(2), 172–178. doi:10.1097/00000658-192887020-00002 PMID:17865827

Stookey, B., & Ransohoff, J. (1959). *Trigeminal Neuralgia: Its History & Treatment*. Springfield, IL: Charles C Thomas.

Sun, T., Saito, S., Nakai, O., & Ando, T. (1994). Long-term results of microvascular decompression for trigeminal neuralgia with reference to probability of recurrence. *Acta Neurochirurgica*, *126*(2–4), 144–148. doi:10.1007/BF01476425 PMID:8042547

Sweet, W. H., Cushing, H., Adson, A. W., Grant, F. C., Jefferson, G., Horrax, G., ... Orley, A. (1950). Trigeminal injection with radiographic control. *Journal of the American Medical Association*, *142*(6), 392. doi:10.1001/jama.1950.02910240010003 PMID:15402380

Sweet, W. H., Poletti, C. E., & Macon, J. B. (1981). Treatment of trigeminal neuralgia and other facial pains by retrogasserian injection of glycerol. *Neurosurgery*, *9*(6), 647–653. doi:10.1227/00006123-198112000-00006 PMID:6976524

Sweet, W. H., & Wepsic, J. G. (1974). Controlled thermocoagulation of trigeminal ganglion and rootlets for differential destruction of pain fibers. *Journal of Neurosurgery*, *40*(2), 143–156. doi:10.3171/jns.1974.40.2.0143 PMID:4587949

Taarnhøj, P. (1952). Decompression of the Trigeminal Root and the Posterior Part of the Ganglion as Treatment in Trigeminal Neuralgia. *Journal of Neurosurgery*, *9*(3), 288–290. doi:10.3171/jns.1952.9.3.0288 PMID:14939059

Taarnhøj, P. (1982). Decompression of the posterior trigeminal root in trigeminal neuralgia. *Journal of Neurosurgery*, *57*(1), 14–17. doi:10.3171/jns.1982.57.1.0014 PMID:7086492

Taha, J. M., & Tew, J. M. Jr. (1996). Comparison of surgical treatments for trigeminal neuralgia: Reevaluation of radiofrequency rhizotomy. *Neurosurgery*, *38*(5), 865–871. doi:10.1097/00006123-199605000-00001 PMID:8727810

Theodros, D., Rory Goodwin, C., Bender, M. T., Zhou, X., Garzon-Muvdi, T., De la Garza-Ramos, R., ... Lim, M. (2016). Efficacy of primary microvascular decompression versus subsequent microvascular decompression for trigeminal neuralgia. *Journal of Neurosurgery*, 1–7. doi:10.3171/2016.5.JNS151692 PMID:27419826

Trojnik, T., & Ŝmigoc, T. (2012). Percutaneous trigeminal ganglion balloon compression rhizotomy: Experience in 27 patients. *TheScientificWorldJournal*, *328936*. doi:10.1100/2012/328936 PMID:22545013

Watson, C. P. N. (2012). Trigeminal Neuralgia. *Pain Research & Management : The Journal of the Canadian Pain Society*, *17*(4), 297–298. doi:10.1155/2012/742324

Wei, Y., Pu, C., Li, N., Cai, Y., Shang, H., & Zhao, W. (2016). Long-term therapeutic effect of microvascular decompression for trigeminal neuralgia: Kaplan-meier analysis in a consecutive series of 425 patients. *Turkish Neurosurgery*. doi:10.5137/1019-5149.JTN.18322-16.1 PMID:27593849

Wiffen, P. J., McQuay, H. J., Edwards, J. E., & Moore, R. A. (2005). Gabapentin for acute and chronic pain. *Cochrane Database of Systematic Reviews, 20*(3), CD005452. doi:10.1002/14651858.CD005452 PMID:16034978

Wiffen, P. J., McQuay, H. J., & Moore, R. A. (2005). Carbamazepine for acute and chronic pain. *Cochrane Database of Systematic Reviews, 3*(3), CD005451. doi:10.1002/14651858.CD005451 PMID:16034977

Wilkins, R. H. (1963). Neurosurgical Classic—XIV. *Journal of Neurosurgery, 20*(12), 1090–1099. doi:10.3171/jns.1963.20.12.1090 PMID:14186111

Wilkins, R. H. (2002). Trigeminal Neuralgia: historical overview, with emphasis on surgical treatment. In K. J. Burchiel (Ed.), *Surgical Management of Pain* (pp. 288–301). New York: Thieme.

Wilkinson, H. A. (1999). Trigeminal nerve peripheral branch phenol/glycerol injections for tic douloureux. *Journal of Neurosurgery, 90*(5), 828–832. doi:10.3171/jns.1999.90.5.0828 PMID:10223447

Woodhall, B., & Odom, G. L. (1956). Stilbamidine treatment of tic douloureux. *Transactions of the American Neurological Association*, 110–4. Retrieved from http://www.ncbi.nlm.nih.gov/pubmed/13312016

Xia, L., Zhong, J., Zhu, J., Wang, Y.-N., Dou, N.-N., Liu, M.-X., ... Li, S.-T. (2014). Effectiveness and Safety of Microvascular Decompression Surgery for Treatment of Trigeminal Neuralgia. *The Journal of Craniofacial Surgery, 25*(4), 1413–1417. doi:10.1097/SCS.0000000000000984 PMID:24978453

Xu-Hui, W., Chun, Z., Guang-Jian, S., Min-Hui, X., Guang-Xin, C., Yong-Wen, Z., & Lun-Shan, X. (2011). Long-term outcomes of percutaneous retrogasserian glycerol rhizotomy in 3370 patients with trigeminal neuralgia. *Turkish Neurosurgery, 21*(1), 48–52. Retrieved from http://www.ncbi.nlm.nih.gov/pubmed/21294091 PMID:21294091

Zakrzewska, J. M., & Linskey, M. E. (2014). Trigeminal neuralgia. *BMJ (Clinical Research Ed.)*, 348. PMID:24534115

Chapter 2
Classification Systems for Trigeminal Neuralgia and Quantification of Facial Pain

Michael G. Brandel
University of California – San Diego, USA

David R. Santiago-Dieppa
University of California – San Diego, USA

Kevin Porras
University of California – San Diego, USA

Vincent J. Cheung
University of California – San Diego, USA

Jeffrey A. Steinberg
University of California – San Diego, USA

Brian R. Hirshman
University of California – San Diego, USA

Robert C. Rennert
University of California – San Diego, USA

Jeffrey Scott Pannell
University of California – San Diego, USA

Arvin R. Wali
University of California – San Diego, USA

John F. Alksne
University of California – San Diego, USA

Alexander A. Khalessi
University of California – San Diego, USA

ABSTRACT

Trigeminal neuralgia is a rare syndrome classically described as brief paroxysms of severe, lancinating facial pain along a unilateral trigeminal nerve distribution. Numerous clinical presentations of trigeminal neuralgia exist, with various distinct etiologies. Several classification schemes have been designed for clinical and research

DOI: 10.4018/978-1-5225-5349-6.ch002

purposes. However, varying terminology and inconsistent utilization of these systems can lead to diagnostic confusion and ungeneralizable research findings. Similarly, multiple pain scales have been used for trigeminal neuralgia with differing degrees of granularity, validity, and reliability. This chapter provides an overview of the commonly used classification systems and pain scales in the context of their evolution and utilization. Furthermore, the authors provide recommendations for application of these systems to clinical and research practice.

INTRODUCTION

Trigeminal neuralgia (TN) is a rare type of facial pain, occurring in approximately 4-5 in 100,000 people (Katusic, Williams, Beard, Bergstralh, & Kurland, 1991; Khan, Nishi, Hassan, Islam, & Gan, 2017), and typically involves brief paroxysms of intense, shock-like pain along the trigeminal nerve distribution that can be triggered by benign stimuli. The symptoms are almost always unilateral, and may coincide with autonomic symptoms such as lacrimation or eye redness.

The etiology of TN is most commonly due to compression of the trigeminal nerve at the root entry zone to the pons (Love & Coakham, 2001). At least 80 percent of cases involve compression by a blood vessel (Hamlyn, 1997; Hilton, Love, Gradidge, & Coakham, 1994), mainly by the superior cerebellar artery (Jannetta, 1985). However, a subset of TN may also be caused by masses including cerebellopontine angle tumors, aneurysms, and arteriovenous malformations, or demyelination of the trigeminal nerve nuclei or nerve itself such which can occur with multiple sclerosis (Cheng, Cascino, & Onofrio, 1993; Figueiredo, Brock, De Oliveira, & Prill, 1989; Ildan et al., 1996; Linskey, Jho, & Jannetta, 1994).

BACKGROUND

Several classification systems have been used to distinguish between clinical and etiologic subtypes of trigeminal neuralgia. These systems are used as diagnostic criteria in the evaluation of facial pain, and play a critical role in research seeking to create and compare treatments. Furthermore, clinicians utilize these systems and results from therapeutic trials when selecting treatments for their patients. Therefore, study results, available treatment options, and ultimately, treatments pursued may vary based on which classification system is utilized for diagnosis. Additionally, multiple methods of grading facial pain are used in conjunction with classification systems for research and clinical practice. Therefore, confusion may also arise due to the inconsistent use of pain terminology. This chapter provides an overview of

TN classification systems and methods for quantifying facial pain, in addition to a discussion of controversy regarding these schemas and recommendations for clinicians and researchers.

CLASSIFICATION SYSTEMS FOR TRIGEMINAL NEURALGIA

The original clinical classification scheme for trigeminal neuralgia was the delineation of Typical (Classic) TN or Atypical TN (Giovanelli, Marini, & Marossero, 1963; Hughes, 1950). Typical TN is the TN presentation best-recognized by physicians, involving brief paroxysms of severe, shock-like pain along one or more unilateral divisions of the trigeminal nerve. The pain may be triggered by light touching of the face, or by other activities such as speaking, chewing, or swallowing (other classic ones are brushing teeth or even wind blowing against face). Furthermore, neurological deficits are almost always absent, and pain-free intervals between attacks are common. In contrast, Atypical TN is used as an umbrella term to classify TN that does not fit the presentation of Typical TN. The timing may be prolonged or constant rather than paroxysmal, and the characteristics of the pain may be aching, dull, sharp, throbbing, or burning in contrast to the classic lancinating pain. The presence of neurological deficits or bilateral pain, particularly in the absence of an identifiable anatomic etiology such as compression of the trigeminal nerve root, suggests a diagnosis of Atypical TN and further workup should be considered.

Etiologic classifications of trigeminal neuralgia have additionally been created. Essential, Classical, Primary, and Idiopathic TN are terms that have been used interchangeably to describe TN due to vascular compression or an unidentifiable cause (Apfelbaum, 1977; Guidetti, 1950; Kaess, 1951; Strandjord, 1973). In contrast, Secondary and Symptomatic TN have been used synonymously to label trigeminal neuralgia caused by tumors, multiple sclerosis, or other discernable anomalies (Elster, 1951; Obrador & Boixados, 1955).

In the early 2000's, Burchiel and Eller et al. published a new classification system for trigeminal neuralgia that expanded upon the Typical and Atypical clinical categories, linking objective natural history and pathophysiology to these classifications schemes (Burchiel, 2003; Eller, Raslan, & Burchiel, 2005). Typical TN is classified as TN1, whereas TN2 is described similarly to Atypical TN, with predominant constant background pain as an additional feature. Both TN1 and TN2 are considered idiopathic. TN1 can theoretically progress to TN2, and TN2 is more commonly associated with an underlying posterior fossa tumor or vascular malformation. Facial pain mediated by the trigeminal nerve that is secondary to trauma or denervation is considered Trigeminal Neuropathic Pain rather than trigeminal neuralgia. Additional categories include Symptomatic TN secondary to trigeminal demyelination in MS patients, Postherpetic TN due to a facial herpes zoster outbreak, and Atypical Facial Pain solely in patients with a somatoform pain disorder that involves multiple pain complaints throughout the body.

Published in 2013, the International Classification of Headache Disorders 3rd edition (ICHD-3) has two broad categories describing facial pain: Classical Trigeminal Neuralgia (CTN) and Painful Trigeminal Neuropathy (PTN) (Headache Classification Committee of the International Headache, 2013).

Classical trigeminal neuralgia is defined as trigeminal neuralgia for which neurovascular compression is the only apparent cause. Diagnostic criteria include at least three attacks of unilateral facial pain that are confined to the trigeminal distribution (typically in the second or third divisions), are not better accounted for by another ICHD-3 diagnosis, and meet at least three of the following four criteria:

- Paroxysmal episodes lasting up to two minutes
- Severe intensity
- Shooting, lancinating, electric shock-like
- Triggered by mild stimuli to the face on the affected side

The ICHD-3 states that classical trigeminal neuralgia may be purely paroxysmal, in which patients are asymptomatic between episodes, or may be accompanied or preceded by prolonged background pain in the affected area. Additionally, classical trigeminal neuralgia is absent of any clinically evident neurologic deficit. In the presence of neurologic deficits such as hypoesthesia/hypoalgesia, which indicate axonal damage, criteria are met for Painful Trigeminal Neuropathy.

Painful trigeminal neuropathy (PTN) is associated with several etiologies. PTN may be attributed to acute herpes zoster, in which a herpetic eruption has occurred in the trigeminal nerve distribution and/or varicella zoster virus DNA is detectable in the CSF by polymerase chain reaction (PCR). The pain is preceded by the herpetic eruption by less than 7 days, lasts less than three months, is more common in immunocompromised patients, and affects the ophthalmic division in over 80% of patients. Post-herpetic PTN may also occur in patients with a history of acute Herpes zoster affecting the trigeminal nerve, in which the pain persists or recurs for at least three months. The pain has a burning and itching quality, with variable sensory abnormalities, and is most common in the elderly. Another etiology is post-traumatic PTN, also known as *anesthesia dolorosa*, which may occur as a complication of rhizotomy or thermocoagulation to treat trigeminal neuralgia (Elahi & Ho, 2014), or within 3-6 months of other mechanical, thermal, chemical, or radiation trauma to the trigeminal nerve. PTN may also be associated with a multiple sclerosis (MS) plaque affecting the trigeminal nerve root or a space-occupying lesion making contact with the trigeminal nerve, both of which must be demonstrated by imaging for diagnosis.

Cruccu et al. (2016) developed a new definition and diagnostic scheme for TN that relies on both diagnostic certainty and clinical/etiologic features (Cruccu et al., 2016). In this system, emphasis is placed on the distinction between idiopathic and etiologically established TN. Within the latter category, the diagnosis of Classical TN requires MRI evidence of vascular compression and morphologic changes of the trigeminal nerve root. Secondary TN requires evidence of a major neurologic disease, such as a cerebellopontine angle tumor or MS, causing the trigeminal neuralgia. In contrast, a clinical diagnosis of TN that lacks etiologic evidence is termed Idiopathic TN.

QUANTIFICATION OF FACIAL PAIN

Numerous methods have been used to quantify pain in patients with trigeminal neuralgia. Two broad classes of pain scales exist: single measure scales and composite scales. Single measure pain scales measure only the intensity of the pain. Composite pain scales combine the measurement of pain intensity and the patient's response to the pain with regards to changes in medication usage.

One of the most frequently used single measure pain scales is the Visual Analog Scale (VAS). The VAS is a 10 centimeter (cm) linear scale that asks the patient to rank their current pain from 0 cm, representing no pain, to 10 cm, representing the most excruciating pain. However, pain is subjective and levels on the VAS do not necessarily correlate between patients. Despite obvious difficulties with standardizing this scale, it has been used for degenerative joint disease (Averbuch & Katzper, 2004), cancer (Jensen, 2003), and rheumatologic disorders (Langley & Sheppeard, 1985), where it has been shown to be reproducible. For trigeminal neuralgia, the VAS has been used as a measure of the efficacy of pharmaceutical therapies such as sumatriptan, nalbuphine and naloxone (Kanai, Suzuki, Osawa, & Hoka, 2006; Schmidt, Gear, & Levine, 2003), and surgical treatments such as microvascular decompression (Sandell & Eide, 2008).

Composite scales, such as the Barrow Neurological Institute Pain Intensity Score (BNIPIS) (Rogers et al., 2000), combine the measurements of both pain intensity and medication usage into a single score. The BNIPIS is a scale with the following five discrete categories:

I: No pain and no medications
II: Occasional pain with no medications required
III: Some pain that is adequately controlled with medications

IV: Some pain that is not adequately controlled with medications
V: Severe pain or no pain relief

Whereas the VAS was difficult to standardize due to the subjective nature of pain, the BNIPIS's categorical descriptions are more amenable to a standardized evaluation of pain. The BNIPIS has been frequently utilized for assessing treatment response of trigeminal neuralgia pain to gamma knife radiosurgery (Kondziolka et al., 1996; Rogers et al., 2000; Young, Vermulen, & Posewitz, 1998). Although the BNIPIS is less subjective than the VAS, it lacks a description of the pain characteristics and does not reflect the impact that the pain has on patients' lives.

A more comprehensive scale is the McGill Pain Questionnaire (MPQ), which addresses several qualities of pain, including sensory, affective, and evaluative descriptors. It contains a series of 78 descriptive words, separated into 20 groups. Groups 1-10 assess the sensory quality of the pain. Groups 11-15 assess the affective quality of the pain. Group 16 assesses the intensity of the pain. Groups 17-20 assess qualities of the pain, such as radiation, numbness, changes in temperature associated with the pain, nausea, etc. Patients circle the descriptor from each set of words that most represents their pain for all 20 groups. A point value is assigned to each word based on its location in that word set, i.e. the third descriptor in a word set is worth 3 points, the fourth descriptor is worth 4 points. The sum of these scores is the Pain Rating Index (PRI). The final section of the MPQ is the present pain intensity (PPI) and is a subjective, discrete 0 to 5 scale of the patient's current pain, where 0 is no pain and 5 is excruciating pain. The MPQ has enabled differentiation between patients with typical trigeminal neuralgia and those with atypical facial pain (Melzack, Terrence, Fromm, & Amsel, 1986). However, the time required to complete the questionnaire and its reliance on complex vocabulary may hinder its use and reproducibility.

In 2010, Chen & Lee (Chen & Lee, 2010) reviewed existing pain scales for trigeminal neuralgia by the standards recommended by the Initiative on Methods, Measurement, and Pain Assessment in Clinical Trials (IMMPACT). The IMMPACT identified 6 core domains of pain that should be used to standardize and directly compare data on chronic pain management. These core domains were: pain intensity, physical functioning, emotional function, improvement and satisfaction with treatment, symptoms and adverse effects, and adherence to treatment regimens (Turk et al., 2003). The authors found that trigeminal neuralgia pain scales in the neurosurgical literature 1) typically had been 1-dimensional, measuring only pain intensity *or* pain improvement, but not both, and 2) had not been carefully tested for their psychometric properties in trigeminal neuralgia patients (Chen & Lee, 2010). In this context, Chen & Lee developed the Brief Pain Inventory (BPI) – Facial scale (now called the Penn Facial Pain Scale; PFPS). This 18-item questionnaire focuses on 2 core domains recommended by the IMMPACT, pain intensity and physical functioning. Patients rank pain intensity at various times and the degree to which pain interferes with general and face-specific activities on a scale from 0 to 10. The authors found their scale to be highly reliable and valid on psychometric testing (Chen & Lee, 2010). The PFPS represents a major advance in the field of pain measurement of trigeminal neuralgia given its efficient administration and face-specific questions that directly apply to trigeminal neuralgia.

Issues, Controversies, Problems

As discussed, numerous systems exist for the classification of trigeminal neuralgia subtypes and for the quantification of pain. Classification systems have been plagued by inconsistent usage and vague terminology, in addition to the contrast between etiologic versus clinical schemes of categorization. Pain scales have been just as varied, if not more so. Their utilization demonstrates a tradeoff between specificity and efficiency, as some pain scales are comprehensive but burdensome to use, whereas others are succinct and generalizable to varied types of pain but lack meaningful sophistication.

SOLUTIONS AND RECOMMENDATIONS

In the context of the burgeoning field of neurosurgical interventions for trigeminal neuralgia, the authors favor classification systems that account for etiology, rather than just clinical presentation. For example, the American Academy of Neurology's system developed by Cruccu et al. (Cruccu et al., 2016) allows clear categorization of patients that may benefit from therapies directed towards correcting aberrant vasculature (e.g., microvascular decompression) versus those that need disease-specific therapy (e.g., tumor resection, multiple sclerosis drugs, etc.) or those with no known etiology and may require purely symptomatic pain therapy. 3D high-resolution MRI has proven to be a reliable method for detecting neurovascular conflict in trigeminal neuralgia, with some recent studies reporting 95-97% sensitivity and 100% specificity (Chun-Cheng, Qing-Shi, Ji-Qing, & Zhi-Gang, 2009; Han, Zhang, Chen, & Hou, 2016; Leal et al., 2010; Leal et al., 2011). Therefore, MRI findings are appropriate for integration into the classification of TN.

For pain scales, the authors recommend methods that account for how the pain affects behavior (e.g., medication usage) rather than simply a subjective intensity. These scales, including the BNIPIS, MPQ, and PFPS, may be more amenable for demonstrating how an intervention meaningfully impacts patient lives.

FUTURE RESEARCH DIRECTIONS

The newest classification system and pain scale for trigeminal neuralgia discussed in this chapter are the American Academy of Neurology guidelines and the Penn Facial Pain Scale, respectively. While these systems have resolved, in theory, some of issues with prior methods, they have yet to be broadly vetted in research or practice. Future studies may provide external validation for these systems, and use them to measure or compare the effects of novel therapeutics.

CONCLUSION

Because many different classification systems and pain scales are used to characterize trigeminal neuralgia, communication issues may arise among physicians and researchers. This chapter summarizes the most commonly used methods for characterizing trigeminal neuralgia and highlights their various strengths and limitations.

REFERENCES

Apfelbaum, R. I. (1977). A comparision of percutaneous radiofrequency trigeminal neurolysis and microvascular decompression of the trigeminal nerve for the treatment of tic douloureux. *Neurosurgery*, *1*(1), 16–21. doi:10.1227/00006123-197707000-00004 PMID:615946

Averbuch, M., & Katzper, M. (2004). Assessment of visual analog versus categorical scale for measurement of osteoarthritis pain. *Journal of Clinical Pharmacology*, *44*(4), 368–372. doi:10.1177/0091270004263995 PMID:15051743

Burchiel, K. J. (2003). A new classification for facial pain. *Neurosurgery*, *53*(5), 1164–1166, discussion 1166–1167. doi:10.1227/01.NEU.0000088806.11659.D8 PMID:14580284

Chen, H. I., & Lee, J. Y. (2010). The measurement of pain in patients with trigeminal neuralgia. *Clinical Neurosurgery*, *57*, 129–133. PMID:21280505

Cheng, T. M., Cascino, T. L., & Onofrio, B. M. (1993). Comprehensive study of diagnosis and treatment of trigeminal neuralgia secondary to tumors. *Neurology*, *43*(11), 2298–2302. doi:10.1212/WNL.43.11.2298 PMID:8232946

Chun-Cheng, Q., Qing-Shi, Z., Ji-Qing, Z., & Zhi-Gang, W. (2009). A single-blinded pilot study assessing neurovascular contact by using high-resolution MR imaging in patients with trigeminal neuralgia. *European Journal of Radiology*, *69*(3), 459–463. doi:10.1016/j.ejrad.2007.10.010 PMID:18035511

Cruccu, G., Finnerup, N. B., Jensen, T. S., Scholz, J., Sindou, M., Svensson, P., ... Nurmikko, T. (2016). Trigeminal neuralgia: New classification and diagnostic grading for practice and research. *Neurology*, *87*(2), 220–228. doi:10.1212/WNL.0000000000002840 PMID:27306631

Elahi, F., & Ho, K. W. (2014). Anesthesia dolorosa of trigeminal nerve, a rare complication of acoustic neuroma surgery. *Case Reports in Neurological Medicine*, *496794*. doi:10.1155/2014/496794 PMID:25328729

Eller, J. L., Raslan, A. M., & Burchiel, K. J. (2005). Trigeminal neuralgia: Definition and classification. *Neurosurgical Focus*, *18*(5), E3. doi:10.3171/foc.2005.18.5.4 PMID:15913279

Elster, P. (1951). Symptoms and diagnosis of trigeminal neuralgia and conclusions regarding essential and symptomatic trigeminal neuralgia. *Psychiatrie, Neurologie, und Medizinische Psychologie*, *3*(4), 86–93. PMID:14844533

Figueiredo, P. C., Brock, M., De Oliveira, A. M. J., & Prill, A. (1989). Arteriovenous malformation in the cerebellopontine angle presenting as trigeminal neuralgia. *Arquivos de Neuro-Psiquiatria*, *47*(1), 61–71. doi:10.1590/S0004-282X1989000100008 PMID:2669692

Giovanelli, M., Marini, G., & Marossero, F. (1963). Typical Trigeminal Neuralgia in the Presence of Macroscopic Organic Lesions of the Central Nervous System. *Minerva Neurochirurgica*, *54*, 124–130. PMID:14125306

Guidetti, B. (1950). Essential trigeminal neuralgia; section of the descending bulbar trigeminal tract according to Sjoqvist's method. *Sistema Nervoso*, *2*(4), 247–257. PMID:14809416

Hamlyn, P. J. (1997). Neurovascular relationships in the posterior cranial fossa, with special reference to trigeminal neuralgia. 2. Neurovascular compression of the trigeminal nerve in cadaveric controls and patients with trigeminal neuralgia: Quantification and influence of method. *Clinical Anatomy (New York, N.Y.)*, *10*(6), 380–388. doi: PMID:9358968

Han, K. W., Zhang, D. F., Chen, J. G., & Hou, L. J. (2016). Presurgical visualization of the neurovascular relationship in trigeminal neuralgia with 3D modeling using free Slicer software. *Acta Neurochirurgica, 158*(11), 2195–2201. doi:10.100700701-016-2936-8 PMID:27543280

Headache Classification Committee of the International Headache S. (2013). The International Classification of Headache Disorders, 3rd edition (beta version). Cephalalgia, 33(9), 629-808. doi:10.1177/0333102413485658

Hilton, D. A., Love, S., Gradidge, T., & Coakham, H. B. (1994). Pathological findings associated with trigeminal neuralgia caused by vascular compression. *Neurosurgery, 35*(2), 299–303, discussion 303. doi:10.1227/00006123-199408000-00017 PMID:7969838

Hughes, B. (1950). Atypical trigeminal neuralgia. *British Dental Journal, 89*(11), 243–249. PMID:14791847

Ildan, F., Gocer, A. I., Bagdatoglu, H., Uzuneyupoglu, Z., Tuna, M., & Cetinalp, E. (1996). Isolated trigeminal neuralgia secondary to distal anterior inferior cerebellar artery aneurysm. *Neurosurgical Review, 19*(1), 43–46. doi:10.1007/BF00346609 PMID:8738365

Jannetta, P. J. (1985). Microsurgical management of trigeminal neuralgia. *Archives of Neurology, 42*(8), 800. doi:10.1001/archneur.1985.04210090068018 PMID:4026617

Jensen, M. P. (2003). The validity and reliability of pain measures in adults with cancer. *The Journal of Pain, 4*(1), 2–21. doi:10.1054/jpai.2003.1 PMID:14622723

Kaess, M. (1951). Etiology and treatment of idiopathic trigeminal neuralgia. *Munchener Medizinische Wochenschrift, 93*(7), 330–335. PMID:14826732

Kanai, A., Suzuki, A., Osawa, S., & Hoka, S. (2006). Sumatriptan alleviates pain in patients with trigeminal neuralgia. *The Clinical Journal of Pain, 22*(8), 677–680. doi:10.1097/01.ajp.0000210917.18536.0d PMID:16988562

Katusic, S., Williams, D. B., Beard, C. M., Bergstralh, E. J., & Kurland, L. T. (1991). Epidemiology and clinical features of idiopathic trigeminal neuralgia and glossopharyngeal neuralgia: Similarities and differences, Rochester, Minnesota, 1945-1984. *Neuroepidemiology, 10*(5-6), 276–281. doi:10.1159/000110284 PMID:1798430

Khan, M., Nishi, S. E., Hassan, S. N., Islam, M. A., & Gan, S. H. (2017). Trigeminal Neuralgia, Glossopharyngeal Neuralgia, and Myofascial Pain Dysfunction Syndrome: An Update. *Pain Research & Management, 7438326*. doi:10.1155/2017/7438326 PMID:28827979

Kondziolka, D., Lunsford, L. D., Flickinger, J. C., Young, R. F., Vermeulen, S., Duma, C. M., ... Lindquist, C. (1996). Stereotactic radiosurgery for trigeminal neuralgia: A multiinstitutional study using the gamma unit. *Journal of Neurosurgery*, *84*(6), 940–945. doi:10.3171/jns.1996.84.6.0940 PMID:8847587

Langley, G. B., & Sheppeard, H. (1985). The visual analogue scale: Its use in pain measurement. *Rheumatology International*, *5*(4), 145–148. doi:10.1007/BF00541514 PMID:4048757

Leal, P. R., Hermier, M., Froment, J. C., Souza, M. A., Cristino-Filho, G., & Sindou, M. (2010). Preoperative demonstration of the neurovascular compression characteristics with special emphasis on the degree of compression, using high-resolution magnetic resonance imaging: A prospective study, with comparison to surgical findings, in 100 consecutive patients who underwent microvascular decompression for trigeminal neuralgia. *Acta Neurochirurgica*, *152*(5), 817–825. doi:10.100700701-009-0588-7 PMID:20108106

Leal, P. R., Hermier, M., Souza, M. A., Cristino-Filho, G., Froment, J. C., & Sindou, M. (2011). Visualization of vascular compression of the trigeminal nerve with high-resolution 3T MRI: A prospective study comparing preoperative imaging analysis to surgical findings in 40 consecutive patients who underwent microvascular decompression for trigeminal neuralgia. *Neurosurgery*, *69*(1), 15–25, discussion 26. doi:10.1227/NEU.0b013e318212bafa PMID:21346659

Linskey, M. E., Jho, H. D., & Jannetta, P. J. (1994). Microvascular decompression for trigeminal neuralgia caused by vertebrobasilar compression. *Journal of Neurosurgery*, *81*(1), 1–9. doi:10.3171/jns.1994.81.1.0001 PMID:8207508

Love, S., & Coakham, H. B. (2001). Trigeminal neuralgia: Pathology and pathogenesis. *Brain*, *124*(Pt 12), 2347–2360. doi:10.1093/brain/124.12.2347 PMID:11701590

Melzack, R., Terrence, C., Fromm, G., & Amsel, R. (1986). Trigeminal neuralgia and atypical facial pain: Use of the McGill Pain Questionnaire for discrimination and diagnosis. *Pain*, *27*(3), 297–302. doi:10.1016/0304-3959(86)90157-0 PMID:3808740

Obrador, S., & Boixados, J. R. (1955). Secondary trigeminal neuralgia due to basilar impression and platybasia. *Revista Clínica Española*, *58*(4), 232–234. PMID:13281048

Rogers, C. L., Shetter, A. G., Fiedler, J. A., Smith, K. A., Han, P. P., & Speiser, B. L. (2000). Gamma knife radiosurgery for trigeminal neuralgia: The initial experience of The Barrow Neurological Institute. *International Journal of Radiation Oncology, Biology, Physics*, *47*(4), 1013–1019. doi:10.1016/S0360-3016(00)00513-7 PMID:10863073

Sandell, T., & Eide, P. K. (2008). Effect of microvascular decompression in trigeminal neuralgia patients with or without constant pain. *Neurosurgery*, *63*(1), 93–99, discussion 99–100. doi:10.1227/01.NEU.0000335075.16858.EF PMID:18728573

Schmidt, B. L., Gear, R. W., & Levine, J. D. (2003). Response of neuropathic trigeminal pain to the combination of low-dose nalbuphine plus naloxone in humans. *Neuroscience Letters*, *343*(2), 144–146. doi:10.1016/S0304-3940(03)00356-2 PMID:12759184

Strandjord, R. (1973). Medicinal treatment planning in primary trigeminal neuralgia. *Tidsskrift for den Norske lageforening: tidsskrift for praktisk medicin, ny rakke*, *93*(30), 2251-2252.

Turk, D. C., Dworkin, R. H., Allen, R. R., Bellamy, N., Brandenburg, N., Carr, D. B., ... Witter, J. (2003). Core outcome domains for chronic pain clinical trials: IMMPACT recommendations. *Pain*, *106*(3), 337–345. doi:10.1016/j.pain.2003.08.001 PMID:14659516

Young, R. F., Vermulen, S., & Posewitz, A. (1998). Gamma knife radiosurgery for the treatment of trigeminal neuralgia. *Stereotactic and Functional Neurosurgery*, *70*(Suppl 1), 192–199. doi:10.1159/000056422 PMID:9782251

KEY TERMS AND DEFINITIONS

Atypical Trigeminal Neuralgia: Trigeminal neuralgia that does not fit the presentation of typical trigeminal neuralgia; for example, having prolonged or constant pain, pain that is aching, dull, sharp, or throbbing, neurological deficits, or bilateral pain.

Barrow Neurological Institute Pain Intensity Score (BNIPIS): A five-tier pain scale for trigeminal neuralgia that combines the measurements of pain intensity and medication usage into a single composite score.

Classical Trigeminal Neuralgia: Trigeminal neuralgia with MRI evidence of vascular compression and morphologic changes of the trigeminal nerve root.

Idiopathic Trigeminal Neuralgia: Trigeminal neuralgia for which there is no known etiology.

McGill Pain Questionnaire (MPQ): A comprehensive pain scale for trigeminal neuralgia that contains a series of 78 descriptive words used to characterize the pain, in addition to a 0-5 pain intensity ranking.

Painful Trigeminal Neuropathy: Trigeminal neuralgia with concurrent neurological deficits such as hypoesthesia/hypoalgesia; associated with several potential etiologies including herpes zoster infection, trauma, space-occupying lesions, and multiple sclerosis.

Penn Facial Pain Scale (PFPS): An 18-item questionnaire used to rate pain from trigeminal neuralgia which focuses on pain intensity and physical functioning.

Secondary/Symptomatic Trigeminal Neuralgia: Trigeminal neuralgia caused by a major neurologic disease such as a cerebellopontine angle tumor or multiple sclerosis.

Trigeminal Neuralgia: A rare type of facial pain, typically involving brief paroxysms of intense, shock-like pain along the unilateral trigeminal nerve distribution that can be triggered by benign stimuli, which may coincide with autonomic symptoms such as lacrimation or eye redness.

Typical Trigeminal Neuralgia: The most common clinical presentation of trigeminal neuralgia, involving brief paroxysms of severe, shock-like pain along one or more divisions of the unilateral trigeminal nerve triggered by benign stimuli, and absent of any neurological deficits.

Chapter 3
Medical Management of Trigeminal Neuralgia

Niushen Zhang
Stanford University, USA

ABSTRACT

The first-line treatment of trigeminal neuralgia can be very effective, but side effects are often difficult for patients to tolerate. This chapter is a guide to the broad selection of medical therapies currently available for the treatment of trigeminal neuralgia which includes oral therapies and other non-surgical methods of treatment such as IV medications, nasal sprays, topical ointments, and injections. The discussion of each treatment includes discussion of its evidence in current literature, its proposed mechanism of action, its dosing and appropriate setting for clinical use, and its side effect profile.

INTRODUCTION

The aim of all trigeminal neuralgia therapies is to modulate the hyperexcitable state of the trigeminal afferents to relieve pain. The first-line treatment of trigeminal neuralgia is oral medication. These medications can be very effective for the treatment of trigeminal neuralgia, but their side effects are often difficult for patients to tolerate. If a patient fails first and second line oral therapies, and if the patient is not a surgical candidate, then the wide array of next-line oral medications and combination therapy should be considered. In addition, there has been exploration into other non-surgical and non-invasive methods of treatment such as IV medications, nasal sprays, topical ointments, and injections. This chapter is a guide to the broad selection of medical therapies currently available for the treatment of trigeminal

DOI: 10.4018/978-1-5225-5349-6.ch003

neuralgia. For each treatment, this chapter will cover multiple aspects including 1) discussion of its evidence in current literature; 2) its proposed mechanism of action; 3) its dosing and appropriate setting for clinical use; and 4) its side effect profile.

PART 1: FIRST-LINE THERAPY

Treatment of trigeminal neuralgia should begin with either carbamazepine or with oxcarbazepine, as agreed upon by the American Academy of Neurology and the European Federation of Neurological Societies (Cruccu & Truini, 2013). When a patient does not respond to either carbamazepine or oxcarbazepine, or if the patient cannot take these medications because of contraindications or intolerable side effects, then the patient is defined as having refractory trigeminal neuralgia (Cruccu, 2013).

Carbamazepine

Carbamazepine has level A evidence and is the first line therapy for initial and long-term treatment of trigeminal neuralgia (Gronseth et al., 2008; Chesire, 2015). Patients who respond to the medication will often experience pain relief within a few days of starting carbamazepine. However, this medication should be used cautiously, especially in the elderly, because of its many side effects.

Carbamazepine's mechanism for pain relief is unknown. It is an iminostilbene whose structure resembles tricyclic antidepressants and phenytoin. One hypothesis is that it decreases conductance in sodium channels, which results in stabilization of hyper excitable membranes and inhibits ectopic discharges (Tremont-Lukats, Megeff, & Backonja, 2000). The medication usually reaches peak concentration in 2-6 hours. After 2-4 weeks of starting carbamazepine, the half-life decreases from about 30 hours to 13-17 hours because of auto-induction. The drug is excreted by the liver. As an anticonvulsant, the therapeutic drug level is 4-12 mcg/dl. In the context of treating trigeminal neuralgia, there is poor correlation between pain relief and drug concentration (Green & Selman, 1991).

Carbamazepine is the best studied medical treatment for trigeminal neuralgia. There are four, high quality (Class I or II), placebo-controlled studies demonstrating that carbamazepine can, not only reduce the frequency and intensity of painful episodes, but is equally efficacious for spontaneous and trigger-evoked attacks (Gronseth et al., 2008). The dose range for carbamazepine in these studies was 300mg to 2,400mg daily. The treatment response in these trials were very strong, with 58-100% of patients on carbamazepine experiencing complete or near complete pain control, compared to 0-40% of patients on placebo experiencing complete or near complete pain control (Jorns & Zakrzewska, 2007). However, there has only been one study that evaluated the long-term efficacy of carbamazepine over a 16-year period. In this study of 146 patients, there was an initial reported success in 60% of patients. But by 5-16 years, only 22% of participants were still experiencing benefit from carbamazepine. About 44% of patients required additional or alternative treatment (Taylor, Brauer, & Espir, 1981). Observational studies have shown that there is a decrease in efficacy over time, but this may be related more to increased severity of the disease rather than development of tolerance (Zakrzewska & Patsalos, 2002).

Carbamazepine should not be used in patients with a history of bone marrow depression or hypersensitivity to tricyclic compounds such as amitriptyline and nortriptyline (Ferrell & McLeod, 2008). Also, before starting carbamazepine, it is imperative to evaluate the patient's risk for potentially developing carbamazepine-induced Stevens-Johnson syndrome (SJS) and toxic epidermal necrolysis (TEN). Though the occurrence is rare, SJS and TEN are two forms of the same life-threatening skin disease that can cause rash, skin peeling, and sores on the mucous membranes. The HLA-B*1502 allele is highly associated with carbamazepine-induced SJS and TEN. The association has been found mostly in the Han Chinese. The association has not been found in Caucasian patients. The HLA-B*1502 allele frequency is 10.2% in Han Chinese living in Asia and 5% in Asians living in North America (Ferrell & McLeod, 2008). There is a 0.25% (1 in 400) incidence of carbamazepine-induced SJS and TEN in Taiwan. Though the positive predictive value of the test is low, the FDA recommends genotyping all Asian patients for the allele. It is most likely prudent to avoid carbamazepine when patients have tested positive given the availability of other effective medications (Ferrell & McLeod, 2008).

Carbamazepine is usually prescribed as extended-release capsules or tablets. It is available as 200mg tablets, 100mg chewable tablets, and suspension of 100mg/5mL. The usual starting dose is 200mg daily or divided into two doses. For elderly patients and for patients who are particularly sensitive to medication side effects, carbamazepine can be started at 100mg daily. Some patients may experience pain relief with doses as small as 100mg twice to three times a day. Otherwise, the daily dose can be increased by 100mg every 3-4 days until adequate pain relief is achieved, or until the patient experiences any intolerable side effects. The typical maintenance dose range is from 200mg to 1200mg per day, divided into two to four doses (Obermann, 2010). For some patients, frequent dosing can be helpful for breakthrough pain that occurs between doses (Tomson & Ekbom, 1981). Initial efficacy is approximately 80% (Obermann, 2010). As mentioned above, over time, larger doses are typically required to maintain pain control. Carbapamezapine is typically recommended as daily preventive therapy, but based on clinical experience, some patients are able to successfully use carbamazepine as rescue therapy and only take it as needed. There are also patients who take a consistent daily dose but will take additional dose (such as 200mg) on an as needed basis.

Approximately 6-10% of patients cannot tolerate carbamazepine (Taylor et al., 1981). Many of the side effects are dose dependent. Dizziness, lightheadedness, drowsiness, ataxia, diplopia, nystagmus, nausea and vomiting are some of the common side effects. Less common side effects include hypertension, paresthesia, blurred vision, hyponatremia, and increase in transaminases. Rare, but potentially serious side effects include allergic rash, myelosuppression, hepatotoxicity, lymphadenopathy, systemic lupus erythematosus, Stevens-Johnson syndrome, and aplastic anemia (Jorns & Zakrzewska, 2007). Within several weeks after starting the medication, labs for serum sodium, complete blood count, and liver function test should be performed. Carbamazepine also has multiple pharmacologic interactions. It is a CYP450 inducer and may increase clearance and lead to sub-therapeutic levels of many drugs including warfarin, anti-epileptic drugs and mood stabilizers (lamotrigine, phenytoin, valproic acid), benzodiazepines, and birth control pills.

Oxcarbazepine

Oxcarbazepine is a keto-derivative of carbamazepine that has simpler pharmacokinetics. The weaker induction of hepatic enzymes is thought to lead to a better side effect profile compared to carbamazepine. It is predominantly excreted by the kidneys. Patients who are allergic to carbamazepine may also be allergic to oxcarbazepine. Genotyping before primary oxcarbazepine treatment has neither been recommended nor studied. However, Oxcarbazepine is not recommended for patients who are HLA-B*1502 positive because there are reports of cross-reactivity for skin reactions in patients who were already intolerant to carbamazepine (Ferrell & McLeod, 2008).

Although carbamazepine has stronger evidence for efficacy, oxcarbazepine has a better safety profile (Beydoun, 2000). There is one double-blind, crossover trial (Liebel, Menger, & Langohr, 2001). and three multi-center, double-blind, randomized trials comparing efficacy and tolerability of oxcarbazepine (900-2100mg/day) vs. carbamazepine (400-1200mg/day) in patients with trigeminal neuralgia (Beydoun, Schmidt, & D'Souza, 2002). These trials showed a comparable analgesic effect between the two treatments which has led to the conclusion that oxcarbazepine can be used as an effective alternative to carbamazepine for the treatment of trigeminal neuralgia. Oxcarbazepine was found to have significantly fewer adverse effects than carbamazepine, especially fewer incidences of dizziness, ataxia, and fatigue (Jorns & Zakrzewska, 2007).

Oxcarbazepine is available as 150mg, 300mg, and 600mg film-coated tablets. It is also available as a 60mg/mL oral suspension. Starting dose is usually 150mg twice daily. But similar to carbamazepine, it is prudent and reasonable to start at 150mg daily for elderly patients and patients known to be sensitive to medication side effects. If 150mg once a day is tolerated, then increase as tolerated by 150mg every three to four days. The typical maintenance dose is 300-600mg twice a day. Effective dose range is 1200-2400mg each day. In one study, onset of the effect was observed within 24 hours (Zakrzewska & Patsalos, 1989). Common side effects include nausea, vomiting, dizziness, fatigue, tremors. Higher doses (>28-35mg/kg/day) can lead to mild hyponatremia. Similar to carbamazepine, within several weeks after starting oxcarbazepine, labs for serum sodium, complete blood count, and liver function test should be performed.

PART 2: SECOND-LINE THERAPY

Existing evidence has shown that patients who are resistant to a therapeutic dose of carbamazepine or oxcarbazepine will most likely not benefit from another orally administered medication. But many patients simply cannot reach the therapeutic dosage because of intolerance to adverse effects. Second-line therapies are typically add-on therapies but can be used on their own if carbamazepine and oxcarbazepine are contraindicated or cause intolerable side effects, even at low doses.

Baclofen

Baclofen is most commonly used to relieve muscle spasticity. The analgesic effect of the drug has been found to be independent from the impairment of motor activity (Levy & Proudfit, 1977). Baclofen is a GABAB receptor agonist and acts by decreasing excitatory neurotransmission, and therefore, may facilitate segmental inhibition of the trigeminal complex (Green & Selman, 1991). Some data, from in vitro studies, show that baclofen exhibits antagonistic properties against substance P (Saito, Konishi, & Otsuka, 1975). Baclofen reaches peak blood levels in about 2 hours and has a half-life of about 3.5 hours. Within 24 hours after a single dose, more than 85% is excreted unchanged by the kidney (Terrence & Fromm, 1981).

There are several trials from the 1980's that examine the efficacy of baclofen but these were small studies with poor methodology. In some of the trials, baclofen was used as monotherapy, and in others, baclofen was an add-on therapy (Parekh, Shah, Kotdawalla, & Gandhi, 1989). In a double-blind study, baclofen was effective in 70% of patients at doses of 10-60mg per day (Fromm, Terrence, & Chattha, 1984). Over one to five years of follow-up of 60 patients, the efficacy was only maintained in 30% of patients and 17% experienced recurrence of pain within 3-6 months, and 22% became refractory after 1-18 months. A second study by the same group compared carbamazepine alone, baclofen and carbamazepine, and baclofen only.

They found the combination therapy appeared to give the best results (Fromm & Terrence, 1987).

Baclofen is most often used in combination with carbamazepine or oxcarbazepine. The starting dose is 5mg twice to three times a day. The dose can be increased by 5-10mg each week. The usual dose taken for maximum pain relief is between 50-60mg per day, divided into three doses. Drowsiness, dizziness, confusion and lethargy, abdominal symptoms. It is important to note that in patients taking baclofen on a long-term basis (many months or more), abrupt discontinuation of baclofen can cause withdrawal seizures and hallucinations. In the cases reported, patients were on 80mg daily or greater. After many months of use, it is strongly advised that baclofen should be gradually tapered by 5-10mg each week. If withdrawal symptoms occur, then the dosage should be raised to prior levels and then resume gradual taper once patient is stable (Terrence & Fromm, 1981).

Lamotrigine

Lamotrigine is best known for its antiepileptic and mood stabilizing properties. Lamotrigine can also be a useful medication to treat trigeminal neuralgia. It is often used as adjunctive therapy to carbamazepine and oxcarbazepine or as monotherapy. Lamotrigine is thought to stabilize neural membranes and inhibits the release of excitatory neurotransmitters by acting on voltage-sensitive sodium channels (Obermann, 2010).

The data for Lamotrigine as add-on therapy has shown mixed results. In a double-blind placebo controlled trial of lamotrigine in combination with other medications (such as gabapentin) for neuropathic pain, Lamotrigine did not show any superiority over placebo in any of the endpoints (Silver, Blum, Grainger, Hammer, & Quessy, 2007). In a small, double-blind, placebo-controlled trial, lamotrigine 400mg daily, as an add-on therapy, was beneficial and more effective than placebo in fourteen patients with trigeminal neuralgia who were refractory to carbamazepine (Zakrzewska, Chaudhry, Nurmikko, Patton, & Mullens, 1997). As for using lamotrigine as monotherapy, there have been previous studies (Canavero & Bonicalzi, 1997), as well as, several more recent studies that have shown promising results. In a crossover trial of lamotrigine vs. carbamazepine, patients were titrated to lamotrigine 400mg and carbamazepine 1,200mg (Shaikh, Yaacob, & Abd Rahman, 2011). Out of a total of twenty-one patients, 62% attained pain relief from lamotrigine and over 90% attained pain relief from carbamazepine. But a greater proportion of patients obtained a complete and greater degree of pain relief with lamotrigine than with carbamazepine. In an open-label study, eleven out of fifteen patients with trigeminal neuralgia experienced pain relief with 400mg of lamotrigine (Lunardi et al., 1997).

In another open label study, lamotrigine was compared with carbamazepine in the efficacy of relieving trigeminal neuralgia pain in eighteen multiple sclerosis (Leandri et al., 2000). These patients were experiencing little or no relief from carbamazepine and could not tolerate the additional CNS side effects from carbamazepine, in addition to their baseline neurological impairments. The patients were tapered off of carbamazepine and were started on a gradual lamotrigine titration. Seventeen out of eighteen patients had complete or nearly complete pain relief on lamotrigine at doses between 75-400mg per day. Patients were much less drowsy on lamotrigine.

Lamotrigine is available as 25mg, 100mg, 150mg, and 200mg tablets. Chewable dispersible tablets and orally disintegrating tables are also available. Because of potential risk for Stevens Johnson Syndrome, a slow titration is recommended. The slower the titration, the less likely that these side effects will occur (Ketter et al., 2005; Obermann, 2010). The recommended starting dose is 25mg daily for one week, then it can be increase by 25mg daily every week until reaching the therapeutic dose range of 200 to 400mg daily. Understandably, some patients find it difficult to undergo a cautious and long titration. This medication is not recommended if symptoms are rapidly progressive and quick pain control is needed. However, based on clinical experience, lamotrigine can be a very effective adjunctive therapy or monotherapy for elderly patients who cannot tolerate the sedation and ataxia caused by carbamazepine and oxcarbazepine.

Common side effects include dizziness, constipation, nausea, and drowsiness. Lamotrigine can cause serious rashes requiring hospitalization. The incidence of these rashes, which can include Stevens-Johnson syndrome is 0.3% (3 in 1,000) in adults who take it for epilepsy. About 7-10% of patients can develop benign skin rash during the first 1-2 months of treatment that often resolves with continued therapy (Wiffen & Rees, 2007). However, it is not possible to predict if a rash will further develop and become life threatening. Therefore, the medication should be discontinued at the first sign of rash that is drug related.

PART 3: NEXT LINE THERAPY

Based on AAN Practice Parameters, there is insufficient evidence to support or refute the efficacy of any of the following therapies for controlling pain in patients with trigeminal neuralgia (Gronseth et al., 2008). However, these are therapies that can often serve as useful adjunctive therapies to help patients gain better pain control. Section one discusses the oral therapies available and section two highlights non-oral therapies that include IV medication, nasal spray, topical ointment, and injections.

Section 1: Oral Therapies

Gabapentin

Gabapentin is a GABA receptor agonist and inhibits release of excitatory neurotransmitters. This medication has many advantages, including faster titration, minimal drug interactions, and usually well-tolerated. Gabapentin has been proven to be effective for neuropathic pain (Serpell, 2002). In a retrospective review of ninety-two patients who took gabapentin for trigeminal neuralgia, forty-three patients reported reduction in facial pain occurring generally within one to three weeks, depending on the rate of dose titration (Chesire, 2002). The effective range of daily dosing was 100-2400mg, divided three times a day (mean dose was 930mg daily). The degree of benefit was complete in 16 patients, nearly complete in 9 patients, moderate in 12 patients, and partial in 6 patients. The medication was well tolerated and no serious side effects were reported. Gabapentin has also been found to be effective, with sustained relief, in multiple sclerosis patients with trigeminal neuralgia (Khan, 1998).

From clinical experience, if a patient is already on combination therapy (such as carbamazepine and lamotrigine), but still does not have adequate pain control, then gabapentin can be considered as an additional therapy to layer on. Typical starting dose is 300mg daily for a week. Then it can be increased by 300mg daily each week. Doses are typically divided into three times a day. A typical maintenance dose is 900-2700mg daily. Gabapentin usually does not interact with other medications and has a favorable side effect profile. Potential side effects include dizziness, sleepiness, diarrhea, confusion, and nausea.

Pregabalin

Pregabalin modulates voltage-gated calcium channels and reduces release of excitatory neurotransmitters and has analgesic, anxiolytic, and anticonvulsant properties. Specifically, it is an alpha2-delta (a sub-unit of voltage-gated calcium channels) binding drug, resembling gabapentin (Obermann et al., 2008). Pregabalin maintains the biological activity of gabapentin but provides improved pharmacokinetics. It is completely absorbed, not metabolized, not bound to plasma proteins, and eliminated unchanged through the kidneys (Obermann et al., 2008). One advantage of pregabalin is that its pharmacokinetic profile allows rapid dose escalation if needed. Placebo-controlled studies have shown that pregabalin has efficacy for pain relief in treatment of diabetic neuropathy and postherpetic neuralgia by improving affective symptoms, sleep, and quality of life (Obermann et al., 2008).

In terms of evidence in treatment of trigeminal neuralgia, a prospective, open-label study, with 53 patients and one-year follow-up, showed that pregabalin 150-600mg daily was effective in reducing pain by over 50% in 74% of patients. There was minor reduction of efficacy over the one-year observational period (Obermann et al., 2008). In a multi-center, observational, prospective 12-week study with 64 patients, there was alleviation of pain in 25% of patients and at least 50% reduction of pain intensity in 49% of patients who took pregabalin 150-600mg daily (mean final dose of 196±105mg/day) (Perez, Navarro, Saldana, Martinez, & Rejas, 2009). Treatment with pregabalin also reduced pain-related comorbid symptoms (anxiety/depression symptoms and difficulty with sleep) and improved disability and quality of life (Perez, Saldana, Navarro, Martinez, & Rejas, 2009). This study suggests that pregabalin can be used in monotherapy or in combination therapy to effectively treat trigeminal neuralgia. And given that patients with trigeminal neuralgia may frequently develop anxiety, depression, and difficulty with sleep, pregabalin can potentially also treat these comorbid conditions in the short-term.

Pregabalin is available in 25mg, 50mg, 75mg, 100mg, 200mg, 225mg, and 300mg capsules. Dosing can be twice daily which provides more convenience for the patient and could lead to higher compliance. However, based on clinical experience, most patients usually need three times a day dosing. Initial dosing starts with 50-75mg daily and can be titrated up by 50-75mg daily each week. A typical maintenance dose is 150mg two to three days daily. The most common side effects of pregabalin are dizziness, somnolence, peripheral edema, dry mouth, weight gain.

Duloxetine

Duloxetine is a serotonin-noradrenaline reuptake inhibitor that has FDA approval for the management of major depressive disorders, fibromyalgia, and diabetic peripheral neuropathic pain (Lunn, Hughes, & Wiffen, 2014). The mechanism of duloxetine for trigeminal neuralgia is thought to be related to modulation of norepinephrine and serotonin and antagonist of NMDA (N-methyl-D-aspartate) receptors. There has been a proposal that duloxetine exerts desynchronizing effects through its NMDA antagonism and thereby modulating the hyperexcitable state of the trigeminal afferents (Bymaster, Lee, Knadler, Detke, & Lyengar, 2005).

An open-label study form 2011 examined the efficacy of duloxetine monotherapy in trigeminal neuralgia and showed promising results (Anand, Khikav, Prasad, & Shewtengna, 2011). Fifteen patients with trigeminal neuralgia were administered duloxetine 40mg daily. Statistically significant pain relief was reported in 9 out of 15 patients. The pain relief was reported as early as in one week and was maintained for 16 weeks. The drug was well tolerated and side effects were mild and reversible. Duloxetine may also be helpful in the setting of trigeminal neuralgia and depression.

A case report from 2014, a patient who was refractory to carbamazepine and surgery was started on duloxetine 30mg daily for management of depression and was then titrated to 60mg daily (Hsu, Chang, Peng, & Liang, 2014). The patient reported remarkable relief of her pain within the first week. Her depressed mood gradually improved in the following 3 weeks. At the 4-year follow-up, her depression and trigeminal neuralgia were well managed on duloxetine 60mg daily and carbamazepine 600mg daily.

Duloxetine is available in 20mg, 30mg, 40mg, and 60mg capsules. Starting dose is typically 20mg twice a day. Within one to two weeks, the dose is usually increased to 30mg twice a day. Maximum dose is 120mg daily. There is lack of evidence for higher dosing. Based on clinical experience, duloxetine is primarily used as an adjuvant in treatment-resistant trigeminal neuralgia. Common side effects include nausea, dry mouth, constipation, diarrhea, fatigue, drowsiness, loss of appetite, agitation, and dizziness. If a patient needs to discontinue duloxetine, then a slow taper is strongly recommended. With an abrupt discontinuation, patients can experience potentially unpleasant withdrawal symptoms such as nightmares, mood swings (irritability and anger), anxiety, insomnia, nausea and vomiting.

Topiramate

Topiramate was first identified as an antiepileptic medication. It acts at different neural transmission levels such as sodium channels and can enhance GABA levels. It has a wide range of uses including treatment of migraine and depression. Topiramate can also be used for trigeminal neuralgia, however, its efficacy remains controversial. A meta-analysis of six randomized controlled trials, with poor methodological quality, that included 354 patients with trigeminal neuralgia, showed that topiramate was more effective than carbamazepine after a treatment duration of two months (Wang, Bai, 2011). However, there was no difference in effectiveness rate after one month of treatment, remission rate after two months of treatment, or in adverse events when comparing topiramate with carbamazepine. All initial dosing was 25mg twice a day and then gradually increased. Maximum dose range was 200-600mg daily. Duration of trials ranged from one to two months.

In practice, topiramate is usually started at 25mg daily and then increased by 25mg daily each week. In the treatment of migraine, doses beyond 100mg daily do not show greater benefit but do cause more side effects. There is no data that supports a specific upper limit to dosing of topiramate for the treatment of trigeminal neuralgia. Some case series found that topiramate 100-400mg daily can be effective (Domingues, Kuster, & Aquino, 2007). Dose titration should be based on pain control and side effects that the patient experiences. Common side effects include, paresthesia, word-finding difficulty, confusion, fatigue, loss of appetite, weight loss. More serious adverse effects include development of kidney stones.

Phenytoin

Phenytoin, similar to carbamazepine, blocks the sodium channels of excitatory membranes and therefore blocks action potentials. It depresses excitatory transmission at the synaptic level (Green & Selman, 1991). Braham and Saiz first recommended the use of phenytoin for the treatment of trigeminal neuralgia in 1960 (Braham & Saiz, 1960). The existing studies of phenytoin in the treatment of trigeminal neuralgia continue to be limited to those studies that were done in the1960's which showed that 54-70% of patients experienced partial or complete pain relief (Blom, 1962; Blom, 1963; Braham & Saiz, 1960). In terms of dosing, the existing studies used 300-600mg daily or 400-800mg daily. In clinical practice, oral phenytoin is rarely used for long-term treatment of trigeminal neuralgia because the evidence is poor and because of its side effect profile. Common side effects included nausea, vertigo, nystagmus tremor, and ataxia. More worrisome, long-term side effects include liver dysfunction, osteoporosis, and gingival hyperplasia. In "Non-oral Therapies" section, there will be further discussion regarding IV fosphenytoin for the treatment of trigeminal neuralgia.

Levetiracetam

The exact mechanism of action of levetiracetam is unknown. Its pharmacokinetics are linear and predictable and reaches peak plasma concentration within 1.5 hours, which is very useful when a rapid response is needed. Unlike carbamazepine and other antiepileptic medications, it does not affect the hepatic cytochrome P450 system. In an open-label prospective study, ten patients with trigeminal neuralgia were started on levetiracetam 1,000mg twice a day and titrated up by 500mg daily (Jorns, Johnston, & Zakrzewska, 2009). Maximum dose range was 3,000-5,000mg daily, which is higher than the recommended dose for epilepsy patients (3,000mg daily). Such a high dose was targeted because patients failed to respond to lower doses. After ten weeks, four patients, on higher doses of 4,000mg/day, had less pain compared with baseline (50-90% improvement). But four other patients actually felt worse after treatment. The final results showed that levetiracetam, at high doses, was only partially effective for trigeminal neuralgia pain relief, but it was very well tolerated. Another study with twenty-three patients showed that there was a 62% reduction of daily attacks when levetiracetam was used as an add-on therapy (Mitsikostas et al. 2010). The advantages of levetiracetam is that it does not interact with other medications and it is usually well tolerated. Common side effects include irritability, aggressive behavior, and change in personality.

Other Oral Therapies

There are other oral therapies that have been tried in the treatment of trigeminal neuralgia (Zhang, Yang, & Zhou 2013; Yang, Zhou, He, Chen, & Zakrzewska, 2011). However, the evidence is poor, or there are no dedicated studies to trigeminal neuralgia, such as sodium valproate and tricyclic antidepressants, respectively (Derry, Wiffen, Aldrington, & Moore, 2015; Peiris, Perera, Devendra, & Lionel, 1980). Pimozide, tizanidine, and clonazepam are certainly oral options to consider if a patient has refractory trigeminal neuralgia but they all have significant limitations.

Pimozide is an anti-psychotic that blocks dopamine receptors. It is primarily used in the treatment of Tourette syndrome. In a randomized trial of 48 patients with trigeminal neuralgia, pimozide (2-12mg daily) was reported to be more effective than carbamazepine but more people experienced adverse effects with pimozide than with carbamazepine (Lechin et al., 1989). Adverse effects included hand tremors, memory impairment, and involuntary movements. Clinically, pimozide is rarely used for the treatment of trigeminal neuralgia because of potentially long-term, extrapyramidal symptoms such as akasthesia, tremor, and slow or shuffling gait.

Tizanidine, an antispasmodic, is a centrally acting alpha-adrenergic agonist that may also have antinociceptive properties. It has proven efficacy in a double-blind crossover study in patients with refractory trigeminal neuralgia, in which eight out of ten patients had fewer painful paroxysms while taking tizanidine 2mg three times a day for 3 days and then 4mg three times a day for 4 days (Fromm, Aumentado, & Terrence, 1993). All patients that were followed-up after 1-3 months experienced recurrence of pain. However, another study found that tizanidine (up to 18mg/day) vs. carbamazepine (up to 900mg/day) had no significant effect on the number of people with relief of pain after treatment for 3 weeks (Vilming, Lyberg, & Latase, 1986). Overall, tizanidine has mixed results and limited efficacy for treating trigeminal neuralgia. Common side effects are dizziness, drowsiness, fatigue, and dry mouth.

Clonazepam is a benzodiazepine that facilitates and enhances GABA transmission in the brain. In a preliminary trial of 19 patients, 68.4% showed excellent or good improvement with no serious side effects (Chandra, 1976). In an open-label study, twenty-five patients with trigeminal neuralgia were treated with 1mg twice to three times a day, titrated up to 6-8mg total each day, over a period of ten days (Court & Kase, 1976). The medication was continued for six to nine weeks if it was effective after the initial ten-day trial. Reported clinical effectiveness was 65%, with 40% of patients achieving complete pain control and 23.3% were much improve. However, side effects of somnolence, confusion, and unsteadiness of gait was present in greater than 80% of the patients. In patients older than 60 years old, the unsteadiness was so severe they had to stay in bed. In clinical practice, clonazepam is not a preferred treatment for daily and long-term use because of withdrawal symptoms and risk of developing dependency and addiction.

Section 2: Non-Oral Therapies

IV Fosphenytoin

Intravenous fosphenytoin is a rapid onset, short-term treatment in select patients with acute, severe episodes of rigeminal neuralgia crisis. Compared to phenytoin, fosphenytoin has the advantage of better tolerability and ease of administration with faster infusion rates and lower risk for hypotension and hemodynamic instability. In a case series of three patients presenting with trigeminal neuralgia crisis who were refractory to oral medications, intravenous fosphenytoin was urgently used for treatment (Cheshire, 2001). Fosphenytoin was diluted to 5-10mg phenytoin sodium equivalents (PE)/mL in 5% dextrose with 0.45% NaCl and injected through an intravenous catheter. Hemodynamic parameters were monitored by electrocardiogram and sphygomomanometer during the infusions. Mean dose of 14mg/kg. In all cases, complete relief of pain was achieved for two days. The reported side effects included mild tinnitus, transient paresthesias, hypotension, and dizziness and ataxia that resolved the following day. As the author of the study points out, this therapy can be considered for cases of acute and sustained exacerbations of chronic recurrent trigeminal neuralgia that is refractory to other medications or serve as a short-term option for patient awaiting surgical intervention. Achieving urgent control of pain can provide a window of time when other medication and therapeutic options can be optimized.

Topical Capsaicin

Capsaicin is a secondary metabolite produced by chili peppers. By enhancing release and inhibiting reuptake of substance P, it selectively stimulates and then blocks nociceptive function of C-fiber afferents. Repeated application of capsaicin has been used to treat localized pain syndromes Data for the treatment of trigeminal neuralgia with capsaicin is mixed and poor.

In an open-label study, twelve patients with trigeminal neuralgia applied 1g of cream, containing 0.05% capsaicin, to the cutaneous area corresponding to the affected distribution of the trigeminal branch (excluding the eyelid or periocular regions), three times a day for several days (Fusco & Allessandri, 1992). Treatment was stopped when the patient no longer experienced burning sensation with application of the capsaicin. Six patients had complete relief of pain, four patients had partial relief of pain, and two patients had no relief of pain. Of the ten patients who were responsive to capsaicin, four had relapses of pain in 95-149 days. There were no relapses following the second therapy for the rest of the year. In a case series of 24 patients with chronic oral pain (five had a diagnosis of trigeminal neuralgia), capsaicin cream (0.025%) was applied to the site of discomfort four times a day for four weeks (Epstein & Marcoe, 1994). There was complete remission of neuropathic pain in 31.6% of patients. Trigeminal neuralgia with intraoral trigger was less responsive, only one out of five trigeminal neuralgia patients reported improvement. Common side effects include burning at the time of application. Patients should not apply capsaicin on the eyelid or in the periocular regions. Contact with the conjunctiva or other ocular tissues can cause intense irritation or even permanent damage in these structures.

Intranasal Lidocaine

Just posterior to the middle turbinate, the second division of the trigeminal nerve passes through the sphenopalatine ganglion. The anatomic location of the SPG allows access for administration of topical anesthetic. For transient analgesia of second-division trigeminal neuralgia, intranasal lidocaine can be used. Nose spray is a preferred method of administration because of ease of administration by the patient. In a randomized controlled study of twenty-five patients with second-division trigeminal neuralgia, patients received two sprays (0.2mL) of either lidocaine 8% or saline placebo in the affected nostril using a metered-dose spray (Kanai, Suzuki, Kobayashi, & Hoka, 2006). Intranasal lidocaine 8% spray resulted in a significant decrease of VAS score whereas placebo spray did not. Pain was described as moderate or better by twenty-three patients of the lidocaine spray group and by one patient of the placebo group. The effect of treatment lasted for an average of 4.3 hours (range was 0.5-24 hours). Over half of the patients reported stinging or burning sensation in the nasal mucosa, but there were no other reported serious adverse effects. In terms of limitations of this treatment, it is restricted to patients with pain in the second trigeminal division and the benefits are very short-lasting.

Sumatriptan

In the setting of trigeminal neuralgia, sumatriptan (a serotonin 5-HT 1B/1D receptor agonist) can potentially inhibit neurogenic inflammation and vasodilation near the irritated trigeminal root. In a randomized controlled trial, 24 patients with classical TN, refractory to previous treatment, received either 3mg of subcutaneous sumatriptan or saline (Kanai, Saito, & Hoka, 2006). After seven days, patients crossed over to receive the alternative treatment. Fifteen minutes after injection of sumatriptan, the baseline pain score decreased significantly; whereas the pain score did not decrease for the placebo group. The number of patients who benefited from sumatriptan was 20 whereas only one patient reported improvement after placebo. The mean duration of pain relief was 7.9 hours. In a second trial by the same group, 15 patients were first treated with subcutaneous injection of sumatriptan 3mg and then with one-week oral administration of sumatriptan (50mg twice daily) (Kanai, Suzuki, Osawa, & Hoka, 2006). At the end of oral treatment, pain scores were significantly decreased and this beneficial reduction persisted for another week after treatment discontinuation.

Adverse effects associated with oral sumatriptan were fatigue, nausea, chest discomfort. Patients with known coronary artery disease or uncontrolled hypertension should not use sumatriptan. In clinical practice, sumatriptan is rarely is used for the treatment of trigeminal neuralgia because there is concern for cardiovascular side effects from daily use of sumatriptan. But the above studies do seem to suggest that sumatriptan could be potentially be considered for use as a short-term preventive of trigeminal neuralgia.

Nerve Blocks

A potential adjunctive treatment is the combination of an antiepileptic drug with an analgesic block for trigeminal neuralgia trigger points. Local anesthetics at low doses block anomalous membrane excitability and potentially lead to improved control of the instability of membrane potential. Nerve block of trigger points with ropivacaine has been used to improve the therapeutic effect of gabapentin in the treatment of trigeminal neuralgia. In a four-week long, randomized trial of thirty-six patients, once a week nerve block with ropivacaine together with oral gabapentin resulted in a greater reduction of pain scores than gabapentin alone or ropivacaine alone at seven and twenty-eight days after treatment, an effect that was still present six and twelve months later (Lemos, Flores, Oliveira, & Almeida, 2008). Also, the patients on combination therapy were able to stay on lower daily doses of gabapentin (mean dose of 300mg daily) than the patients on gabapentin alone (mean dose of 525mg daily). For the analgesic block, a 27-gauge needle was used for administering subcutaneously 2mL of a 2mg/mL ropivacaine solution in each trigger point that was pointed out by the patient. These points varied for each patient and could be located in the V1, V2, or V3 distribution. Some patients received injections in more than one distribution of the face. Nerve blocks are usually very safe and have minimal side effects.

Acupuncture

The use of acupuncture for treatment of chronic pain is becoming more common and accepted in developed countries. In traditional Chinese medicine, pain is a sign of blockage of the flow of qi (energy, air, or essence). Physiological studies show that acupuncture stimulation can induce changes in the nervous system, particularly in pain inhibitory pathways (Zhao, Stillman, & Rozen, 2005). A review of twelve studies (n=920), with an acupuncture arm and carbamazepine as the control treatment, found four trials in which acupuncture was superior to carbamazepine, whereas the remaining eight trials showed no difference between the treatment and control groups (Zhao et al., 2005). All of the studies were low-quality, hence, meta-analysis was not performed. A systemic review from 2010 suggests that acupuncture is of similar efficacy as carbamazepine but with fewer adverse effects in treatment of trigeminal neuralgia; however, the evidence is weak because of low methodological quality of the reviewed studies (Liu, Li, Xu, Chung, & Zhang, 2010).

Based on clinical experience, acupuncture can be a helpful adjunctive therapy, especially if patients also have other chronic pain syndromes, insomnia, or anxiety. If patients are open to this therapy and would like to try it as an adjunctive therapy, then the recommended frequency is one to two sessions each week for a total of eight to ten sessions. Side effects are usually minimal but can include syncope, bleeding and hematoma.

Botulinum Toxin A

Botulinum toxin A (BTX-A) is a neurotoxin derived from Clostridium botulinum (Morra et al., 2016). BTX-A inhibits the release of acetylcholine at the neuromuscular junction, leading to muscle paralysis. But in the treatment of chronic migraine, the implicated mechanism of BTX-A is inhibition of central and peripheral sensitization, which is a result of blocking of the TRPV1 receptor of unmyelinated C fiber terminals and inhibiting the release of peripheral pain molecules such as substance P, CGRP, and glutamate (Aoki, 2005). In the last fifteen years, there has been a number of studies on BTX-A for the treatment of trigeminal neuralgia (Guardinani, Sadoughi, Blitzer, & Sirois, 2013). A study from 2002 reported successful relief of twitching and pain in a patient with hemifacial spasm associated with trigeminal neuralgia (Micheli, Scorticati, & Raina, 2002). However, the treatment mechanism of BTX-A in trigeminal neuralgia remains unclear. Some studies suggest that BTX-A acts locally or on the trigeminal ganglia (Cui, Khanijou, Rubino, & Aoki, 2004; Xiao et al., 2013). Whereas other studies report a central antinociceptive effect of BTX-A in a rat model of trigeminal neuralgia (Matak, Bach-Rojecky, Fillipovic, & Lackovic, 2011). A 2016 study showed that peripherally applied BTX-A exerts antinociceptive function via reducing central sensitization and inhibiting high expression of nociceptors (Wu et al., 2016).

In a 2016 systematic review and meta-analysis, four randomized controlled trials (n=178) were selected for analysis of safety and efficacy of botulinum toxin type A (BTX-A) for trigeminal neuralgia (Morra et al., 2016). According to the authors, "The evidence from this systematic review suggests that botulinum toxin type A has a clinically significant benefit in treatment of trigeminal neuralgia when compared to placebo in terms of proportion of responders, the mean paroxysms frequency per day, and the VAS score at the end of follow up. These overall outcomes consistently favored BTX-A compared with placebo across studies." One of the studies was a randomized, double-blind, placebo-controlled trial (Wu et al, 2012). Though these results are promising, a careful comparison of the four studies reveals the wide variation of protocols for dosage, site of injections, number of injections, and frequency of injections. For instance, the dosage range amongst the studies was 25 to 100 units and some studies administered the injections subcutaneously, whereas others administered the injections intradermally. Two studies used trigger zones as injection sites (Shehata, El-Tamawy, Shalaby, & Ramzy, 2013; Wu et al, 2016). As for site selection, one study used dermatome and/or mucosa (Zhang et al., 2014). Another study used "various sites, 1cm apart from one another" (Zuniga, Piedimonte, Diaz, & Micheli, 2013). The two major reported adverse events were facial asymmetry and edema or hematoma at the site of injection. Both of these adverse effects were generally tolerated and transient. Edema and hematoma resolved within 5-6 days and facial asymmetry recovered within 5-7 weeks.

Overall, the data supporting the use of BTX-A for treatment of trigeminal neuralgia is still limited. Existing studies suggest that BTX-A may be a safe and effective treatment for trigeminal neuralgia. Ongoing study is needed for the mechanism of action of BTX-A in trigeminal neuralgia. Larger randomized controlled trials are needed. And there needs to be a standard protocol for dosage, administration, and duration of treatment.

CONCLUSION

In recent years, there has been an expanding selection of non-surgical treatment options for trigeminal neuralgia. However, carbamazepine remains the first-line treatment. Patients who cannot tolerate the side effects of carbamazepine are usually switched to oxcarbazepine, which is usually just as effective. Unfortunately, there is limited evidence for management of patients who fail first line therapy. As second-line treatment, lamotrigine and baclofen are often added on to first-line therapy for increased benefit and to minimize the dosage of carbamazepine or oxcarbazepine. But there are certainly cases when lamotrigine and baclofen can be used as monotherapy. For patients who are refractory to both first and second-line treatments (and are not surgical candidates), it is necessary to try next-line therapies that include, not only oral medications, but also nasal spray, topical ointment, intravenous medication, and injections. Finding the optimal combination of therapies is heavily dependent on side effect profile and patient tolerance. Some of these next-line therapies can have potentially advantageous effects on comorbid conditions such as anxiety, depression, insomnia, muscle tension, and migraine.

REFERENCES

Anand, K., Khikav, V., & Prasad, A., & Shewtengna. (2011). Efficacy, safety, and tolerability of duloxetine in idiopathic trigeminal neuralgia. *Journal of the Indian Medical Association*, *109*(4), 264–266. PMID:22187799

Aoki, K. (2005). Review of a proposed mechanism for the antinocicpetive action of botulinum toxin type A. *Neurtoxicology*, *26*(5), 785–793. doi:10.1016/j.neuro.2005.01.017 PMID:16002144

Beydoun, A. (2000). Safety and efficacy of oxcarbazepine: Results of randomized, double-blind trials. *Pharmacotherapy*, *20*(8), 152–158. doi:10.1592/phco.20.12.152S.35254 PMID:10937814

Beydoun, A., Schmidt, D., & D'Souza, J. (2002). Oxcarbazepine versus carbamazepine in trigeminal neuralgia: a meta-analysis of three double blind comparative trials. *Neurology*, *58*(suppl 3).

Blom, S. (1962). Trigeminal neuralgia: Its treatment with a new anticonvulsant drug. *Lancet*, *1*(7234), 839–840. doi:10.1016/S0140-6736(62)91847-0 PMID:13870089

Blom, S. (1963). Tic Douloureux Treated With New Anticonvulsant. *Archives of Neurology*, *9*(3), 285–290. doi:10.1001/archneur.1963.00460090091009 PMID:14049402

Braham, J., & Saiz, A. (1960). Phenytoin in the treatment of trigeminal and other neuralgias. *Lancet*, *2*(7156), 892–893. doi:10.1016/S0140-6736(60)91959-0

Bymaster, F. P., Lee, T. C., Knadler, M. P., Detke, M. K., & Lyengar, S. (2005). The dual transporter inhibitor duloxetine: A review of its preclinical pharmacology, pharmacokinetic profile, and clinical results in depression. *Current Pharmocology Design*, *11*(12), 1475–1493. doi:10.2174/1381612053764805 PMID:15892657

Canavero, S., & Bonicalzi, V. (1997). Lamotrigine control of trigeminal neuralgia: An expanded study. *Journal of Neurology*, *244*(8), 527–532. doi:10.1007004150050137 PMID:9309561

Chandra, B. (1976). The use of clonazepam in the treatment of trigeminal neuralgia. *Proceedings of the Australian Association of Neurologists*, *13*, 119-22.

Cheshire, W. Jr. (2001). Fosphenytoin: An intravenous option for the management of acute trigeminal neuralgia crisis. *Journal of Pain and Symptom Management*, *21*(6), 506–510. doi:10.1016/S0885-3924(01)00269-X PMID:11397609

Cheshire, W. (2015). Cranial Neuralgias. *Confinia Neurologica*, *21*(4), 1072–1085. PMID:26252592

Chesire, W. (2002). Defining the role for gabapentin in the treatment of trigeminal neuralgia: A retrospective study. *The Journal of Pain*, *3*(2), 137–142. doi:10.1054/jpai.2002.122944 PMID:14622800

Court, J. E., & Kase, C. S. (1976). Treatment of tic douloureux with a new anticonvulsant (clonazepam). *Journal of Neurology, Neurosurgery, and Psychiatry*, *39*(3), 297–299. doi:10.1136/jnnp.39.3.297 PMID:932745

Cruccu, G., & Truini, A. (2013). Refractory trigeminal neuralgia. Non-surgical treatment options. *CNS Drugs*, *27*(2), 91–96. doi:10.100740263-012-0023-0 PMID:23225488

Cui, M., Khanijou, S., Rubino, J., & Aoki, K. R. (2004). Subcutaneous administration of botulinum toxin type A reduces formalin-induced pain. *Pain*, *107*(1-2), 125–133. doi:10.1016/j.pain.2003.10.008 PMID:14715398

Derry, S., Wiffen, PJ., Aldrington, D., & Moore, R.A. (2015). Nortriptyline for neuropathic pain in adults. *Cochrane Database Systematic Reviews, 8*(1).

Domingues, R., Kuster, G., & Aquino, C. (2007). Treatment of trigeminal neuralgia with low doses of topiramate. *Arquivos de Neuro-Psiquiatria*, *65*(3b), 792–794. doi:10.1590/S0004-282X2007000500011 PMID:17952282

Epstein, J. B., & Marcoe, J. H. (1994). Topical application of capsaicin for treatment of oral neuropathic pain and trigeminal neuralgia. *Oral Surgery, Oral Medicine, and Oral Pathology*, *77*(2), 135–140. doi:10.1016/0030-4220(94)90275-5 PMID:8139830

Ferrell, P., & McLeod, H. (2008). Carbamazepine, HLA-B*1502 and risk of Stevens-Johnson syndrome and toxic epidermal necrolysis: US FDA recommendations. *Pharmacogenomics*, *9*(10), 1543–1546. doi:10.2217/14622416.9.10.1543 PMID:18855540

Fromm, G., Aumentado, D., & Terrence, C. (1993). A clinical and experimental investigation of the effects of tizanidine in trigeminal neuralgia. *Pain*, *53*(3), 265–271. doi:10.1016/0304-3959(93)90222-B PMID:8351156

Fromm, G., & Terrence, C. (1987). Comparison of L-baclofen and racemic baclofen in trigeminal neuralgia. *Neurology*, *37*(11), 1725–1728. doi:10.1212/WNL.37.11.1725 PMID:3313099

Fromm, G., Terrence, C., & Chattha, A. (1984). Baclofen in the treatment of trigeminal neuralgia: Double-blind study and longer-term follow-up. *Annals of Neurology*, *15*(3), 240–244. doi:10.1002/ana.410150306 PMID:6372646

Fusco, B., & Alessandri, M. (1992). Analgesic Effect of Capsaicin in idiopathic trigeminal neuralgia. *Anesthesia and Analgesia*, *74*(3), 375–377. doi:10.1213/00000539-199203000-00011 PMID:1539818

Green, M., & Selman, J. (1991). Review Article: The Medical Management of Trigeminal Neuralgia. *Headache*, *31*(9), 588–592. doi:10.1111/j.1526-4610.1991.hed3109588.x PMID:1774173

Gronseth, G., Crucu, G., Alksne, J., Argoff, C., Brainin, M., Burchiel, K., ... Zakrzewska, J. (2008). Practice Parameter: The diagnostic evaluation and treatment of trigeminal neuralgia (an evidence-based review). *Neurology*, *71*(15), 1183–1190. doi:10.1212/01.wnl.0000326598.83183.04 PMID:18716236

Guardinani, E., Sadoughi, B., Blitzer, A., & Sirois, D. (2013). A new treatment paradigm for trigeminal neuralgia using botulinum toxin type A. *The Laryngoscope*, *124*(2), 413–417. doi:10.1002/lary.24286 PMID:23818108

Hsu, C., Chang, C., Peng, C., & Liang, C. (2014). Rapid Management of trigeminal neuralgia and comorbid major depressive disorder with duloxetine. *The Annals of Pharmacotherapy*, *48*(8), 1090–1092. doi:10.1177/1060028014532789 PMID:24788987

Jorns, T., Johnston, A., & Zakrzewska, J. (2009). Pilot study to evaluate the efficacy and tolerability of levetiracetam in treatment of patients with trigeminal neuralgia. *European Journal of Neurology*, *16*(6), 740–744. doi:10.1111/j.1468-1331.2009.02585.x PMID:19475723

Jorns, T., & Zakrzewska, J. (2007). Evidence-based approach to the medical management of trigeminal neuralgia. *British Journal of Neurosurgery*, *21*(3), 253–261. doi:10.1080/02688690701219175 PMID:17612914

Kanai, A., Saito, M., & Hoka, S. (2006). Subcutaneous sumatriptan for refractory trigeminal neuralgia. *Headache*, *46*(4), 577–582. doi:10.1111/j.1526-4610.2006.00405.x PMID:16643550

Kanai, A., Suzuki, A., Kobayashi, M., & Hoka, S. (2006). Intranasal lidocaine 8% spray for second-division trigeminal neuralgia. *British Journal of Anaesthesia*, *97*(4), 559–563. doi:10.1093/bja/ael180 PMID:16882684

Kanai, A., Suzuki, A., Osawa, S., & Hoka, S. (2006). Sumatriptan alleviates pain in patients with trigeminal neuralgia. *The Clinical Journal of Pain*, *22*(8), 677–680. doi:10.1097/01.ajp.0000210917.18536.0d PMID:16988562

Ketter, T., Wang, P., Chandler, R., Alarcon, A., Becker, O., Nowakowska, C., ... Schumacher, M. (2005). Dermatology precautions and slower titration yield low incidence of lamotrigine treatment-emergent rash. *The Journal of Clinical Psychiatry*, *66*(05), 642–645. doi:10.4088/JCP.v66n0516 PMID:15889953

Khan, O. (1998). Gabapentin relieves trigeminal neuralgia in multiple sclerosis patients. *Neurology*, *51*(2), 611–614. doi:10.1212/WNL.51.2.611 PMID:9710050

Leandri, M., Lunardi, G., Inglese, M., Messmer-Uccelli, M., Mancardi, G. L., Gottlieb, A., & Solaro, C. (2000). Lamotrigine in trigeminal neuralgia secondary to multiple sclerosis. *Journal of Neurology*, *247*(7), 556–558. doi:10.1007004150070157 PMID:10993501

Lechin, F., van der Dijs, B., Lechin, M., Amat, J., Lechin, A., Cabrera, A., ... Jimenez, V. (1989). Pimozide therapy for trigeminal neuralgia. *Archives of Neurology*, *46*(9), 960–963. doi:10.1001/archneur.1989.00520450030015 PMID:2673161

Lemos, L., Flores, S., Oliveira, P., & Almeida, A. (2008). Gabapentin supplemented with ropivacaine block of trigger points improves pain control and quality of life in trigeminal neuralgia patients when compared with gabapentin alone. *The Clinical Journal of Pain*, *24*(1), 64–75. doi:10.1097/AJP.0b013e318158011a PMID:18180639

Levy, R., & Proudfit, H. (1977). The analgesic action of baclofen (beta-(4-chlorophenyl)-gamma-aminobutyric acid). *The Journal of Pharmacology and Experimental Therapeutics*, *202*, 437–445. PMID:886473

Liebel, J. T., Menger, N., & Langohr, H. (2001). Oxcarbazepine in der Behandlung der Trigeminusneuralgie. *Nervenheilkunde: Zeitschrift für Interdisziplinaere Fortbildung*, *20*, 461–465.

Liu, H., Li, H., Xu, M., Chung, K., & Zhang, S. (2010). A systematic review on acupuncture for trigeminal neuralgia. *The Journal of Alternative Therapies*, *16*(6), 30–35. PMID:21280460

Lunardi, G., Leandri, M., Albano, C., Cultrera, S., Fracassi, M., Rubino, V., & Favale, E. (1997). Clinical effectiveness of lamotrigine and plasma levels in essential and symptomatic trigeminal neuralgia. *Neurology*, *48*(6), 1714–1717. doi:10.1212/WNL.48.6.1714 PMID:9191794

Lunn, M., Hughes, R., & Wiffen, P. (2014). Duloxetine for treating pain neuropathy, chronic pain or fibromyalgia. *Cochrane Database of Systematic Reviews*, *3*(1). PMID:24385423

Matak, I., Bach-Rojecky, L., Fillipovic, B., & Lackovic, Z. (2011). Behavioral and immunohistochemical evidence for central antinocicpetive activity of botulinum toxin A. *Neuroscience*, *186*, 201–207. doi:10.1016/j.neuroscience.2011.04.026 PMID:21539899

Micheli, F., Scorticati, M. C., & Raina, G. (2002). Beneficial effects of botulinum toxin type a for patients with painful tic convulsive. *Clinical Neuropharmacology*, *25*(5), 260–262. doi:10.1097/00002826-200209000-00006 PMID:12410057

Mitsikostas, D. D., Pantes, G. V., Avramidis, T. G., Karageorgiou, K. E., Gartzonis, S. D., & Stathis, P. G. (2010). An observational trial to investigate the efficacy and tolerability of levetiracetam in trigeminal neuralgia. *Headache*, *50*(8), 1371–1377. doi:10.1111/j.1526-4610.2010.01743.x PMID:21044281

Morra, M., Elgebaly, A., Elmaraezy, A., Khalil, A., Altibi, A., Vu, T., ... Hirayama, K. (2016). Therapeutic efficacy and safety of Botulinum Toxin A Therapy in Trigeminal Neuralgia: A systematic review and metaanalysis of randomized controlled trials. *The Journal of Headache and Pain*, *17*(1), 63. doi:10.118610194-016-0651-8 PMID:27377706

Obermann, M. (2010). Treatment options in trigeminal neuralgia. *Therapeutic Advances in Neurological Disorders*, *3*(2), 107–115. doi:10.1177/1756285609359317 PMID:21179603

Obermann, M., Yoon, M., Sensen, K., Maschke, M., Diener, H., & Katsarava, Z. (2008). Efficacy of pregabalin in the treatment of trigeminal neuralgia. *Cephalalgia*, *28*, 174–181. PMID:18039340

Parekh, S., Shah, K., Kotdawalla, H., & Gandhi, I. (1989). Baclofen in carbamazepine resistant trigeminal neuralgia- a double blind clinical trial. *Cephalalgia*, *9*(10_suppl), 392–393. doi:10.1177/0333102489009S10208

Peiris, J. B., Perera, G. L. S., Devendra, S. V., & Lionel, N. D. W. (1980). Sodium valproate in trigeminal neuralgia. *The Medical Journal of Australia*, *2*, 278. PMID:6776393

Perez, C., Navarro, A., Saldana, M. T., Martinez, S., & Rejas, J. (2009). Patient-reported outcomes in subjects with painful trigeminal neuralgia receiving pregabalin: Evidence from medical practice in primary care settings. *Cephalalgia*, *29*(7), 781–790. doi:10.1111/j.1468-2982.2008.01792.x PMID:19522052

Perez, C., Saldana, M. T., Navarro, A., Martinez, S., & Rejas, J. (2009). Trigeminal neuralgia treated with pregabalin in family medicine settings: Its effect on pain alleviation and cost reduction. *Journal of Clinical Pharmacology*, *49*(5), 582–590. doi:10.1177/0091270009333017 PMID:19299534

Saito, K., Konishi, S., & Otsuka, M. (1975). Antagonism between Lioresal and substance P in rat spinal cord. *Brain Research*, *97*(1), 177–180. doi:10.1016/0006-8993(75)90928-2 PMID:1175037

Serpell, M. G. (2002). Neuropathic pain study group. Gabapentin in neuropathic pain syndromes: A randomized, double-blind, placebo-controlled trial. *Pain*, *99*, 557–566. doi:10.1016/S0304-3959(02)00255-5 PMID:12406532

Shaikh, S., Yaacob, H. B., & Abd Rahman, R. B. (2011). Lamotrigine for trigeminal neuralgia: Efficacy and safety in comparison with carbamazepine. *Journal of the Chinese Medical Association*, *74*(6), 243–249. doi:10.1016/j.jcma.2011.04.002 PMID:21621166

Shehata, H., El-Tamawy, M., Shalaby, N., & Ramzy, G. (2013). Botulinum toxin type A: Could it be an effective treatment option in intractable trigeminal neuralgia? *The Journal of Headache and Pain*, *14*(1), 92. doi:10.1186/1129-2377-14-92 PMID:24251833

Silver, M., Blum, D., Grainger, J., Hammer, A., & Quessy, S. (2007). Double-blind, placebo-controlled trial of lamotrigine in combination with other medications for neuropathic pain. *Journal of Pain and Symptom Management*, *34*(4), 446–454. doi:10.1016/j.jpainsymman.2006.12.015 PMID:17662571

Taylor, J., Brauer, S., & Espir, M. (1981). Long-term treatment of trigeminal neuralgia. *Postgraduate Medical Journal*, *57*(663), 16–28. doi:10.1136/pgmj.57.663.16 PMID:7279817

Terrence, C., & Fromm, G. (1981). Complications of Baclofen Withdrawal. *Journal of the American Medical Association*, *38*(9), 588–589. PMID:6791618

Tomson, T., & Ekbom, K. (1981). Trigeminal neuralgia: Time course of pain in relation to carbamazepine dosing. *Cephalalgia, 1*(2), 91–98. doi:10.1111/j.1468-2982.1981.tb00015.x PMID:7346177

Tremont-Lukats, I., Megeff, C., & Backonja, M. M. (2000). Anticonvulsants for neuropathic pain syndromes: Mechanisms of action and place in therapy. *Drugs, 60*(5), 1029–1052. doi:10.2165/00003495-200060050-00005 PMID:11129121

Vilming, S., Lyberg, T., & Latase, X. (1986). Tizanidine in the management of trigeminal neuralgia. *Cephalalgia, 6*(3), 181–182. doi:10.1046/j.1468-2982.1986.0603181.x PMID:3533272

Wang, Q. P., & Bai, M. (2011). Topiramate versus carbamazepine for the treatment of classical trigeminal neuralgia: A meta-analysis. *CNS Drugs, 25*(10), 847–857. doi:10.2165/11595590-000000000-00000 PMID:21936587

Wiffen, P., & Rees, J. (2007). Lamotrigine for acute and chronic pain. *Cochrane Database of Systematic Reviews, 2*, CD006044. PMID:17443611

Wu, C., Lian, Y., Zheng, Y., Zhang, H., Chen, Y., Xie, N., & Wang, L. F. (2012). Botulinum toxin type A for the treatment of trigeminal neuralgia results from a randomized, double-blind, placebo-controlled trial. *Cephalalgia, 32*(6), 443–450. doi:10.1177/0333102412441721 PMID:22492424

Wu, C., Xie, N., Lian, Y., Xu, H., Chen, C., Zheng, Y., ... Zhang, H. (2016). Central antinociceptive activity of peripherally applied botulinum toxin type A in lab rat model of trigeminal neuralgia. *SpringerPlus, 5*(1), 431. doi:10.118640064-016-2071-2 PMID:27104119

Xiao, L., Cheng, J., Zuang, Y., Qu, W., Muir, J., Liang, H., & Zhang, D. (2013). Botulinum toxin type A reduces hyperalgesia and TRPV1 expression in rats with neuropathic pain. *Pain Medicine, 14*(2), 276–286. doi:10.1111/pme.12017 PMID:23301515

Yang, M., Zhou, M., He, L., Chen, N., & Zakrzewska, J. (2011). Non-antiepileptic drugs for trigeminal neuralgia. *Cochrane Database of Systematic Reviews, 1*, CD004029. PMID:21249658

Zakrzewska, J., & Patsalos, P. (1989). Oxcarbazepine: A new drug in the management of intractable trigeminal neuralgia. *Journal of Neurology, Neurosurgery, and Psychiatry, 52*(4), 472–476. doi:10.1136/jnnp.52.4.472 PMID:2738589

Zakrzewska, J., & Patsalos, P. (2002). Long-term cohort study comparing medical (oxcarbazepine) and surgical management of intractable trigeminal neuralgia. *Pain*, *95*(3), 259–266. doi:10.1016/S0304-3959(01)00406-7 PMID:11839425

Zakrzewska, J. M., Chaudhry, Z., Nurmikko, T. J., Patton, D. W., & Mullens, E. L. (1997). Lamotrigine in refractory trigeminal neuralgia: Results from a double-blind placebo controlled crossover trial. *Pain*, *73*(2), 223–230. doi:10.1016/S0304-3959(97)00104-8 PMID:9415509

Zhang, H., Lian, Y., Ma, Y., Chen, Y., He, C., Xie, N., & Wu, C. (2014). Two doses of botulinum toxin type A for the treatment of trigeminal neuralgia: Observation of therapeutic effect from a randomized, double-blind, double-blind, placebo controlled trial. *The Journal of Headache and Pain*, *15*(1), 65. doi:10.1186/1129-2377-15-65 PMID:25263254

Zhang, J., Yang, M., Zhou, M., He, L., Chen, N., & Zakrzewska, J. M. (2013). Non-antiepileptic drugs for trigeminal neuralgia. *Cochrane Database of Systematic Reviews*. doi:10.1002/14651858.CD004029.pub4 PMID:24297506

Zhao, C., Stillman, M., & Rozen, T. (2005). Traditional and evidence-based acupuncture in headache management: Theory, mechanism, and practice. *Headache*, *45*(6), 716–730. doi:10.1111/j.1526-4610.2005.05139.x PMID:15953304

Zuniga, C., Piedimonte, F., Diaz, S., & Micheli, F. (2013). Acute Treatment of Trigeminal Neuralgia with Onabotulinum Toxin A. *Clinical Neuropharmacology*, *36*(5), 146–150. doi:10.1097/WNF.0b013e31829cb60e PMID:24045604

Chapter 4
Open Microvascular Decompression

James Pan
Stanford University, USA

Lily H. Kim
Stanford School of Medicine, USA

Allen Ho
Stanford University, USA

Eric S. Sussman
Stanford School of Medicine, USA

Arjun V. Pendharkar
Stanford School of Medicine, USA

Terry C. Burns
Mayo Clinic School of Medicine, USA

ABSTRACT

Microvascular decompression (MVD) is a neurosurgical procedure used to treat various neuralgias of the cranial nerves. The clinical presentation, natural history, pathophysiology, and medical management of trigeminal neuralgia, hemifacial spasm, glossopharyngeal neuralgia, and nervus intermedius neuralgia is reviewed. A thorough discussion on the retrosigmoid approach for decompression of cranial nerves is presented, along with newer techniques and controversies on adjuvant therapies and neuromonitoring. The surgical outcomes of MVD are discussed, along with alternative techniques to open MVD.

DOI: 10.4018/978-1-5225-5349-6.ch004

INTRODUCTION

Microvascular decompression (MVD) is a microneurosurgical procedure used to treat various neuralgias of the cranial nerves. Originally developed for patients suffering from trigeminal neuralgia (TN), MVD has found increasing utility in the surgical management of other cranial nerve neuropathies such as hemifacial spasm (HFS), glossopharyngeal neuralgia (GN), nervus intermedius neuralgia (NIN), and refractory positional vertigo or tinnitus. A brief history of the procedure, conditions where MVD is shown to provide benefit, surgical technique and outcomes, and alternative treatments are reviewed.

HISTORY OF THE PROCEDURE

Walter Dandy was pivotal in the development of the MVD procedure by performing the first retrosigmoid approach to access the cerebellopontine angle, which was subsequently used by future surgeons to manipulate nerves at the cranial base (Dandy, 1932). In describing the pathophysiology of TN, Dandy was the first to realize that the trigeminal nerve was often impinged by a nearby blood vessel in patients with the disorder, thereby causing the prototypical shock-like pain of the face. This was observed during the very first treatments for TN which involved sectioning the fifth nerve near the brainstem (DANDY, 1929). Although division of the trigeminal nerve resulted in relief of symptoms, permanent sensory loss was an unavoidable side effect. It was not until the 1960s when the first MVD operations for TN (GARDNER & MIKLOS, 1959) and HFS (Gardner & Sava, 1962) was described by Gardner and later popularized by Jannetta (Jannetta, 2007).

OPERATIVE INDICATIONS

Trigeminal Neuralgia

Trigeminal neuralgia was first described in 1773 by John Fothergill as brief, sudden bursts of sharp, excruciating pain, triggered by light touch or eating (Fothergill, 1776). Also known as *tic douloureux*, this was a syndrome defined by paroxysms of severe facial pain, often described as electric, lancinating pain with an abrupt onset and termination, with each episode lasting a few seconds to minutes (Prasad & Galetta, 2009). These episodes are often exacerbated by minor stimuli such as chewing, a breeze across the face, touching the upper lip, or brushing the teeth. Severe pain can also cause facial muscle spasms ("tics"). The pain was often so debilitating that Harvey Cushing ascribed TN as the "suicide disease" as patients were known to kill themselves to end their suffering (Adams et al., 2011).

TN is a relatively rare condition which affects women at a rate of 1.5-1.7 times more than men (Katusic, Beard, Bergstralh, & Kurland, 1990; Maarbjerg, Gozalov, Olesen, & Bendtsen, 2014) (Table 1). The annual incidence of TN is estimated at 4 to 13 per 100,000 people (Katusic, Williams, Beard, Bergstralh, & Kurland, 1991a; MacDonald, 2000). There is also evidence that there is an increased risk of TN among those with hypertension (El-Tallawy et al., 2013; Pan, Yen, Chiu, Chen, & Chen, 2011) and migraines (Lin, Chen, Fuh, & Wang, 2015). The International Classification of Headache Disorders, 3rd edition (ICHD-3) classifies TN into "classic" cases caused by neurovascular compression and painful neuropathy caused by a number of other etiologies (Headache Classification Committee of the International Headache Society (IHS), 2013). The various etiologies of TN are summarized in Table 2.

Table 1. Epidemiology of various cranial nerve neuropathies

Disorder	Incidence	Predisposing Factors
Trigeminal Neuralgia	4-13 per 100,000	Women, increasing age, hypertension, migraine
Hemifacial Spasm	0.78 per 100,000	Women, increasing age
Glossopharyngeal Neuralgia	0.7-0.8 per 100,000	

Table 2. Possible etiologies of TN and other cranial nerve neuropathies

Category	Causes	Workup
Mass Effect	Neurovascular Compression	MRI, MRA
	Aneurysm, arteriovenous malformation	MRI, MRA, Angiogram
	Tumors (i.e. meningioma, schwannoma, epidermoid, chordoma)	MRI with and without contrast
Inflammatory	Multiple sclerosis	MRI, CSF analysis, clinical history
	Neurosarcoidosis	CSF analysis, MRI
Infectious	Herpes Zoster	Clinical history and examination
	Lyme disease	Clinical history and examination, serology
	Postherpetic Neuralgia	Clinical history
Other	Trauma	Clinical history and examination
	Idiopathic	Clinical history and examination

Classic TN is most often due to compression of the trigeminal nerve root entry zone. In 80-90% of cases, compression is due to an aberrant loop of an artery or vein (Love & Coakham, 2001). However, less common causes of TN such as demyelinating disease or structural lesions including tumors must be considered in the workup. Magnetic resonance imaging (MRI) of the brain with and without contrast is crucial in the diagnosis of TN as this can initially rule in or out obvious structural lesions such as meningioma, aneurysms, epidermoid tumors, vestibular schwannoma, or cavernomas (T. M. Cheng, Cascino, & Onofrio, 1993; El-Ghandour, 2010; Ildan et al., 1996; Matthies & Samii, 1997; Mohanty et al., 1997). Magnetic resonance angiography (MRA) can identify ectopic vascular structures impinging on the nerve root. Anatomic changes of the trigeminal nerve such as atrophy, distortion, flattening, or demyelination were also found by MR imaging in up to 53% of symptomatic patients with neurovascular compression (Antonini et al., 2014). If no mass effect lesion is identified, it may be prudent to examine white matter tracts with MR imaging which can reveal lesions consistent with multiple sclerosis. Other causes of TN can include acute herpes zoster, or postherpetic neuralgia. Trauma to the trigeminal nerve can often be revealed through history and examination alone; and in some cases, no etiology is identified (Headache Classification Committee of the International Headache Society (IHS), 2013)

Initial treatment of TN consists of medical therapy. Carbamazepine has been the best studied treatment for TN and is usually the first-line medication. Relief with carbamazepine usually occurs in the first 24-48 hours of initiating treatment. A systematic review showed that 58-100% of patients demonstrated complete or near complete pain control compared to 0-40% of patients on placebo (Gronseth et al., 2008). Although the number needed to treat was <2, the side effect profile of carbamazepine, which includes drowsiness, dizziness, nausea, vomiting, blood dyscrasias, and various drug interactions, raised the concern of the number needed to harm for minor and severe adverse events of 3 and 24, respectively. Other drugs that have shown possible efficacy for the treatment of TN include oxcarbazepine, baclofen, lamotrigine, and pimozide. Treatments such as botulinum toxin injections, clonazepam, gabapentin, phenytoin, tocainide, tinzanidine, and valproate have shown limited use in the management of TN. Typically, failure of one first line medical therapy, usually carbamazepine, at an effective dose is considered ample justification for surgery. However, a failed trial of a single less efficacious medications, such as gabapentin is not considered adequate to claim failure of conservative therapy.

It has been estimated that 25-50% patients with TN will eventually fail medical management and will require surgery (Dalessio, 1982). Careful patient selection is crucial to ensure optimal benefit from MVD. Improvement of symptoms with carbamazepine is considered diagnostic of true trigeminal neuralgia and a positive predictor of success with MVD (BLOM, 1962; Oesman & Mooij, 2011). The overall health of the patient should be evaluated as MVD is considered a major neurosurgical operation. Patients who have undergone prior procedures such as radiofrequency rhizotomy, peripheral nerve sections, radiosurgery, or prior MVD have less successful outcomes (Barker, Jannetta, Bissonette, Larkins, & Jho, 1996), although other studies suggest that prior radiosurgery or MVD do not affect operative difficulty and outcomes (Huang, Chuang, Tu, & Chou, 2006; Theodros et al., 2016). MVD provides most benefit in cases of "classic trigeminal neuralgia" with an identified neurovascular compression. For example, in a study of 179 patients who had undergone MVD for TN, outcomes were significantly better with patients presenting with symptoms of "classic" TN consisting of preponderance of shock-like pain (J. P. Miller, Magill, Acar, & Burchiel, 2009). At 3 years follow-up after MVD, pain-free rates were 66% for patients with classic TN compared to 32% of patients with atypical TN.

Hemifacial Spasm

HFS manifests as a segmental myoclonus of the muscles innervated by the facial nerve. Patients usually present in the fifth or sixth decade of life, and is usually unilateral. This disorder usually begins as brief clonic or twitching movements of the obicularis oculi and spreads to other facial muscles over a period of years to decades. Though the spasms themselves are not painful, constant stimulation and irritation of the muscle may result in a pain syndrome. In contrast to other movement disorders, HFS can continue during sleep and patients cannot suppress these movements (N.-C. Tan, Chan, & Tan, 2002).

The incidence of HFS is estimated to be approximately 0.78 per 100,000 (Auger & Whisnant, 1990). The disorder is slightly more common in women. One study suggests that the peak age with highest prevalence was between 40 and 59 years (Auger & Whisnant, 1990) whereas another showed a continual increase in the prevalence as a function of age (Nilsen, Le, & Dietrichs, 2004).

This etiology of HFS is believed to be due to irritation of the facial nerve nucleus or the proximal nerve root (Møller, 1991). Similar to TN, compressive lesions such as aberrant blood vessels, tumors, aneurysms, and arteriovenous malformations in addition to non-compressive lesions such as strokes and multiple sclerosis contribute to the pathogenesis of this disease. Therefore, in addition to a detailed history and clinical examination, MRI is essential in the workup of HFS, especially if mass effect is suspected. Electromyography (EMG) can reveal high frequency discharges and variable synkinesis (i.e. involuntary movements of the orbicularis oculi muscles following voluntary movements) on blink reflex testing. These features are useful for ruling out essential blepharospasm, dystonia, or seizures. Needle EMG can reveal irregular, brief, high-frequency bursts of motor unit potentials which correspond to clinically observed facial spasms. MRA is indicated for patients planning to undergo surgical intervention, after failure of medical management.

Due to the relative rarity of HFS, there is a paucity of clinical trials to determine the optimal medication regimen for treatment. However, a list of drugs, similar to those used to treat TN, have found utility in the management of HFS including anticonvulsants such as carbamazepine, clonazepam, and gabapentin, and others such as baclofen, anticholinergics, and haloperidol (Yaltho & Jankovic, 2011). These medications, which unlike for TN, are largely limited by their inconsistent efficacy and side effect profile (Chaudhry, Srivastava, & Joshi, 2015). Botulinum toxin injections remains the most widely used non-surgical treatment modality as the potent biological toxin derived from *Clostridium botulinum* prevents the presynaptic calcium-mediated release of acetylcholine at the neuromuscular junction. The most widely used preparation is onabotulinumtoxinA which has been reported to result in symptomatic improvements in up to 75-100% of individuals (Costa et al., 2005; Defazio et al., 2002; Jost & Kohl, 2001). However, botulinum therapy is limited by the cost of therapy and the need for repeated injections at an interval of three to six months. Side effects can also include mild facial paresis, diplopia, and ptosis (Batisti et al., 2017).

For patients who has failed medical management or botulinum toxin therapy, surgery can offer a complete cure to the disease, which unlike toxin therapy, addresses the underlying cause. The goal of surgery, in most cases, is to remove compression of the facial nerve by an offending blood vessel. Prior botulinum injections does not decrease the efficacy of MVD for hemifacial spasm (X. Wang et al., 2013). However, prior botulinum use has been reported to result in higher lateral spread response during intraoperative neuromonitoring and should be considered in the preoperative evaluation (Habeych et al., 2011).

Nervus Intermedius Neuralgia

NIN is a neuropathic pain syndrome characterized by paroxysmal episodes of shock-like pain felt deeply in the auditory canal. This sharp or burning pain is occasionally associated with a trigger-zone in the posterior wall of the ear canal, and can radiate from the auditory canal to the parieto-occipital region or to parts of the face in a trigeminal-like distribution (Smith, Robertson, Garza, & Cutrer, 2013). The origin of the pain is thought to be due to compromise of the nervus intermedius (also known as the intermediate nerve of Wrisberg), a small sensory branch of the facial nerve. The sensory afferent cell bodies are located in the geniculate ganglion, and the peripheral axons provide sensation to the inner ear, the middle ear, the mastoid air cells, the eustachian tube, and parts of the pinna of the ear.

The exact pathophysiology of NIN is debated; however, some believe that compression of the nerve by an aberrant blood vessel is a possible mechanism (Sakas et al., 2007; Yeh & Tew, 1984). However, multiple cranial nerves innervate the sensory afferents in the ear, and it is difficult to differentiate otalgia secondary to compromise of the nervus intermedius, and/or a combination of cranial nerves VII and VIII. It has been previously reported that decompression of multiple cranial nerves, potentially including some combination of V, VII, VIII, IX, X and/or XI may be necessary to obviate symptoms (Bruyn, 1984). However, similar to the workup of other cranial nerve neuropathies, a history and examination, in addition to MRI/MRA should be performed to investigate secondary causes of nerve compromise. Infection is the most common cause of secondary nervus intermedius neuropathy; therefore, a thorough history should be obtained to rule out the Ramsay Hunt syndrome which can also cause ear pain, ipsilateral facial paresis, and vesicular eruption in the auditory canal and auricle.

If the diagnosis of NIN is made, medical management is similar to that of TN. Surgery is considered when pharmacotherapy fails or cannot be tolerated. Because the etiology of NIN is more complex than that of other cranial nerve neuropathies, the neurosurgeon must anticipate the need for exploration and decompression of multiple nerves.

Glossopharyngeal Neuralgia

GN manifests as paroxysmal pain in areas innervated by the ninth and tenth cranial nerve, resulting in severe, stabbing pain involving the ear, tonsillar fossa, base of the tongue, or beneath the angle of the mandible (Khan, Nishi, Hassan, Islam, & Gan, 2017). The pain is exacerbated by chewing, coughing, yawning, talking, and swallowing, and typically lasts for seconds to minutes (Minagar & Sheremata, 2000). Due to the nonspecific nature of its presenting symptoms and the relative rarity of the condition (0.7-0.8 per 100,000) (Katusic, Williams, Beard, Bergstralh, & Kurland, 1991b; Koopman et al., 2009)., patients will often present years after symptom onset, and with extensive workup by other specialists such as otolaryngologists, dentists, and neurologists. There is no significant gender bias, and overall incidence increased slightly with age (Katusic, Williams, Beard, Bergstralh, & Kurland, 1991b).

As with other cranial nerve neuralgias, GN can be idiopathic or secondary to tumors, demyelinating lesions, peritonsilar abscesses, carotid aneurysms, and Eagle syndrome, wherein the ninth nerve is compressed laterally against an ossified stylohyoid ligament. Compression by an aberrant artery is most commonly due to the posterior inferior cerebellar artery or vertebral artery at the nerve root entry zone (Gaul, Hastreiter, Duncker, & Naraghi, 2011; Laha & Jannetta, 1977). These patients should be evaluated with a thorough history, with careful attention to trigger factors and nocturnal awakening. Local disease such as lesions within the neck and oral cavity should be excluded by an otolaryngologist. Plain skull films may reveal an ossified stylohyoid ligament consistent with Eagle syndrome, and MRI/MRA is essential in completing a comprehensive workup.

Medical treatment for GN is similar to that of TN, with carbamazepine, gabapentin, and pregabalin as first-line pharmacological agents. Application of local anesthetics and/or nerve block of the oropharynx may prove to be both diagnostic and therapeutic. Surgical decompression is indicated for patients who fail or cannot tolerate medical management.

SURGICAL TECHNIQUE

Patient Positioning and Anesthesia

The patient can be positioned in the lateral decubitus or supine position with shoulder bump, with the head pinned in three-point fixation and facing away from the surgeon. The neck should not be excessively rotated to avoid compression of the jugular vein which may compromise venous return and brain relaxation. Slight downward tilt of the head creates additional valuable space for the surgeon away from the shoulder. Gentle neck extension can improve exposure of the lower cranial nerves, whereas an MVD for TN is comfortably performed with otherwise relatively neutral neck positioning or slight flexion. Patient positioning with upper back and shoulder at the edge of the table towards the surgeon minimizes reach; ensuring the foot of the operative table is away from the head creates room to operate bipolar pedal. Neuroanesthesia techniques such as mannitol administration and/or titration of end-tidal CO2, in conjunction with reverse Trendelenburg are used to facilitate brain relaxation as needed. Note that in decompression for HFS, monitoring of the facial nerve is necessary, therefore, these patients cannot be paralyzed. Some advocate use of a lumbar drain to facilitate relaxation, but early controlled release of CSF from the cerebellopontine cistern or cisterna magna should obviate need for lumbar CSF release.

Neuromonitoring

Intraoperative neuromonitoring (IOM) is essential to prevent inadvertent injury to the cranial nerves which can result in deficits such as hearing loss. Appropriate cranial nerve electromyogram (EMG) and brainstem auditory evoked potential (BAEP) is routinely monitored. During the retrosigmoid approach for all cranial nerve manipulations, CN VIII is the most prone to mechanical manipulation due to its location at the lateral cerebellopontine angle (Hanakita & Kondo, 1988; Jannetta, 1974). If extensive exposure is indicated, it is also possible to release cerebrospinal fluid (CSF) from the cisterna magna. Patience in waiting for optimal CSF removal to achieve optimal brain relaxation can often enable the surgery to be performed with minimal use of retraction, which is the most common cause of CN VIII injury (Barker et al., 1996; Gubian & Rosahl, 2017). Changes in BAEP can be due to injury to the nerve or excessive retraction, however, in the latter case, release of retraction will usually restore BAEP to baseline levels.

For decompression of the trigeminal nerve, more experienced neurosurgeons can opt to forego IOM (Cohen-Gadol, 2011) although no formal studies have compared the rates of major deficits in cases with or without IOM. However, there is evidence to suggest that BAEP monitoring was useful in identifying surgical maneuvers that may compromise hearing, which is of particular utility to the neurosurgeon-in-training (Brock, Scaioli, Ferroli, & Broggi, 2004).

Special considerations must be made for IOM for HFS. EMGs for the facial nerve in patients with HFS are notable for the lateral spread phenomenon caused by abnormal dispersion of action potentials through the various branches of CN VII. The resolution of lateral spread is used to determine the adequacy of decompression (Møller & Jannetta, 1987), as opposed to other procedures where the disappearance of EMG activity serves as a warning for potential nerve injury.

The role of IOM for HFS operations has also been debated. In 114 consecutive patients receiving MVD without the use of neurophysiological monitoring, no major deficits were reported and the outcomes, rates of hearing loss, and other complications were comparable to those reported in series where neuromonitoring was used (Dannenbaum, Lega, Suki, Harper, & Yoshor, 2008). Other studies have also questioned the role of IOM as the persistence of the lateral spread response (LSR) may not always correlate with poor outcome (Wei et al., 2017).

Retrosigmoid Craniotomy

Considerable attention should be made to bony and surface landmarks to delineate the location of the transverse and sigmoid sinus. The asterion is the prototypical landmark for the transverse and sigmoid sinus junction, though this is only seen in 60-80% of patients (Sheng et al., 2012; Ucerler & Govsa, 2006). A parallel line to the zygomatic arch or external acoustic meatus, which extended posteriorly generally marks the location of the transverse sinus. Neuronavigation, when available, can also aid in locating the precise location of the junction and to limit bony opening. Pre-operative imaging should be inspected carefully to evaluate the anatomy of the sinus, cerebellum, and any anomalous veins as these can vary considerably in patients with hindbrain malformations (i.e. Chiari malformations) or small posterior fossa. Since MRI is almost always obtained as part of the diagnostic workup, routine inclusion of high-resolution stereotactic images in such diagnostic scans can permit intra-operative registration via facial tracing. This obviates the need for any additional pre-operative MRI scans and should enable sufficient accuracy to localize significant variations in the transverse-sigmoid junction anatomy, if desired.

After the patient is positioned, a vertical or curvilinear incision that crosses over the asterion is made approximately two finger breadths posterior to the mastoid process. The incision can also be made 1cm posterior to the digastric groove, another surface landmark to approximate the location of the sigmoid sinus. The scalp is then dissected off the skull, and bleeding, usually from an emissary vein is controlled using bipolar cautery or bonewax. The mastoid air cells should also be waxed thoroughly to prevent CSF leak.

The goal of the craniotomy should be to adequately expose the lower margin of the transverse sinus, the posterior margin of the sigmoid sinus, and the inferior portion of the squamous portion of the occipital bone. A small craniotomy or burr hole is placed inferior and posterior to the junction of the transverse and sigmoid sinuses. A single burrhole is typically sufficient to separate the underlying dura. Some surgeons find sufficient exposure for MVD for TN using a small craniectomy scarcely larger than a burr hole; a small craniotomy can provide a wider exposure. The edge of the sigmoid sinus should be exposed to provide an optimal approach to the CP angle with minimal retraction. Exposure may include bone removal more inferiorly for optimal access to the lower cranial nerves.

Neuroanesthesia and positioning techniques as described previously are used to ensure adequate relaxation prior to opening dura. The cerebellum is then gently retracted from the inferior and lateral aspect and the operating microscope is brought in to visualize the cerebellomedullary cistern. The cistern is opened with an arachnoid knife and cerebrospinal fluid is aspirated to further relax the cerebellum. With patience and CSF aspiration, very little retraction should be needed; however a retractor can be used to help gently support the cerebellar hemisphere away from the surgical corridor if needed. Dynamic retraction may also be sufficient. The surgeon should remain aware that excessive retraction can cause traction injury to the vestibulocochlear nerve, and relive retraction if any latency changes are detected on BAEPs.

Few, if any, bridging veins should be encountered along the surgical corridor between the petrous bone and the cerebellum. The superior petrosal vein (of Dandy) is exposed by dissection along the junction of the tentorium and the petrous bone. Most surgeons coagulate and divide this with impunity during trigeminal MVD, thereby minimizing risk of inadvertent avulsion. However isolated reports of venous infarct from a sacrificed Dandy's vein prompt some to think twice before dividing a particularly large vein. If divided, coagulation closer to the brain rather than the sinus junction minimizes risk of sinus injury. At this point, the cranial nerves, along with associated arteries should be visualized and identified.

Decompression of CN V

To better visualize the trigeminal nerve, a retractor can be placed superiorly and laterally on the cerebellum, superior to the vestibulocochlear nerve. The most common offending vessel is a loop of the superior cerebellar artery (SCA), most commonly compressing the rostral or rostral medial aspect of the trigeminal nerve. The SCA often has two branches in this location, and either or both branches can compress the trigeminal nerve. Inspection with a neuroendoscope can be of value as the trigeminal vein can also come into contact with the posterior and caudal aspect of the trigeminal nerve. The endoscope can also aid with visualization anterior towards Meckel's cave. After vessels are identified, arachnoid should be dissected from the nerve root to Meckel's cave to allow complete mobilization of the nerve without traction on other structures. The vessel and the nerve are then mobilized away from each other, and small teflon felt pledgets are placed between the two. Generous irrigation can be used to ensure plegets are securely positioned. Some surgeons also advocate for internal neurolysis of the trigeminal nerve, which can take the form of simple manipulation of the nerve during decompression up to systematic division of the nerve longitudinally along its fibers into 5-10 bundles from the root entry zone up to the petrous bone. Portio minor and major can both be included in this neurolysis as portio minor has been shown to carry the unmyelinated fibers implicated in pathological facial pain (Tubbs, Griessenauer, Hogan, Loukas, & Cohen-Gadol, 2014). This maneuver has been shown to be both safe and effective for ensuring post-operative relief of symptoms. In the event there is no clear offending vessel loop, internal neurolysis alone is recommended. (Ko, Ozpinar, et al., 2015b)

Overall, SCA compression is the most common (up to 88%) followed by AICA compression (<25%) (Sindou, Howeidy, & Acevedo, 2002). AICA compression can also occur with SCA compression and both vessels must be mobilized and held away from the nerve. These vessels usually compress the nerve in the superomedial portion in up to 60% of cases (Sindou et al., 2002). Other vessels (Haller et al., 2016) known to cause compression include the posterior inferior cerebellar artery (PICA), basilar artery, vertebral artery (Becker, Kohler, Vargas, Viallon, & Delavelle, 2008; Borges & Casselman, 2010), and in less common cases, an ecstatic or fusiform basilar artery aneurysm, arteriovenous malformations (de Bondt, Stokroos, & Casselman, 2007), or venous structures.

Decompression of CN VII

The facial nerve originates from the ventrolateral surface of the brainstem, just rostral to the pontomedullary junction. It is slightly anterior to the origin of CN VIII and superior to the roots of the CN IX, X, and XI complex. The choroid plexus emanating from the foramen of Luschka is an important intraoperative landmark and is located immediately posterior and inferior to the root entry zone of the facial nerve. The flocculus of the cerebellum is also located immediately posterior to CN VII. Vessels commonly compressing CN VII include the AICA (43%), PICA (31%), VA (23%), veins, and/or a combination of these structures (Campos-Benitez & Kaufmann, 2008). Published reports have varied widely on ehe site of compression, which can occur either at the root entry zone (10-96%), adjacent cisternal segment (up to 64%), transition zone (22%), or other cisternal portions (3%) (Haller et al., 2016).

Arteries compressing CN VII must be mobilized away carefully using a Rhoton microdissector taking care to avoid disruption of any brainstem perforators. The AICA and PICA can be held in place away from the nerve using Teflon pledgets, however, if involved, an ectatic VA often cannot be decompressed using Teflon alone. The VA can be dissected and moved anterior to CNs IX and X and tacked up to the dura anterior to the jugular foramen using 8-0 braided silk or nylon sutures. Offending veins can be mobilized away from the nerve and selectively coagulated with bipolar cautery.

Neuromonitoring can be utilized to help assess the adequacy of decompression. The automatism of HFS recorded by electromyography often disappears during arachnoid dissection and retraction of the cerebellum and cannot be used as a reliable marker of adequate decompression (Møller & Jannetta, 1987). Instead, disappearance of lateral spread can indicate successful decompression of the nerve and should be communicated by the neuromonitoring team (Hatem, Sindou, & Vial, 2001).

Decompression of the Nervus Intermedius

The role of MVD for nervus intermedius neuralgia is less well-defined, with evidence limited to case reports. Yeh et al. performed the first MVD for a patient with a combination of NIN and HFS caused by vascular compression (Yeh & Tew, 1984). A retromastoid craniotomy was performed to gain access to the cerebellopontine angle and the right anterior inferior cerebellar artery was mobilized away from CN VII and VIII. The patient tolerated the procedure well, had no postoperative complications, and no recurrence of otalgia or facial spasm was observed at four years follow-up. Other case reports have described a retrosigmoid approach similar to that for HFS surgery where an aberrant loop of the AICA was mobilized away from the sensory branches of CN VII using Teflon pledgets (Bellotti et al., 1988; Inoue, Shima, Hirai, Suzuki, & Matsuda, 2017; Saers, Han, & de Ru, 2011; Sakas et al., 2007; Younes, Capelle, & Krauss, 2010).

If no neurovascular compromise is identified intraoperatively, the nervus intermedius can be sectioned. This branch of CN VII is observed as one or two fascicles running between CN VII and CN VIII. The nervus intermedius can be revealed with gentle retraction of CN VII and mobilized using rhoton microdissecting instruments or fine blunt hook. A small segment is excised, and Schirmer's test to assess tear production post-operatively can be used to assess the adequacy of resection.

Decompression of CN IX

Decompression of the glossopharyngeal nerve is performed in a similar manner, though requires a slightly more inferior exposure. The offending vessel, most commonly the PICA or the AICA, is mobilized and held in place typically with Teflon pledgets or rarely stitched to the dura near the jugular foramen (Alafaci et al., 2015; Hiwatashi et al., 2008). Neurovascular compression occurs almost exclusively (95%) in the proximal root entry zone (Haller et al., 2016). If CN IX is not significantly compressed by a vascular structure, the nerve and the upper two fascicles of the vagus nerve can be sectioned and a small segment removed (Ordóñez-Rubiano, García-Chingaté, Rodríguez-Vargas, Cifuentes-Lobelo, & Perilla-Cepeda, 2017; Rey-Dios & Cohen-Gadol, 2013). It is important to note that sectioning of the nerve can result in dysphagia and vocal cord paralysis. Monitoring of the vagus nerve by placing electrodes on the false vocal cords (Taha, Tew, Keith, & Payner, 1994) or the surface of the endotracheal tube (Harries, Dong, & Honey, 2012) can help the surgeon identify critical motor branches and to reduce the morbidity of the procedure.

Other Exploratory Approaches of MVD

MVD of the CN IX-X root entry and exit zone and lateral medullar has also been performed for medically refractory hypertension secondary to neurovascular compression. The surgical procedure is essentially the same as a classical MVD for cranial nerve neuralgias. In 48 patients with neurogenic hypertension who underwent MVD, 28 patients had blood pressures returning to normal, with 14 being able to remain normotensive without any antihypertensive treatment (Sindou, Mahmoudi, & Brînzeu, 2015). Similar decompression has also been performed for type 2 diabetes, with seven out of ten patients showing significant improvement in glucose control after surgery (Jannetta, Fletcher, Grondziowski, Casey, & Sekula, 2010).

Closure

Given the relatively higher pressure placed on dural closures in the posterior fossa and proximity to the pneumatized mastoid bone, water-tight dural closure is important to prevent development of a pseudomeningocele and CSF leakage. The dura is closed under the microscope using interrupted and/or running 4-0 nylon, silk or Gore-Tex® sutures. Small defects in the dura may be oversewn with pieces of muscle or fascia harvested from within the wound. If the dura cannot be reapproximated, an artificial dural graft of piece of pericranium can be used. Fibrin sealant or DuraSeal® can be used for reinforcement. The mastoid air cells are thoroughly re-waxed. The authors prefer replacing the bone flap and any bony defects can be covered with titanium plates or mesh. Some have advocated use of bone cement to reinforce the closure, whilst others use nothing to cover even a craniectomy. The deep muscle and fascial layers are then closed in anatomic layers in a water-tight manner. The subcutaneous tissue and skin is closed in standard fashion.

OUTCOMES AND PROGNOSIS OF MVD

Trigeminal Neuralgia

The first major study addressing the efficacy of microvascular decompression for trigeminal neuralgia examined 1185 patients over a 20-year period. Ten years after surgery, 70% of patients were free from pain without medication and an additional 4% had occasional pain which did not require long-term medication (Barker et al., 1996). The 2008 AAN/EFNS practice guidelines also identified five studies of MVD and concluded that despite initial pain relief being obtained in 90% of patients, relief rates declined to 80%, 75%, and 73% at one, three, and five years respectively (Gronseth et al., 2008). A systematic review covering 26 studies and 6847 distinct patients treated with MVD for TN demonstrated a postoperative success rate of 83.5% (95% CI 79.6-89.1%) at a mean follow-up duration of 35.8 months (95% CI 26.2-56.6). 11.1% of patients had symptomatic recurrence and were re-operated during the follow-up period (Xia et al., 2014). The efficacy of primary MVD versus repeat MVD is mixed, with one study showing that second operations were less successful (Barker et al., 1996); however another study reports that the efficacy of primary MVD versus repeat MVD does not seem to differ with similar control and failure rates, although repeat MVDs tend to be associated with older age, and longer duration of symptoms (Theodros et al., 2016).

The mortality of the MVD operation has been estimated to be from 0.1-0.2% (Gronseth et al., 2008; Xia et al., 2014). Major adverse events such as cerebrospinal fluid leaks, infarction, or hematoma has been reported in up to 4% of patients. Aseptic meningitis was the most common complication seen in 11% of patients, long term hearing loss occurred in 1.51-10%, and sensory loss in the trigeminal distribution was seen in 2.3-7% (Gronseth et al., 2008) (Gubian & Rosahl, 2017).

Hemifacial Spasm

Several case series have addressed the role of MVD in the treatment of HFS. In a study of 194 Hispanic patients treated for HFS, 79.9% of patients achieved complete remission of symptoms at mean follow-up of 51 months (Soriano-Baron, Vales-Hidalgo, Arvizu-Saldana, Moreno-Jimenez, & Revuelta-Gutierrez, 2015). Another study which examined 189 consecutive HFS patients who underwent MVD showed that 68% achieved complete resolution at six years of follow-up (Lv, Deng, Long, & Liu, 2017). A systematic review across 22 studies representing 5685 patients published from 2000-2012 showed that 91.1% of patients had complete resolution of symptoms at 2.9-years follow-up (L. E. Miller & Miller, 2012). Repeat MVD for those who fail their initial surgery can also be effective, with complete success rates of 70.6% and near-complete success rates of 23.5% (Engh, Horowitz, Burkhart, Chang, & Kassam, 2005).

Glossopharyngeal Neuralgia

MVD has also shown excellent control for glossopharyngeal neuralgia. A literature review of 14 studies examining the efficacy of MVD for GN has shown long-term relief from pain in 84.7% of patients, with a recurrence rate of 7% at mean 4.9 years follow-up (Rey-Dios & Cohen-Gadol, 2013). Transient CN X dysfunction such as dyaphagia and/or hoarseness occurred in 13.2% of cases, and permanent deficits occurred in 5.5% of cases.

ALTERNATIVES TO MVD

Stereotactic Radiosurgery

Stereotactic radiosurgery (SRS) can be a viable alternative for treatment of TN and HFS, especially for patients who have multiple medical comorbidities or are poor surgical candidates. In addition, many of these neuralgias exist on a spectrum, with some presenting with atypical pain, and others having neuralgias secondary to causes other than vascular or mass effect compression. SRS is a noninvasive method which involves irradiating the proximal trigeminal nerve near the pons. The first studies investigating the Gamma Knife (GK) for treatment of medication-resistant TN demonstrated that 77% of patients maintained at least a 50% reduction in pain at mean 18 months follow-up (Kondziolka, Perez, Flickinger, Habeck, & Lunsford, 1998). More recent case series have demonstrated control rates of 60%, 41%, 34%, and 22% at 1, 3, 5, and 7 years respectively (Anil A Dhople et al., 2009). Another study has shown significant pain relief rates of 73% at 1 year, 65% at 2 years, and 41% at 5 years (Douglas et al., 2010). Because SRS involves lesioning the nerve, side effects such as persistent hyperthesias and anesthesia dolorosa may be expected with rates of 20.4% at 5 years, and 21.1% at 7 years follow-up (Douglas et al., 2010).

Multiple retrospective studies have compared efficacy rates for MVD vs. SRS for treatment of TN. In a study of 24 patients treated with MVD versus 61 with GK, complete pain relief at 12 months was observed in 68% of the MVD cohort compared with 24% of the GK group (Brisman, 2007) A systematic review across 53 studies and 13,805 patients has shown that initial success rates for MVD was 86.9% compared to 71.1% for SRS (Gubian & Rosahl, 2017). At >5 year follow-up, MVD maintained control rates of 84% compared to 63.8% for SRS. SRS was also associated with a higher rate of recurrence (25% vs 11%), cranial nerve palsies (3.31% vs 0.66%), and facial dysesthesias (28.08% vs 2.30%) compared to MVD. SRS, however, does offer the advantage of reducing the risk of injury to CN VIII as the rates of vertigo and hearing loss was significant lower (1.76% vs 3.53%, and 0.74% vs 1.51% respectively). Another systematic review across 57 studies and 8,484 cases modeled pain relief and complication outcomes to assign health-related quality of life (QOL) values for MVD versus SRS. At seven years follow-up, MVD outcomes (6.009 ± 0.173 QALYs) were significantly higher than that of SRS (5.411 ± 0.132 QALYs) (Berger et al., 2017).

The role of SRS for the treatment of HFS is less well-defined. A small case series of three patients has shown complete resolution of symptoms in one patient and marked improvement of symptoms in the other two patients at mean follow-up of 24 months (M. F. Fraioli, Moschettoni, Fraioli, & Strigari, 2010) Although no adverse events was observed in this case series, there is a theoretical risk of late-presenting facial weakness which should be considered in the treatment plan. Treatment of HFS secondary to cerebellopontine angle tumors such as meningiomas and vestibular schwannomas can also be achieved by targeting the tumor itself (C.-S. Chang et al., 2012). Glossopharyngeal neuralgia also appears to be amenable to treatment with SRS with few case reports and series demonstrating satisfactory control (Martínez-

Álvarez, Martínez-Moreno, Kusak, & Rey-Portolés, 2014; Pollock & Boes, 2011; Pommier et al., 2017; B. J. Williams, Schlesinger, & Sheehan, 2010; Yomo, Arkha, Donnet, & Régis, 2009).

Ablative Therapies

If no vascular structure is identified compressing a nerve intraoperatively, other methods to manipulate the nerve can be considered. A retrospective review of 156 patients with TN undergoing posterior fossa exploration revealed that 27 patients had no identifiable neurovascular compromise. TN which occur in the absence of neurovascular compromise tend to be observed in younger and female patients and suggests that a vascular etiology is neither sufficient nor necessary for the development of classic TN (Ko, Lee, et al., 2015a). It is estimated that 3.1-28% of TN have no vascular compromise (Lee, McCartney, Burbidge, Raslan, & Burchiel, 2014; Revuelta-Gutierrez, López-González, & Soto-Hernández, 2006; Revuelta-Gutierrez, Martinez-Anda, Coll, Campos-Romo, & Perez-Peña, 2013; Sindou, Chiha, & Mertens, 1994).

Internal neurolysis, or "brushing" or "combing" of the nerve, is a procedure in which all or portions of the trigeminal nerve are manipulated longitudinally by physically separating nerve fascicles between the pons and Meckel's cave. This method was investigated in a group of 27 patients with classical symptoms of TN but in whom no neurovascular compromise was identified either with imaging or surgical inspection (i.e. these patients were not suitable candidates for MVD) (Ko, Ozpinar, et al., 2015b). Immediate postoperative results were similar to that of MVD with 85% of patients free of pain, and 96% of patients with reduction of pain. However, control rates at 1 and 5 years were 58% and 47% respectively— lower than that expected following MVD. Another study demonstrated that neurocombing resulted in immediate relief in 94.6% of patients, and continued relief in 86.5% and 83.3% at one and three year follow-up, respectively (Liang et al., 2017). However, immediate post-operative facial numbness was reported in 91.9% of patients, with 67.5% having persistent hypoesthesia after 6 months.

Glycerol rhizotomy via a retrosigmoid approach has also been explored as a complementary surgical approach involving direct injection of the trigeminal nerve with glycerin in the cisternal portion of the nerve. In a series of 14 patients with TN and no identifiable neurovascular compromise, glycerol rhizotomy provided immediate pain relief in 100% of patients, and four patients reported a 50-80% decrease in pain at three month follow-up (Goodwin et al., 2013). No neurological deficits as a complication of the procedure was reported. This is in contrast to percutaneous trigeminal rhizotomy in which injection of glycerol into the trigeminal cistern (Meckel's cave) and not the nerve itself selectively ablates A-delta and

C-fibers while sparing A-alpha and beta fibers. Such a strategy can provide pain relief, but these patients have been reported to require multiple interventions over time (Fujimaki, Fukushima, & Miyazaki, 1990) since it is unclear as to whether this method has altered the nerve directly.

Other ablative methods such as radiofrequency ablation, peripheral neurectomy, and partial sensory rhizotomy has also been explored. The 2008 AAN/EFNS practice guidelines found that techniques such as radiofrequency thermocoagulation, peripheral glycerol rhizotomy, and balloon compression achieved immediate pain relief in 90% of patients. However, long-term control rates ranged from 68-85% at one year, 54-64% at three years, and 50% at five years (Gronseth et al., 2008). A more recent review has shown similar long term control rates of 54-66% for balloon compression, glycerol rhizotomy, and radiofrequency thermocoagulation (J. S. Cheng, Lim, Chang, & Barbaro, 2014). For patients with pain primarily in the maxillary branch of the trigeminal nerve, a pterygopalatine fossa segment neurectomy of the maxillary nerve through the maxillary sinus has demonstrated complete relief in 73% of patients at 2 year follow-up (Zhu, Rong, Chen, & Li, 2013). Because ablative procedures physically damage the nerve, there is a risk of sensory loss, dysesthesias, and anesthesia dolorosa, that are avoided with open MVD. In addition, there is a small but non-zero risk of carotid injury that can be fatal with percutaneous approaches to Meckels cave (Emril & Ho, 2010).

SAMPLE CASES

Case 1: 69-Year-Old With Trigeminal Neuralgia

A 69-year-old woman presented with a 10-year history of left V2-V3 trigeminal pain. She had failed medical management with oxcarbazapine and carbamazapine, and her current regimen of oxycodone and pregabalin poorly controlled the pain. The pain was described as intermittent, electric shock-like, and was triggered by touch and wind to the face. A MRI of the brain demonstrated a vascular loop near the trigeminal nerve in the cerebellopontine cistern (Figure 1). Due to failure of multiple medications, she elected to undergo a microvascular decompression.

Intraoperatively, two veins were found along the inferior and superior aspect of the nerve. Two teflon pledgets were placed in this recess to separate the inferior vein further away from the nerve. A single teflon pledget was also placed in between the superior vein and the nerve. The patient tolerated the procedure well and was noted to have immediate resolution of the facial pain after surgery. At one month follow-up, the patient reports that she feels well and remains pain free.

Figure 1. Axial high resolution FIESTA MRI with vascular loop abutting the left trigeminal nerve in the cerebellopoontine cistern

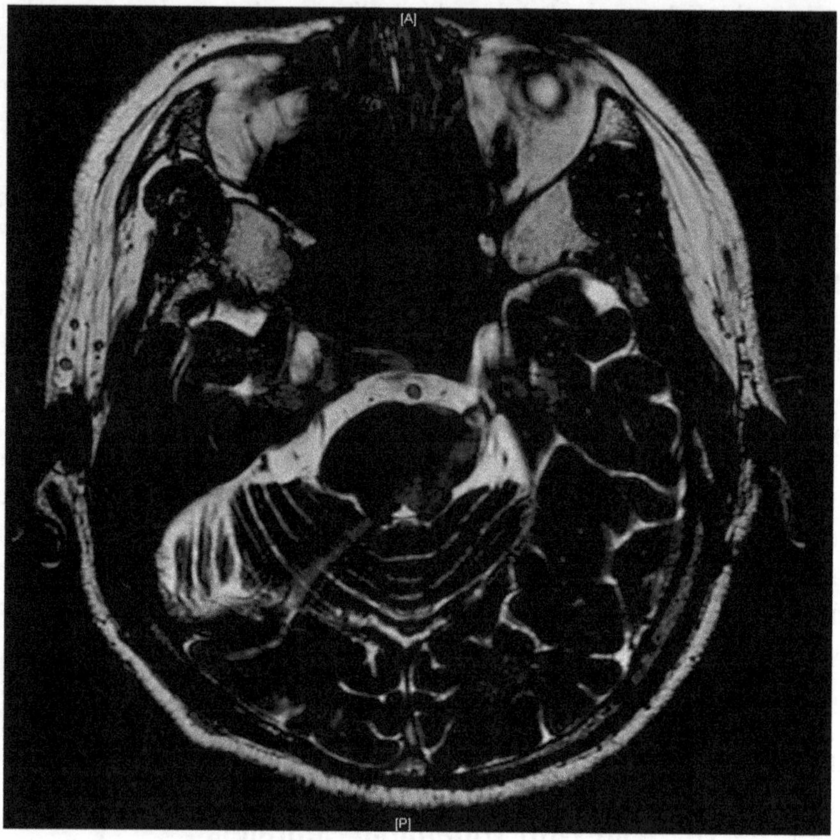

Case 2: 41-Year-Old With Trigeminal Neuralgia and Nervus Intermedius Neuralgia

A 41-year-old woman with a history of migraine, anxiety, and depression who developed sudden onset left-sided electric shock-like pain in the V2 distribution from the posterior maxilla radiating to the lateral nasal media orbital nasal region. Her pain had been episodic, random, unpredictable, and was described as a hot, stinging, electric shock-like sensation. The pain also radiated from the upper lip into the eyes and nose, and was triggered by brushing teeth, eating, or washing the face. The patient also described a constant crushing pain in the left V2 distribution, with a sense of pressure on her cheek bone and eye. She was managed initially with carbamazepine, but experienced significant cognitive side effects.

The examination was non-focal with limited examination of the face due to fear of exacerbating pain. A high-resolution FIESTA MRI revealed a blood vessel abutting the trigeminal nerve on the left side (Figure 2). She elected to undergo a microvascular decompression for definitive management. Intraoperatively, a branch of the superior cerebellar artery was found compressing the lateral aspect of the trigeminal nerve, which was mobilized and held away with a single Teflon pledget. Two veins were also encountered along the root entry zone of the trigeminal nerve and both were cauterized and divided. The patient tolerated the procedure well.

At her first 1-week follow-up, she reported approximately 75% resolution of her trigeminal neuralgia symptoms, but continued to have left-sided achy facial pain

Figure 2. Axial high resolution FIESTA MRI with blood vessel abutting the trigeminal nerve on the left side

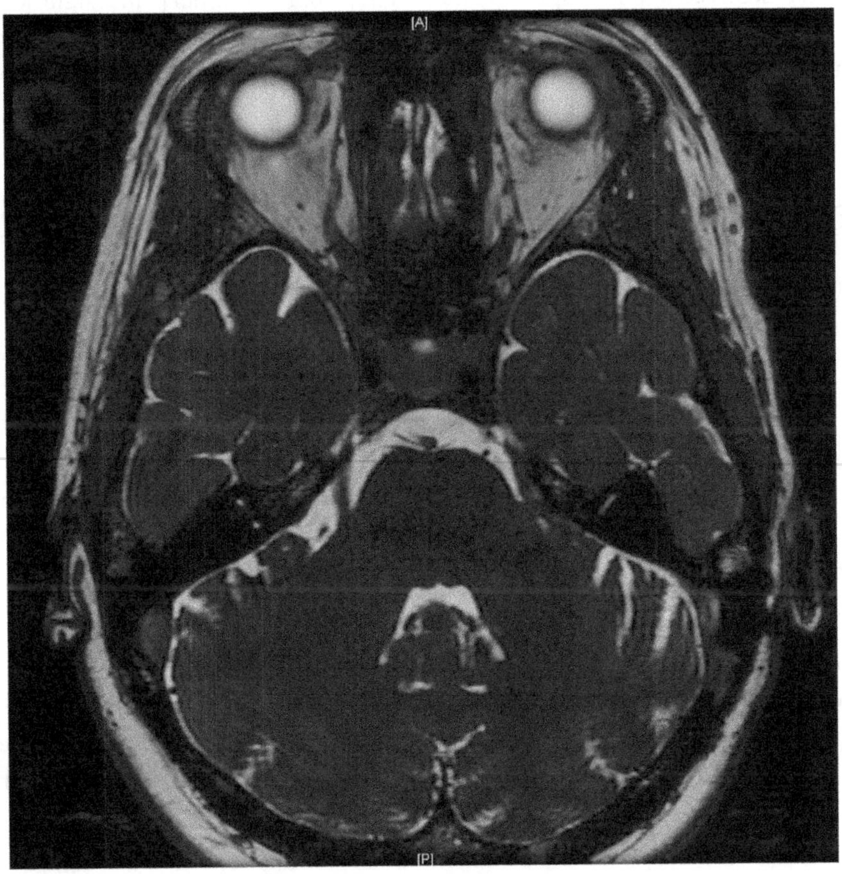

symptoms and developed also left ear pain. Two weeks after surgery, the patient was urgently seen for worsening pain behind and inside her ear. A MRI was performed which revealed stable post-surgical changes. With a reassuring ENT consult and normal audiology findings, the pain was presumed to be related to surgical inflammation and the patient was given two courses of steroids. At three-weeks follow-up, the ear pain was not relieved with steroids and required maximal doses for gabapentin and oxycontin for relief. At this point, a diagnosis of geniculate neuralgia was suspected, and she was recommended to undergo another microvascular decompression of the left side.

During her second MVD operation, the nervus intermedius was identified and separated from the motor branch of the facial nerve. The nervus intermedius was then stimulated, no motor potentials were identified, and was subsequently divided. The patient otherwise tolerated the procedure without complication. Post-operatively, she experienced immediate improvement in her ear pain.

At her most recent follow-up two years after decompression, her pain is significantly better prior to her second surgery. She continues to see a pain management specialist for her original intermittent left-sided facial pain, but shows overall symptomatic improvement and radiographic stability.

REFERENCES

Adams, H., Pendleton, C., Latimer, K., Cohen-Gadol, A. A., Carson, B. S., & Quinones-Hinojosa, A. (2011). Harvey Cushing's case series of trigeminal neuralgia at the Johns Hopkins Hospital: a surgeon's quest to advance the treatment of the 'suicide disease'. In *Acta neurochirurgica* (Vol. 153, pp. 1043–1050). Academic Press. doi:10.1007/s00701-011-0975-8

Alafaci, C., Granata, F., Cutugno, M., Marino, D., Conti, A., & Tomasello, F. (2015). Glossopharyngeal neuralgia caused by a complex neurovascular conflict: Case report and review of the literature. *Surgical Neurology International*, *6*(1), 19. doi:10.4103/2152-7806.150810 PMID:25709856

Antonini, G., Di Pasquale, A., Cruccu, G., Truini, A., Morino, S., Saltelli, G., ... Bozzao, A. (2014). Magnetic resonance imaging contribution for diagnosing symptomatic neurovascular contact in classical trigeminal neuralgia: A blinded case-control study and meta-analysis. *Pain*, *155*(8), 1464–1471. doi:10.1016/j.pain.2014.04.020 PMID:24785270

Auger, R. G., & Whisnant, J. P. (1990). Hemifacial spasm in Rochester and Olmsted County, Minnesota, 1960 to 1984. *Archives of Neurology*, *47*(11), 1233–1234. doi:10.1001/archneur.1990.00530110095023 PMID:2241620

Barker, F. G., Jannetta, P. J., Bissonette, D. J., Larkins, M. V., & Jho, H. D. (1996). The long-term outcome of microvascular decompression for trigeminal neuralgia. *The New England Journal of Medicine*, *334*(17), 1077–1083. doi:10.1056/NEJM199604253341701 PMID:8598865

Batisti, J. P. M., Kleinfelder, A. D. F., Galli, N. B., Moro, A., Munhoz, R. P., & Teive, H. A. G. (2017). Treatment of hemifacial spasm with botulinum toxin type a: Effective, long lasting and well tolerated. *Arquivos de Neuro-Psiquiatria*, *75*(2), 87–91. doi:10.1590/0004-282x20160191 PMID:28226076

Becker, M., Kohler, R., Vargas, M. I., Viallon, M., & Delavelle, J. (2008). Pathology of the trigeminal nerve. *Neuroimaging Clinics of North America*, *18*(2), 283–307. doi:10.1016/j.nic.2007.11.002

Bellotti, C., Medina, M., Oliveri, G., Ettorre, F., Barrale, S., Sturiale, C., & Melcarne, A. (1988). Neuralgia of the intermediate nerve combined with trigeminal neuralgia: Case report. *Acta Neurochirurgica*, *91*(3-4), 142–143. doi:10.1007/BF01424571 PMID:2457298

Berger, I., Nayak, N., Schuster, J., Lee, J., Stein, S., & Malhotra, N. R. (2017). Microvascular Decompression Versus Stereotactic Radiosurgery for Trigeminal Neuralgia: A Decision Analysis. *Cureus*, *9*(1), e1000. doi:10.7759/cureus.1000 PMID:28280653

Blom, S. (1962). Trigeminal neuralgia: Its treatment with a new anticonvulsant drug (G-32883). *Lancet (London, England)*, *1*(7234), 839–840. PMID:13870089

Borges, A., & Casselman, J. (2010). Imaging the trigeminal nerve. *European Journal of Radiology*, *74*(2), 323–340. doi:10.1016/j.ejrad.2010.02.006 PMID:20227216

Brisman, R. (2007). Microvascular decompression vs. gamma knife radiosurgery for typical trigeminal neuralgia: Preliminary findings. *Stereotactic and Functional Neurosurgery*, *85*(2-3), 94–98. doi:10.1159/000097925 PMID:17167238

Brock, S., Scaioli, V., Ferroli, P., & Broggi, G. (2004). Neurovascular decompression in trigeminal neuralgia: Role of intraoperative neurophysiological monitoring in the learning period. *Stereotactic and Functional Neurosurgery*, *82*(5-6), 199–206. doi:10.1159/000082446 PMID:15583464

Bruyn, G. W. (1984). Nervus intermedius neuralgia (Hunt). *Cephalalgia: an International Journal of Headache*, *4*(1), 71–78. doi:10.1046/j.1468-2982.1984.0401071.x PMID:6370459

Campos-Benitez, M., & Kaufmann, A. M. (2008). Neurovascular compression findings in hemifacial spasm. *Journal of Neurosurgery*, *109*(3), 416–420. doi:10.3171/JNS/2008/109/9/0416 PMID:18759570

Chang, C.-S., Chuang, C.-C., Wu, M.-F., Liu, W.-S., Tu, H.-T., & Huang, C.-F. (2012). Gamma Knife surgery for hemifacial spasm related to cerebellopontine angle tumors. *Journal of Neurosurgery*, *117*(Suppl), 170–174. doi:10.3171/2012.7.GKS12999 PMID:23205806

Chaudhry, N., Srivastava, A., & Joshi, L. (2015). Hemifacial spasm: The past, present and future. *Journal of the Neurological Sciences*, *356*(1-2), 27–31. doi:10.1016/j.jns.2015.06.032 PMID:26111430

Cheng, J. S., Lim, D. A., Chang, E. F., & Barbaro, N. M. (2014). A review of percutaneous treatments for trigeminal neuralgia. *Neurosurgery*, *10*(1), 25–33. doi:10.1227/NEU.0000000000001687

Cheng, T. M., Cascino, T. L., & Onofrio, B. M. (1993). Comprehensive study of diagnosis and treatment of trigeminal neuralgia secondary to tumors. *Neurology*, *43*(11), 2298–2302. doi:10.1212/WNL.43.11.2298 PMID:8232946

Cohen-Gadol, A. A. (2011). Microvascular decompression surgery for trigeminal neuralgia and hemifacial spasm: Naunces of the technique based on experiences with 100 patients and review of the literature. *Clinical Neurology and Neurosurgery*, *113*(10), 844–853. doi:10.1016/j.clineuro.2011.06.003 PMID:21752534

Costa, J., Espírito-Santo, C., Borges, A., Ferreira, J. J., Coelho, M., Moore, P., & Sampaio, C. (2005). Botulinum toxin type A therapy for hemifacial spasm. *The Cochrane Database of Systematic Reviews*, *40*(1). doi:10.1002/14651858.CD004899.pub2

Dalessio, D. J. (1982). Trigeminal neuralgia. A practical approach to treatment. *Drugs*, *24*(3), 248–255. doi:10.2165/00003495-198224030-00005 PMID:7128480

Dandy, W. (1929). An operation for the cure of tic douloureux: Partial section of the sensory root at the pons. *Archives of Surgery*, *18*(2), 687–734. doi:10.1001/archsurg.1929.04420030081005

Dandy, W. E. (1932). The treatment of trigeminal neuralgia by the cerebellar route. *Annals of Surgery, 96*(4), 787–795. doi:10.1097/00000658-193210000-00026 PMID:17866870

Dannenbaum, M., Lega, B. C., Suki, D., Harper, R. L., & Yoshor, D. (2008). Microvascular decompression for hemifacial spasm: Long-term results from 114 operations performed without neurophysiological monitoring. *Journal of Neurosurgery, 109*(3), 410–415. doi:10.3171/JNS/2008/109/9/0410 PMID:18759569

de Bondt, B.-J., Stokroos, R., & Casselman, J. (2007). Persistent trigeminal artery associated with trigeminal neuralgia: Hypothesis of neurovascular compression. *Neuroradiology, 49*(1), 23–26. doi:10.100700234-006-0150-8 PMID:17089114

Defazio, G., Abbruzzese, G., Girlanda, P., Vacca, L., Currà, A., De Salvia, R., ... Berardelli, A. (2002). Botulinum toxin A treatment for primary hemifacial spasm: A 10-year multicenter study. *Archives of Neurology, 59*(3), 418–420. doi:10.1001/archneur.59.3.418 PMID:11890846

Dhople, Adams, Maggio, Naqvi, Regine, & Kwok. (2009). *Long-term outcomes of Gamma Knife radiosurgery for classic trigeminal neuralgia: implications of treatment and critical review of the literature.* Academic Press. doi:10.3171/2009.2.JNS08977

El-Ghandour, N. M. F. (2010). Microvascular decompression in the treatment of trigeminal neuralgia caused by vertebrobasilar ectasia. *Neurosurgery, 67*(2), 330–337. doi:10.1227/01.NEU.0000371978.86528.60 PMID:20644418

El-Tallawy, H. N., Farghaly, W. M., Rageh, T. A., Shehata, G. A., Abdel Hakeem, M. N., Badry, R., & Kandil, M. R. (2013). Prevalence of trigeminal neuralgia in Al-Quseir city (Red sea Governorate), Egypt. *Clinical Neurology and Neurosurgery, 115*(9), 1792–1794. doi:10.1016/j.clineuro.2013.04.014 PMID:23692870

Emril, D. R., & Ho, K.-Y. (2010). Treatment of trigeminal neuralgia: Role of radiofrequency ablation. *Journal of Pain Research, 3*, 249–254. doi:10.2147/JPR.S14455 PMID:21311718

Engh, J. A., Horowitz, M., Burkhart, L., Chang, Y.-F., & Kassam, A. (2005). Repeat microvascular decompression for hemifacial spasm. *Journal of Neurology, Neurosurgery, and Psychiatry, 76*(11), 1574–1580. doi:10.1136/jnnp.2004.056861 PMID:16227555

Fothergill, J. (1776). *Of a painful affection of the face*. Academic Press.

Fraioli, M. F., Moschettoni, L., Fraioli, C., & Strigari, L. (2010). Treatment of idiopathic hemifacial spasm with radiosurgery or hypofractionated stereotactic radiotherapy: Preliminary results. *Minimally Invasive Neurosurgery: MIN*, *53*(1), 34–36. doi:10.1055-0030-1247584 PMID:20376743

Fujimaki, T., Fukushima, T., & Miyazaki, S. (1990). Percutaneous retrogasserian glycerol injection in the management of trigeminal neuralgia: Long-term follow-up results. *Journal of Neurosurgery*, *73*(2), 212–216. doi:10.3171/jns.1990.73.2.0212 PMID:2195139

Gardner, W. J., & Miklos, M. V. (1959). Response of trigeminal neuralgia to decompression of sensory root; discussion of cause of trigeminal neuralgia. *Journal of the American Medical Association*, *170*(15).

Gardner, W. J., & Sava, G. A. (1962). Hemifacial Spasm—a Reversible Pathophysiologic State. *Journal of Neurosurgery*, *19*(3), 240–247. doi:10.3171/jns.1962.19.3.0240

Gaul, C., Hastreiter, P., Duncker, A., & Naraghi, R. (2011). Diagnosis and neurosurgical treatment of glossopharyngeal neuralgia: Clinical findings and 3-D visualization of neurovascular compression in 19 consecutive patients. *The Journal of Headache and Pain*, *12*(5), 527–534. doi:10.100710194-011-0349-x PMID:21567138

Goodwin, C. R., Yang, J. X., Bettegowda, C., Hwang, B., James, C., Biser, A., ... Lim, M. (2013). Glycerol rhizotomy via a retrosigmoid approach as an alternative treatment for trigeminal neuralgia. *Clinical Neurology and Neurosurgery*, *115*(12), 2454–2456. doi:10.1016/j.clineuro.2013.09.009 PMID:24161889

Gronseth, G., Cruccu, G., Alksne, J., Argoff, C., Brainin, M., & Burchiel, K. (2008, October 7). Practice parameter: the diagnostic evaluation and treatment of trigeminal neuralgia (an evidence-based review): report of the Quality Standards Subcommittee of the American Academy of Neurology and the European Federation of Neurological Societies. In *Neurology*. Lippincott Williams & Wilkins. doi:10.1212/01.wnl.0000326598.83183.04

Gubian, A., & Rosahl, S. K. (2017). Meta-Analysis on Safety and Efficacy of Microsurgical and Radiosurgical Treatment of Trigeminal Neuralgia. *World Neurosurgery*, *103*, 757–767. doi:10.1016/j.wneu.2017.04.085 PMID:28435111

Habeych, M. E., Shah, A. C., Nikonow, T. N., Balzer, J. R., Crammond, D. J., Thirumala, P. D., ... Horowitz, M. (2011). Effect of botulinum neurotoxin treatment in the lateral spread monitoring of microvascular decompression for hemifacial spasm. *Muscle & Nerve*, *44*(4), 518–524. doi:10.1002/mus.22104 PMID:21826681

Haller, S., Etienne, L., Kövari, E., Varoquaux, A. D., Urbach, H., & Becker, M. (2016). Imaging of Neurovascular Compression Syndromes: Trigeminal Neuralgia, Hemifacial Spasm, Vestibular Paroxysmia, and Glossopharyngeal Neuralgia. *AJNR. American Journal of Neuroradiology*, *37*(8), 1384–1392. doi:10.3174/ajnr.A4683 PMID:26892985

Hanakita, J., & Kondo, A. (1988). Serious complications of microvascular decompression operations for trigeminal neuralgia and hemifacial spasm. *Neurosurgery*, *22*(2), 348–352. doi:10.1227/00006123-198802000-00012 PMID:3352885

Harries, A. M., Dong, C. C. J., & Honey, C. R. (2012). Use of endotracheal tube electrodes in treating glossopharyngeal neuralgia: Technical note. *Stereotactic and Functional Neurosurgery*, *90*(3), 141–144. doi:10.1159/000335714 PMID:22508038

Hatem, J., Sindou, M., & Vial, C. (2001). Intraoperative monitoring of facial EMG responses during microvascular decompression for hemifacial spasm. Prognostic value for long-term outcome: A study in a 33-patient series. *British Journal of Neurosurgery*, *15*(6), 496–499. doi:10.1080/02688690120105101 PMID:11814001

Headache Classification Committee of the International Headache Society (IHS). (2013). The International Classification of Headache Disorders (3rd ed.). Cephalalgia: An International Journal of Headache, 33(9), 629–808. doi:10.1177/0333102413485658

Hiwatashi, A., Matsushima, T., Yoshiura, T., Tanaka, A., Noguchi, T., Togao, O., ... Honda, H. (2008). MRI of glossopharyngeal neuralgia caused by neurovascular compression. *AJR. American Journal of Roentgenology*, *191*(2), 578–581. doi:10.2214/AJR.07.3025 PMID:18647935

Huang, C.-F., Chuang, J.-C., Tu, H.-T., & Chou, M.-C. (2006). Microsurgical outcomes after failed repeated Gamma Knife surgery for refractory trigeminal neuralgia. *Journal of Neurosurgery*, *105*(Suppl), 117–119. doi:10.3171up.2006.105.7.117 PMID:18503343

Ildan, F., Göçer, A. I., Bağdatoğlu, H., Uzuneyüpoğlu, Z., Tuna, M., & Cetinalp, E. (1996). Isolated trigeminal neuralgia secondary to distal anterior inferior cerebellar artery aneurysm. *Neurosurgical Review*, *19*(1), 43–46. doi:10.1007/BF00346609 PMID:8738365

Inoue, T., Shima, A., Hirai, H., Suzuki, F., & Matsuda, M. (2017). Nervus Intermedius Neuralgia Treated with Microvascular Decompression: A Case Report and Review of the Literature. *NMC Case Report Journal*, *4*(3), 75–78. doi:10.2176/nmccrj.cr.2016-0261 PMID:28840083

Jannetta, P. J. (1974). Letter: Complications from microsurgical treatment of tic douloureux. *Journal of Neurosurgery*, *40*(5), 675. PMID:4817815

Jannetta, P. J. (2007). Arterial compression of the trigeminal nerve at the pons in patients with trigeminal neuralgia. 1967. *Journal of Neurosurgery*, *107*, 216–219. doi:10.3171/JNS-07/07/0216

Jannetta, P. J., Fletcher, L. H., Grondziowski, P. M., Casey, K. F., & Sekula, R. F. (2010). Type 2 diabetes mellitus: A central nervous system etiology. *Surgical Neurology International*, *1*(1), 31. doi:10.4103/2152-7806.66460 PMID:20847912

Jost, W. H., & Kohl, A. (2001). Botulinum toxin: Evidence-based medicine criteria in blepharospasm and hemifacial spasm. *Journal of Neurology*, *248*(S1), 21–24. doi:10.1007/PL00007813 PMID:11357234

Katusic, S., Beard, C. M., Bergstralh, E., & Kurland, L. T. (1990). Incidence and clinical features of trigeminal neuralgia, Rochester, Minnesota, 1945-1984. *Annals of Neurology*, *27*(1), 89–95. doi:10.1002/ana.410270114 PMID:2301931

Katusic, S., Williams, D. B., Beard, C. M., Bergstralh, E., & Kurland, L. T. (1991b). Incidence and clinical features of glossopharyngeal neuralgia, Rochester, Minnesota, 1945-1984. *Neuroepidemiology*, *10*(5-6), 266–275. doi:10.1159/000110283 PMID:1798429

Katusic, S., Williams, D. B., Beard, C. M., Bergstralh, E. J., & Kurland, L. T. (1991a). Epidemiology and clinical features of idiopathic trigeminal neuralgia and glossopharyngeal neuralgia: Similarities and differences, Rochester, Minnesota, 1945-1984. *Neuroepidemiology*, *10*(5-6), 276–281. doi:10.1159/000110284 PMID:1798430

Khan, M., Nishi, S. E., Hassan, S. N., Islam, M. A., & Gan, S. H. (2017). Trigeminal Neuralgia, Glossopharyngeal Neuralgia, and Myofascial Pain Dysfunction Syndrome: An Update. *Pain Research & Management*, (3): 7438326–18. doi:10.1155/2017/7438326 PMID:28827979

Ko, A. L., Lee, A., Raslan, A. M., Ozpinar, A., McCartney, S., & Burchiel, K. J. (2015a). Trigeminal neuralgia without neurovascular compression presents earlier than trigeminal neuralgia with neurovascular compression. *Journal of Neurosurgery*, *123*(6), 1519–1527. doi:10.3171/2014.11.JNS141741 PMID:26047411

Ko, A. L., Ozpinar, A., Lee, A., Raslan, A. M., McCartney, S., & Burchiel, K. J. (2015b). Long-term efficacy and safety of internal neurolysis for trigeminal neuralgia without neurovascular compression. *Journal of Neurosurgery*, *122*(5), 1048–1057. doi:10.3171/2014.12.JNS14469 PMID:25679283

Kondziolka, D., Perez, B., Flickinger, J. C., Habeck, M., & Lunsford, L. D. (1998). Gamma Knife Radiosurgery for Trigeminal Neuralgia: Results and Expectations. *Archives of Neurology*, *55*(12), 1524–1529. doi:10.1001/archneur.55.12.1524 PMID:9865796

Koopman, J. S. H. A., Dieleman, J. P., Huygen, F. J., de Mos, M., Martin, C. G. M., & Sturkenboom, M. C. J. M. (2009). Incidence of facial pain in the general population. *Pain*, *147*(1-3), 122–127. doi:10.1016/j.pain.2009.08.023 PMID:19783099

Laha, R. K., & Jannetta, P. J. (1977). Glossopharyngeal neuralgia. *Journal of Neurosurgery*, *47*(3), 316–320. doi:10.3171/jns.1977.47.3.0316 PMID:894337

Lee, A., McCartney, S., Burbidge, C., Raslan, A. M., & Burchiel, K. J. (2014). Trigeminal neuralgia occurs and recurs in the absence of neurovascular compression. *Journal of Neurosurgery*, *120*(5), 1048–1054. doi:10.3171/2014.1.JNS131410 PMID:24506241

Liang, X., Dong, X., Zhao, S., Ying, X., Du, Y., & Yu, W. (2017). A retrospective study of neurocombing for the treatment of trigeminal neuralgia without neurovascular compression. *Irish Journal of Medical Science*, *40*(1), 39–7. doi:10.100711845-016-1547-y PMID:28063126

Lin, K.-H., Chen, Y.-T., Fuh, J.-L., & Wang, S.-J. (2015). Increased risk of trigeminal neuralgia in patients with migraine: A nationwide population-based study. *Cephalalgia: an International Journal of Headache*, *36*(13), 1218–1227. doi:10.1177/0333102415623069 PMID:26692399

Love, S., & Coakham, H. B. (2001). Trigeminal neuralgia: Pathology and pathogenesis. *Brain, 124*(Pt 12), 2347–2360. doi:10.1093/brain/124.12.2347 PMID:11701590

Lv, M.-Y., Deng, S.-L., Long, X.-F., & Liu, Z.-L. (2017). Long-term outcome of microvascular decompression for hemifacial spasm. *British Journal of Neurosurgery, 31*(3), 322–326. doi:10.1080/02688697.2017.1297368 PMID:28288523

Maarbjerg, S., Gozalov, A., Olesen, J., & Bendtsen, L. (2014). Trigeminal neuralgia-a prospective systematic study of clinical characteristics in 158 patients. *Headache, 54*(10), 1574–1582. doi:10.1111/head.12441 PMID:25231219

MacDonald, B. K. (2000). The incidence and lifetime prevalence of neurological disorders in a prospective community-based study in the UK. *Brain, 123*(4), 665–676. doi:10.1093/brain/123.4.665 PMID:10733998

Martínez-Álvarez, R., Martínez-Moreno, N., Kusak, M. E., & Rey-Portolés, G. (2014). Glossopharyngeal neuralgia and radiosurgery. *Journal of Neurosurgery, 121*(Suppl), 222–225. doi:10.3171/2014.8.GKS141273 PMID:25434956

Matthies, C., & Samii, M. (1997). Management of 1000 vestibular schwannomas (acoustic neuromas): clinical presentation. *Neurosurgery, 40*(1), 1–9.

Miller, J. P., Magill, S. T., Acar, F., & Burchiel, K. J. (2009). Predictors of long-term success after microvascular decompression for trigeminal neuralgia. *Journal of Neurosurgery, 110*(4), 620–626. doi:10.3171/2008.9.17660 PMID:19231931

Miller, L. E., & Miller, V. M. (2012). Safety and effectiveness of microvascular decompression for treatment of hemifacial spasm: A systematic review. *British Journal of Neurosurgery, 26*(4), 438–444. doi:10.3109/02688697.2011.641613 PMID:22168965

Minagar, A., & Sheremata, W. A. (2000). Glossopharyngeal neuralgia and MS. *Neurology, 54*(6), 1368–1370. doi:10.1212/WNL.54.6.1368 PMID:10746612

Mohanty, A., Venkatrama, S. K., Rao, B. R., Chandramouli, B. A., Jayakumar, P. N., & Das, B. S. (1997). Experience with cerebellopontine angle epidermoids. *Neurosurgery, 40*(1), 24–9.

Møller, A. R. (1991). The cranial nerve vascular compression syndrome: II. A review of pathophysiology. *Acta Neurochirurgica, 113*(1-2), 24–30. doi:10.1007/BF01402110 PMID:1799140

Møller, A. R., & Jannetta, P. J. (1987). Monitoring facial EMG responses during microvascular decompression operations for hemifacial spasm. *Journal of Neurosurgery*, *66*(5), 681–685. doi:10.3171/jns.1987.66.5.0681 PMID:3572493

Nilsen, B., Le, K.-D., & Dietrichs, E. (2004). Prevalence of hemifacial spasm in Oslo, Norway. *Neurology*, *63*(8), 1532–1533. doi:10.1212/01.WNL.0000142080.85228.E8 PMID:15505186

Oesman, C., & Mooij, J. J. A. (2011). Long-term follow-up of microvascular decompression for trigeminal neuralgia. *Skull Base: Official Journal of North American Skull Base Society*, *21*(5), 313–322. doi:10.1055/s-0031-1284213

Ordónez-Rubiano, E. G., García-Chingaté, C. C., Rodríguez-Vargas, S., Cifuentes-Lobelo, H. A., & Perilla-Cepeda, T. A. (2017). Microvascular Decompression for a Patient with a Glossopharyngeal Neuralgia: A Technical Note. *Cureus*, *9*(7), e1494. doi:10.7759/cureus.1494 PMID:28948114

Pan, S.-L., Yen, M.-F., Chiu, Y.-H., Chen, L.-S., & Chen, H.-H. (2011). Increased risk of trigeminal neuralgia after hypertension: A population-based study. *Neurology*, *77*(17), 1605–1610. doi:10.1212/WNL.0b013e3182343354 PMID:21998318

Pollock, B. E., & Boes, C. J. (2011). Stereotactic radiosurgery for glossopharyngeal neuralgia: Preliminary report of 5 cases. *Journal of Neurosurgery*, *115*(5), 936–939. doi:10.3171/2011.5.JNS1133 PMID:21740122

Pommier, B., Touzet, G., Lucas, C., Vermandel, M., Blond, S., & Reyns, N. (2017). Glossopharyngeal neuralgia treated by Gamma Knife radiosurgery: Safety and efficacy through long-term follow-up. *Journal of Neurosurgery*, 1–8. doi:10.3171/2017.3.JNS162542 PMID:28621622

Prasad, S., & Galetta, S. (2009). Trigeminal neuralgia: Historical notes and current concepts. *The Neurologist*, *15*(2), 87–94. doi:10.1097/NRL.0b013e3181775ac3 PMID:19276786

Revuelta-Gutierrez, R., López-González, M. A., & Soto-Hernández, J. L. (2006). Surgical treatment of trigeminal neuralgia without vascular compression: 20 years of experience. *Surgical Neurology*, *66*(1), 32–6. doi:10.1016/j.surneu.2005.10.018

Revuelta-Gutierrez, R., Martinez-Anda, J. J., Coll, J. B., Campos-Romo, A., & Perez-Peña, N. (2013). Efficacy and safety of root compression of trigeminal nerve for trigeminal neuralgia without evidence of vascular compression. *World Neurosurgery*, *80*(3-4), 385–389. doi:10.1016/j.wneu.2012.07.030 PMID:22889619

Rey-Dios, R., & Cohen-Gadol, A. A. (2013). Current neurosurgical management of glossopharyngeal neuralgia and technical nuances for microvascular decompression surgery. *Neurosurgical Focus*, *34*(3), E8. doi:10.3171/2012.12.FOCUS12391 PMID:23451790

Saers, S. J. F., Han, K. S., & de Ru, J. A. (2011). Microvascular decompression may be an effective treatment for nervus intermedius neuralgia. *The Journal of Laryngology and Otology*, *125*(5), 520–522. doi:10.1017/S0022215110002677 PMID:21223630

Sakas, D. E., Panourias, I. G., Stranjalis, G., Stefanatou, M. P., Maratheftis, N., & Bontozoglou, N. (2007). Paroxysmal otalgia due to compression of the intermediate nerve: A distinct syndrome of neurovascular conflict confirmed by neuroimaging. Case report. *Journal of Neurosurgery*, *107*(6), 1228–1230. doi:10.3171/JNS-07/12/1228 PMID:18077963

Sheng, B., Lv, F., Xiao, Z., Ouyang, Y., Lv, F., Deng, J., ... Liu, N. (2012). Anatomical relationship between cranial surface landmarks and venous sinus in posterior cranial fossa using CT angiography. *Surgical and Radiologic Anatomy*, *34*(8), 701–708. doi:10.100700276-011-0916-5 PMID:22160178

Sindou, M., Howeidy, T., & Acevedo, G. (2002). Anatomical observations during microvascular decompression for idiopathic trigeminal neuralgia (with correlations between topography of pain and site of the neurovascular conflict). Prospective study in a series of 579 patients. *Acta Neurochirurgica, 144*(1), 1–12. doi:10.1007/s007010200000

Sindou, M., Mahmoudi, M., & Brînzeu, A. (2015). Hypertension of neurogenic origin: Effect of microvascular decompression of the CN IX-X root entry/exit zone and ventrolateral medulla on blood pressure in a prospective series of 48 patients with hemifacial spasm associated with essential hypertension. *Journal of Neurosurgery*, *123*(6), 1405–1413. doi:10.3171/2014.12.JNS141775 PMID:26230479

Sindou, M. P., Chiha, M., & Mertens, P. (1994). Anatomical findings observed during microsurgical approaches of the cerebellopontine angle for vascular decompression in trigeminal neuralgia (350 cases). *Stereotactic and Functional Neurosurgery*, *63*(1-4), 203–207. doi:10.1159/000100316 PMID:7624636

Smith, J. H., Robertson, C. E., Garza, I., & Cutrer, F. M. (2013). Triggerless neuralgic otalgia: A case series and systematic literature review. *Cephalalgia: an International Journal of Headache*, *33*(11), 914–923. doi:10.1177/0333102413477743 PMID:23444079

Soriano-Baron, H., Vales-Hidalgo, O., Arvizu-Saldana, E., Moreno-Jimenez, S., & Revuelta-Gutierrez, R. (2015). Hemifacial spasm: 20-year surgical experience, lesson learned. *Surgical Neurology International*, *6*(1), 83. doi:10.4103/2152-7806.157443 PMID:26015871

Taha, J. M., Tew, J. M. Jr, Keith, R. W., & Payner, T. D. (1994). Intraoperative monitoring of the vagus nerve during intracranial glossopharyngeal and upper vagal rhizotomy: Technical note. *Neurosurgery*, *35*(4), 775–777. doi:10.1227/00006123-199410000-00032 PMID:7808629

Tan, N.-C., Chan, L.-L., & Tan, E.-K. (2002). Hemifacial spasm and involuntary facial movements. *QJM: Monthly Journal of the Association of Physicians*, *95*(8), 493–500. doi:10.1093/qjmed/95.8.493 PMID:12145388

Theodros, D., Goodwin, C. R., Bender, M. T., Zhou, X., & Garzon-Muvdi, T. (2016). Efficacy of primary microvascular decompression versus subsequent microvascular decompression for trigeminal neuralgia. *Journal of Neurosurgery*, *126*(5), 1691–1697. doi:10.3171/2016.5.JNS151692 PMID:27419826

Tubbs, R. S., Griessenauer, C. J., Hogan, E., Loukas, M., & Cohen-Gadol, A. A. (2014). Neural interconnections between portio minor and portio major at the porus trigeminus: Application to failed surgical treatment of trigeminal neuralgia. *Clinical Anatomy (New York, N.Y.)*, *27*(1), 94–96. doi:10.1002/ca.22299 PMID:23943366

Ucerler, H., & Govsa, F. (2006). Asterion as a surgical landmark for lateral cranial base approaches. *Journal of Cranio-Maxillo-Facial Surgery: Official Publication of the European Association for Cranio-Maxillo-Facial Surgery*, *34*(7), 415–420. doi:10.1016/j.jcms.2006.05.003 PMID:16963269

Wang, X., Thirumala, P. D., Shah, A., Gardner, P., Habeych, M., Crammond, D. J., ... Horowitz, M. (2013). Effect of previous botulinum neurotoxin treatment on microvascular decompression for hemifacial spasm. *Neurosurgical Focus*, *34*(3), E3. doi:10.3171/2012.11.FOCUS12373 PMID:23452316

Wei, Y., Yang, W., Zhao, W., Pu, C., Li, N., Cai, Y., & Shang, H. (2017). Microvascular decompression for hemifacial spasm: Can intraoperative lateral spread response monitoring improve surgical efficacy? *Journal of Neurosurgery*, 1–6. doi:10.3171/2016.11.JNS162148 PMID:28498061

Williams, B. J., Schlesinger, D., & Sheehan, J. (2010). Glossopharyngeal neuralgia treated with gamma knife radiosurgery. *World Neurosurgery*, *73*(4), 413–417. doi:10.1016/j.wneu.2010.01.007 PMID:20849803

Xia, L., Zhong, J., Zhu, J., Wang, Y.-N., Dou, N.-N., Liu, M.-X., ... Li, S.-T. (2014). Effectiveness and safety of microvascular decompression surgery for treatment of trigeminal neuralgia: A systematic review. *The Journal of Craniofacial Surgery*, *25*(4), 1413–1417. doi:10.1097/SCS.0000000000000984 PMID:24978453

Yaltho, T. C., & Jankovic, J. (2011). The many faces of hemifacial spasm: Differential diagnosis of unilateral facial spasms. *Movement Disorders: Official Journal of the Movement Disorder Society*, *26*(9), 1582–1592. doi:10.1002/mds.23692 PMID:21469208

Yeh, H. S., & Tew, J. M. (1984). Tic convulsif, the combination of geniculate neuralgia and hemifacial spasm relieved by vascular decompression. *Neurology*, *34*(5), 682–683. doi:10.1212/WNL.34.5.682 PMID:6538661

Yomo, S., Arkha, Y., Donnet, A., & Régis, J. (2009). Gamma Knife surgery for glossopharyngeal neuralgia. *Journal of Neurosurgery*, *110*(3), 559–563. doi:10.3171/2008.8.17641 PMID:19025360

Younes, W. M., Capelle, H.-H., & Krauss, J. K. (2010). Microvascular decompression of the anterior inferior cerebellar artery for intermediate nerve neuralgia. *Stereotactic and Functional Neurosurgery*, *88*(3), 193–195. doi:10.1159/000313873 PMID:20431332

Zhu, S., Rong, Q., Chen, S., & Li, X. (2013). Pterygopalatine fossa segment neurectomy of maxillary nerve through maxillary sinus route in treating trigeminal neuralgia. *Journal of Cranio-Maxillo-Facial Surgery: Official Publication of the European Association for Cranio-Maxillo-Facial Surgery*, *41*(7), 652–656. doi:10.1016/j.jcms.2013.01.002 PMID:23375531

Zorro, Lobato-Polo, Hideyuki, Flannery, Flickinger, & Lunsford. (2010). *Gamma Knife stereotactic radiosurgery for idiopathic trigeminal neuralgia*. Academic Press. doi:10.3171/2009.7.JNS09694

KEY TERMS AND DEFINITIONS

Glossopharyngeal Neuralgia: Paroxysmal pain in areas innervated by the ninth and tenth cranial nerve, resulting in severe, stabbing pain involving the ear, tonsillar fossa, base of the tongue, or beneath the angle of the mandible.

Hemifacial Spasm: A segmental myoclonus of the muscles innervated by the facial nerve.

Nervus Intermedius Neuralgia: Pain syndrome characterized by paroxysmal episodes of shock-like pain felt deeply in the auditory canal.

Neurolysis: Application of surgical manipulation (e.g., combing), physical agents (e.g., heat or cold), or chemicals (e.g., glycerol) to cause degradation of nerve fibers, thereby interrupting pain signals.

Retrosigmoid Craniotomy: Surgical approach involving an incision behind the ear and opening of the skull behind the mastoid bone to expose the cranial nerves after relaxation or retraction of the cerebellum.

Stereotactic Radiosurgery: Non-surgical radiation therapy using precisely focused beams of radiation to alter the function of nerves involved in various pain syndromes.

Trigeminal Neuralgia: A pain syndrome characterized by paroxysms of severe facial pain, often described as electric, lancinating pain with an abrupt onset and termination.

Chapter 5
Microsurgical Nuances in the Management of Trigeminal Neuralgia

Robert C. Rennert
University of California – San Diego, USA

David R. Santiago-Dieppa
University of California – San Diego, USA

Jeffrey A. Steinberg
University of California – San Diego, USA

Jeffrey Scott Pannell
University of California – San Diego, USA

Keiko M. Kang
University of California – San Diego, USA

John F. Alksne
University of California – San Diego, USA

Arvin R. Wali
University of California – San Diego, USA

Alexander A. Khalessi
University of California – San Diego, USA

ABSTRACT

Microvascular decompression (MVD) is a highly effective surgical treatment for patients with trigeminal neuralgia (TN) caused by arterial compression. In cases of TN without arterial compression of the nerve, however, a variety of other surgical treatments can be effective for pain relief including neurolysis, nerve section, and placement of a tentorial sling. In this chapter, the authors discuss the nuances of surgical interventions for TN outside of standard MVDs. They also explore recent innovations in MVD surgery for TN.

DOI: 10.4018/978-1-5225-5349-6.ch005

INTRODUCTION AND BACKGROUND

Trigeminal neuralgia (TN) is a severe, lancinating pain most often caused by arterial compression at the trigeminal nerve root entry zone. Microvascular decompression (MVD) surgery is one of the most common surgical treatments for TN, and demonstrates high rates of short- and long-term pain relief (Wang et al., 2017). The goal of this procedure is separation of the compressive artery from the nerve root entry zone, which is classically achieved by placement of a piece of Teflon between the two structures. However, up to 30% of TN cases occur in the absence of a compressive lesion (Bederson & Wilson, 1989; Zhao, Zhang, Tang, & Li, 2017). This finding may only be evident upon exploration of the posterior fossa and requires consideration of other causative pathologies and treatments. In these situations, venous compression or intraneural vessels are sometimes encountered, and can be surgically addressed to provide pain relief (Hong et al., 2011; Matsushima, Huynh-Le, & Miyazono, 2004). In the absence of an identifiable intraoperative pathology, alternative treatments to relieve nerve pain, such as internal neurolysis or partial/complete sectioning have also demonstrated efficacy and can be considered (Ko et al., 2015; Zhao et al., 2017; Zhou et al., 2016). Even in cases without atypical intraoperative findings, neurosurgeons should also be aware of the ongoing development and applications of novel operative techniques for TN, such as the use of a tentorial sling to transpose compressive arteries (Steinberg et al, 2017), and intra-operative nerve monitoring to assess cranial nerve function in real time (Brock, Scaioli, Ferroli, & Broggi, 2004; C. C. Lee et al., 2014). A thorough understanding of the indications and operative considerations for revision surgeries is also critical when assessing cases of recurrent TN following an MVD.

In this chapter, we discuss the operative nuances of MVD surgery for TN, including the intra-operative considerations and treatment options available in the absence of a compressive artery. The role of MVD-related surgical innovations for TN, such as tentorial slings and intra-operative nerve monitoring, are also reviewed. Finally, the practices and pitfalls related to revision procedures for TN are explored.

OPERATIVE NUANCES OF MICROVASCULAR DECOMPRESSION

Surgical Options for Atypical Vascular Pathology or Non-Compressive Cases of TN

TN From Atypical or Non-Compressive Arteries

Due to its anatomic proximity to the trigeminal nerve, the most common compressive artery associated with TN is the superior cerebellar artery (SCA). When performing a MVD, however, surgeons should be aware of the other compressive arteries that can be encountered to ensure a complete understanding of the involved anatomy and decide how best to decompress the nerve without risking arterial kinking and subsequent ischemia. While the second most common offending artery is the anterior inferior cerebellar artery (AICA), anomalous arteries causing TN have also been reported such as a persistent trigeminal artery or its variants/branches (S. H. Lee, Koh, & Lee, 2011; Morita, Fukushima, Miyazaki, Shimizu, & Atsuchi, 1989; Park, Choi, Lee, & Rhee, 2014; Yamada, Kondo, & Tanabe, 2006), as well as a rarely seen artery supplying the anterolateral pons, the trigeminal nerve root, the middle cerebellar peduncle, and the petrosal surface of the cerebellum, termed the trigeminocerebellar artery (Amagasaki, Abe, Watanabe, Naemura, & Nakaguchi, 2014; Marinković, Gibo, & Nikodijević, 1996). As described in one case report, a megadolichoectatic basilar artery can also be the cause of TN (Banczerowski, Czigléczki, & Nyáry, 2014). In all such cases, the goal of safely relieving any identifiable arterial compression from the nerve should be pursued, as this pathologic finding is most likely to be the cause of the patients' TN (G. Q. Chen, Wang, Wang, & Zheng, 2014). In MVD surgeries where trigeminal nerve irritation is caused by atypical arterial compression, separation of the artery and nerve using a standard Teflon implant can be considered if the involved structures are anatomically amenable. A multitude of other techniques have also been described in situations where the caliber or course of the atypical compressive artery precludes simple decompression, including the use of slings, glues, or titanium plates (Banczerowski et al., 2014; Ichikawa et al., 2011; Masuoka et al., 2015; Masuoka et al., 2011).

In cases where no arterial compression is identified, arteries in contact or close to the nerve are significantly less likely to be causative of TN (G. Q. Chen et al., 2014). Arterial transposition using the sling method described later in this chapter is nonetheless considered in this scenario by some authors who suggest intraoperative cerebrospinal fluid drainage can impact the position of potentially compressive arteries relative to the nerve and confound a surgeons ability to accurately assess its potential as a causative TN vessel (Toda, Goto, & Iwasaki, 2015). Independent of the decision to pursue a sling in this situation, surgeons should not focus on the removal of arachnoid adhesions if they are encountered, as these are unlikely to be causative of TN outside of revision operations (G. Q. Chen et al., 2014).

Venous Compression of the Nerve Root

In the absence arterial compression, veins have also been described as causative agents of TN (Hong et al., 2011; Matsushima et al., 2004). The transverse pontine vein is the most common offending vessel (Hong et al., 2011; Matsushima et al., 2004; Sato, Kanazawa, & Kokunai, 1979)), although symptomatic compression from the superior petrosal vein, the pontotrigeminal vein, the vein of the cerebellopontine fissure, and venous combinations/plexuses have also been described (Hong et al., 2011; Kimura, Sako, Tohyama, & Yonemasu, 1999). In this scenario, coagulation and transection of the involved vein(s) are typically preferred over decompression, as it is considered to be highly efficacious for pain relief with little risk of recurrence. This approach is nonetheless associated with a moderate risk of facial numbness as a result of coagulation injury. While reported case numbers are limited, in one series of 15 patients, nearly 75% achieved high levels of pain relief following the coagulation and transection of compressive veins that were the only identifiable lesion on exploration of the trigeminal nerve. Post-operative facial numbness occurred in 4 patients (26%) (Hong et al., 2011).

Trigeminal Neuralgia Caused by Intraneural Vessels

Rarely, intraneural arteries or veins can be the cause of TN, with the close association of the vessels to the nerve complicating treatment. In one small series of eight patients, the authors describe using a similar approach for the treatment of intraneural arteries and veins, respectively, as that described above for extraneural vessels (Zheng et al., 2012). Intraneural arteries were wrapped with thin pieces of Teflon to insulate the arterial pulsations from the nerve, while intraneural veins were carefully coagulated and divided. Ten of the eleven patients (91%) in the series experienced excellent or good pain relief with such techniques, yet facial numbness (without corneal numbness or loss of corneal reflex) due to coagulation or mechanical injury occurred in three patients (27%). As such, other authors have recommended selective trigeminal nerve rhizotomies (as described below) in similar cases with large intraneural vessels, rather than direct manipulation of the vessel itself (Helbig, Callahan, & Cohen-Gadol, 2009).

Internal Neurolysis/Trigeminal Nerve Massage/Combing

In patients without obvious intraoperative compressive anatomy causing TN, other treatment options aside from MVD must be considered. One such method is internal neurolysis (IN), also referred to as "nerve combing," "trigeminal massage," or "nerve brushing." The goal of IN is the disruption of axon continuity to dampen but not destroy the electrical excitability of afferent fibers, rendering it a less destructive option than nerve sectioning.

As part of the IN procedure, the trigeminal nerve is exposed from the nerve root entry zone to Meckels cave. The nerve is then split longitudinally into 2-6 fascicles with a microneedle, blunt tip probe, nerve fiber knife, or other similar instrument (Ko et al., 2015; Zhao et al., 2017; Zhou et al., 2016). IN may be performed along the length of the nerve, or along specific segments in accordance with patient symptoms (Jie et al., 2013). Additionally, Ko et al. describe performing IN on both the sensory and motor roots of the trigeminal nerve, as intracranial connections between the two have been described (Tubbs, Griessenauer, Hogan, Loukas, & Cohen-Gadol).

Several studies have reported successful, long-term pain relief when IN is performed for TN in the absence of vascular compression. Using outcome criteria established by the University of California – San Francisco, Jie et al. report excellent outcomes in 82.1% of patients and a recurrence rate of 3.6% over a more than 48 month follow up period. Similarly, Ma et al. report excellent outcomes in 70% of patients and a recurrence rate of 10% over more than 36 months of follow up. Defining a successful procedure as a 1 or 2 on the Barrow Neurologic Institute Pain Intensity Scale, Ko et al. nonetheless demonstrate significant pain relief with IN in 72% of patients and a recurrence rate of 50% over a 5 year follow up period. These studies suggest that while IN can be an effective surgical option for the treatment of non-arterial TN, pain can recur after this procedure.

The most common adverse effect caused by IN is temporary or permanent facial numbness, with a reported incidence varying widely from 17.9 to 96% (Jie et al., 2013; Ko et al., 2015; Zhao et al., 2017). Ko et al. also describe the development of deafferentiation pain in 16% of patients post IN. Other reported complications related to IN include loss of corneal reflex (10-14%), and dysesthesias (16%), in addition to the commonly reported risks associated with posterior fossa explorations such as diplopia (2-3.6%), permanent or transient hearing loss or tinnitus (2-3.6%), CSF leak (3.6-6%), and meningitis (8%) (Jie et al., 2013; Ko et al., 2015; Ma & Li, 2009; Zhao et al., 2017; Zhou et al., 2016).

Microsurgical Nerve Sectioning

Another option for surgeons to consider in the absence of an intraoperative identifiable cause of TN is complete or partial sectioning of the trigeminal sensory root. While this approach has historically been effective for providing pain relief from non-compressive TN in upwards of 80% of cases (Adams, Kaye, & Teddy, 1982; Bederson & Wilson, 1989), it is generally considered a last resort due to the resulting numbness and potential complications stemming from an altered corneal response. If considered, partial as opposed to complete sectioning of the sensory root may be preferred due to similar rates of pain relief with a lower associated risk of corneal complications. Complete sectioning of the trigeminal nerve proximal to the ganglion in the posterior fossa can also be considered, but risks the above sensory changes as well as the loss of the motor component of the trigeminal nerve relating to the muscles of mastication.

Innovations in the Surgical Treatment of TN

Tentorial Sling for Arterial Transposition From the Nerve Root Entry Zone

In cases where arterial compression of the nerve root entry zone is clear, microvascular decompression is most commonly performed by inserting a foreign material, such as Teflon, between the trigeminal nerve and the site of vascular compression. While this technique can be highly effective, the implantation of a foreign body can lead to granulomatous reactions and scarring at the nerve root entry zone (Bobek & Sagher, 1999; Capelle, Brandis, Tschan, & Krauss, 2010; J. Chen et al., 2000; Masuoka et al., 2011; Matsushima, Yamaguchi, Inoue, Matsukado, & Fukui, 2000; Yang, Jiang, Chen, & Wang, 2015), which may cause recurrent pain and complicate subsequent repeat MVD procedures.

An alternative microsurgical decompressive technique for TN utilizes a tentorial sling for arterial transposition (Steinberg et al, 2017). In this method a standard retrosigmoid craniotomy is performed to access the cerebellopontine angle, exploring for any compressive vessel at the nerve root entry zone. Once an offending artery has been located and dissected free from the nerve, attention is turned to creation of the tentorial sling. The underside of the tentorium is viewed and a 2-4mm horizontal split thickness incision in the tentorium is made using a #15 surgical scalpel or similar instrument. Two perpendicular incisions are then completed tracking deep to the first incision with use of microscissors and a microdissector, forming a split thickness tentorial pedicle. Hemostatic agents and bipolar cautery are utilized during creation of this flap to maintain hemostasis, being careful not to shrink the pedicle with excessive cautery. Once created, the tentorial sling is mobilized around the compressive artery and the free edge is brought up to the proximal portion of the tentorial pedicle. A Weck clip is utilized to secure the tentorial sling to the pedicle or the cut edge of tentorium. Care is taken to ensure perforators are not avulsed and that the compressive vessel is not strangulated.

While this or similar tentorial sling methodologies are typically reserved for cases where an artery is found to be compressing the trigeminal nerve, some authors advocate for artery transposition in cases where a non-compressive artery near the trigeminal nerve is identified intraoperatively with possible additional neurolysis (Toda et al., 2015). Benefits of the tentorial sling method include the avoidance of foreign materials (aside from a Weck clip), and complete transposition of the compressive vessel away from the nerve. This allows for a fully decompressed nerve and may ultimately decrease chances of inflammatory reactions at the nerve root entry zone. Early experience using the tentorial sling on 45 patients undergoing a first time MVD surgery for TN demonstrated approximate rates of immediate pain relief around 80% (Steinberg et al, 2017). Recurrence rates of TN using this approach were less than 10% over a 16 month follow period. While these outcomes are comparable to one of the largest studies on MVD for TN by Barker and Jannetta et al (Barker, Jannetta, Bissonette, Larkins, & Jho, 1996), longer-term data is needed to determine whether the tentorial sling offers more durable long-term pain relief as compared to traditional MVD.

Potential disadvantages of this method include the learning curve of acquiring this new technique, which adds approximately 40 minutes of operative time initially, and 20 minutes of operative time once versed in the procedure. Tentorial bleeding can also be encountered, however, this is typically easily controlled with hemostatic agents and bipolar cautery.

Intraoperative Neuromonitoring During Microvascular Decompression Surgery

Intraoperative neuromonitoring (IONM) is increasingly utilized in skull base surgery to assess cranial nerve function in real time. While typically utilized in MVD operations for hemifacial spasm due to operative manipulation of the facial and vestibulocochlear nerves (Huang, Chang, & Hsu, 2009; Kim et al., 2012; Polo, Fischer, Sindou, & Marneffe, 2004), IONM has also been reported for use in MVD operations of the glossopharyngeal and trigeminal nerves (Brock et al., 2004; C. C. Lee et al., 2014; Motoyama et al., 2016). One described benefit of IONM in TN MVD surgery is for the definitive identification of cranial nerves by novice surgeons (Brock et al., 2004). Others report a utility of IONM, particularly brainstem auditory evoked responses (BAERs), for the prevention of high frequency hearing loss, which has been reported in approximately 1% of MVD surgeries for TN (C. C. Lee et al., 2014). In this scenario, changes in BAERs can potentially alert surgeons to effects of surgical maneuvers on cranial nerve function in real-time, allowing for immediate corrective actions. The effectiveness of IONM for predicting high frequency hearing loss in TN MVD cases has nonetheless been questioned by other authors (Thirumala et al., 2015), and IONM remains an optional adjunct in MVD surgery for TN.

Revision Surgery for TN

Exploratory surgery can be considered in cases of recurrent, refractory TN that develop after an initial MVD surgery, although such procedures are associated with a unique set of challenges. In one study of thirty-one repeat operations for TN, surgical exploration was negative for any causative pathology in more than 50% of patients (Cho et al., 1994). Arterial or venous nerve compression was the next most likely finding, occurring in 22% and 13% of cases, respectively. Although it is considered an inert material, Teflon compression or reactive adhesions were found in the remaining 13% of cases, with other authors describing the development of even more extensive granulomatous tissue formation at the site of Teflon implantation in 1.3% of cases (Premsagar, Moss, & Coakham, 1997). While meticulous surgical technique is required in revision surgeries to avoid nerve injury when dissecting through scar tissues, rates of pain relief as high as 70% have been reported by addressing any identifiable causative pathologies, or performing partial sensory rhizotomies in the absence of causative lesions (Cho et al., 1994). Similar to first time operations, vascular compressions identified during revision surgeries are treated with repeat decompression of arteries or coagulation of veins, and compressive Teflon scars are treated with careful dissection and replacement. If not used in the first surgery, a tentorial sling for vascular decompression can also be considered.

FUTURE RESEARCH DIRECTIONS

As highlighted in this chapter, continual innovations for the surgical treatment of TN are being made in relation to both surgical technique and technical adjuncts to improve the safety and effectiveness of this procedure. Specific areas of future research suggested by this work include an exploration of the long-term efficacy of the tentorial sling for arterial transposition, and further assessments of the utility of IONM during MVDs for TN.

CONCLUSION

Surgery for recurrent trigeminal neuralgia or cases not caused by classically described SCN compression can still result in high rates of pain relief. Operative considerations in such cases discussed in this chapter include use of meticulous surgical technique, exploration for other pathologic vessels, and pursuit of nerve manipulation or sectioning techniques in the absence of compressive lesions. Novel innovations in the microsurgical treatment of typical TN are also explored.

REFERENCES

Adams, C. B., Kaye, A. H., & Teddy, P. J. (1982). The treatment of trigeminal neuralgia by posterior fossa microsurgery. *Journal of Neurology, Neurosurgery, and Psychiatry*, *45*(11), 1020–1026. doi:10.1136/jnnp.45.11.1020 PMID:7175525

Amagasaki, K., Abe, S., Watanabe, S., Naemura, K., & Nakaguchi, H. (2014). Trigeminal neuralgia caused by a trigeminocerebellar artery. *Journal of Neurosurgery*, *121*(4), 940–943. doi:10.3171/2014.6.JNS132292 PMID:25014438

Banczerowski, P., Czigléczki, G., & Nyáry, I. (2014). Long-term effectiveness of an ad hoc tailored titanium implant as a spacer for microvascular decompression in the treatment of trigeminal neuralgia caused by megadolichoectatic basilar artery anomaly: 9-year follow-up. *Journal of Neurosurgery*, *121*(6), 1492–1496. doi:10.3171/2014.8.JNS132445 PMID:25259563

Barker, F. G., Jannetta, P. J., Bissonette, D. J., Larkins, M. V., & Jho, H. D. (1996). The long-term outcome of microvascular decompression for trigeminal neuralgia. *The New England Journal of Medicine*, *334*(17), 1077–1083. doi:10.1056/NEJM199604253341701 PMID:8598865

Bederson, J. B., & Wilson, C. B. (1989). Evaluation of microvascular decompression and partial sensory rhizotomy in 252 cases of trigeminal neuralgia. *Journal of Neurosurgery*, *71*(3), 359–367. doi:10.3171/jns.1989.71.3.0359 PMID:2769387

Bobek, M. P., & Sagher, O. (1999). Aseptic meningitis caused by Teflon implantation for microvascular decompression. Case report. *Journal of Neurosurgery*, *90*(1), 145–147. doi:10.3171/jns.1999.90.1.0145 PMID:10413169

Brock, S., Scaioli, V., Ferroli, P., & Broggi, G. (2004). Neurovascular decompression in trigeminal neuralgia: Role of intraoperative neurophysiological monitoring in the learning period. *Stereotactic and Functional Neurosurgery*, *82*(5-6), 199–206. doi:10.1159/000082446 PMID:15583464

Capelle, H. H., Brandis, A., Tschan, C. A., & Krauss, J. K. (2010). Treatment of recurrent trigeminal neuralgia due to Teflon granuloma. *The Journal of Headache and Pain, 11*(4), 339–344. doi:10.100710194-010-0213-4 PMID:20419329

Chen, G. Q., Wang, X. S., Wang, L., & Zheng, J. P. (2014). Arterial compression of nerve is the primary cause of trigeminal neuralgia. *Neurological Sciences, 35*(1), 61–66. doi:10.100710072-013-1518-2 PMID:23963805

Chen, J., Lee, S., Lui, T., Yeh, Y., Chen, T., & Tzaan, W. (2000). Teflon granuloma after microvascular decompression for trigeminal neuralgia. *Surgical Neurology, 53*(3), 281–287. doi:10.1016/S0090-3019(00)00169-5 PMID:10773262

Cho, D. Y., Chang, C. G., Wang, Y. C., Wang, F. H., Shen, C. C., & Yang, D. Y. (1994). Repeat operations in failed microvascular decompression for trigeminal neuralgia. *Neurosurgery, 35*(4), 665–669, discussion 669–670. doi:10.1227/00006123-199410000-00012 PMID:7808609

Helbig, G. M., Callahan, J. D., & Cohen-Gadol, A. A. (2009). Variant intraneural vein-trigeminal nerve relationships: An observation during microvascular decompression surgery for trigeminal neuralgia. *Neurosurgery, 65*(5), 958–961, discussion 961. doi:10.1227/01.NEU.0000351757.29658.C0 PMID:19834410

Hong, W., Zheng, X., Wu, Z., Li, X., Wang, X., Li, Y., ... Li, S. (2011). Clinical features and surgical treatment of trigeminal neuralgia caused solely by venous compression. *Acta Neurochirurgica, 153*(5), 1037–1042. doi:10.100700701-011-0957-x PMID:21298451

Huang, B. R., Chang, C. N., & Hsu, J. C. (2009). Intraoperative electrophysiological monitoring in microvascular decompression for hemifacial spasm. *Journal of Clinical Neuroscience, 16*(2), 209–213. doi:10.1016/j.jocn.2008.04.016 PMID:19103492

Ichikawa, T., Agari, T., Kurozumi, K., Maruo, T., Satoh, T., & Date, I. (2011). "Double-stick tape" technique for transposition of an offending vessel in microvascular decompression: technical case report. *Neurosurgery, 68*(2 Suppl), 377-382. doi:10.1227/NEU.0b013e318217141c

Jie, H., Xuanchen, Z., Deheng, L., Kun, G., Fengyang, X., Xiang, C., . . . Yiqing, L. (2013). The long-term outcome of nerve combing for trigeminal neuralgia. *Acta Neurochir (Wien), 155*(9), 1703-1708. doi:10.1007/s00701-013-1804-z

Kim, H. J., Park, Y. S., Ryu, J. S., Huh, R., Han, I., Shin, D. A., ... Chung, S. S. (2012). Intraoperative facial electromyography and brainstem auditory evoked potential findings in microvascular decompression for hemifacial spasm: Correlation with postoperative delayed facial palsy. *Stereotactic and Functional Neurosurgery, 90*(4), 260–265. doi:10.1159/000338685 PMID:22777492

Kimura, T., Sako, K., Tohyama, Y., & Yonemasu, Y. (1999). Trigeminal neuralgia caused by compression from petrosal vein transfixing the nerve. *Acta Neurochirurgica, 141*(4), 437–438. doi:10.1007007010050321 PMID:10352756

Ko, A. L., Ozpinar, A., Lee, A., Raslan, A. M., McCartney, S., & Burchiel, K. J. (2015). Long-term efficacy and safety of internal neurolysis for trigeminal neuralgia without neurovascular compression. *Journal of Neurosurgery, 122*(5), 1048–1057. doi:10.3171/2014.12.JNS14469 PMID:25679283

Lee, C. C., Liao, C. H., Lin, C. F., Yang, T. F., Hsu, S. P., Yen, Y. S., & Shih, Y. H. (2014). Brainstem auditory evoked potential monitoring and neuro-endoscopy: Two tools to ensure hearing preservation and surgical success during microvascular decompression. *Journal of the Chinese Medical Association, 77*(6), 308–316. doi:10.1016/j.jcma.2014.02.016 PMID:24768092

Lee, S. H., Koh, J. S., & Lee, C. Y. (2011). Trigeminal neuralgia caused by an anomalous posterior inferior cerebellar artery from the primitive trigeminal artery: Case report. *Cerebellum (London, England), 10*(2), 199–203. doi:10.100712311-011-0249-2 PMID:21279490

Ma, Z., & Li, M. (2009). "Nerve combing" for trigeminal neuralgia without vascular compression: Report of 10 cases. *The Clinical Journal of Pain, 25*(1), 44–47. doi:10.1097/AJP.0b013e31817e138e PMID:19158545

Marinković, S., Gibo, H., & Nikodijević, I. (1996). Trigeminocerebellar artery--anatomy and possible clinical significance. *Neurologia Medico-Chirurgica, 36*(4), 215–219. doi:10.2176/nmc.36.215 PMID:8741249

Masuoka, J., Matsushima, T., Inoue, K., Nakahara, Y., Takase, Y., & Kawashima, M. (2015). Outcome of microvascular decompression for trigeminal neuralgia treated with the stitched sling retraction technique. *Neurosurgical Review, 38*(2), 361–365, discussion 365. doi:10.100710143-015-0607-5 PMID:25663308

Masuoka, J., Matsushima, T., Kawashima, M., Nakahara, Y., Funaki, T., & Mineta, T. (2011). Stitched sling retraction technique for microvascular decompression: Procedures and techniques based on an anatomical viewpoint. *Neurosurgical Review, 34*(3), 373–379, discussion 379–380. doi:10.100710143-011-0310-0 PMID:21347661

Matsushima, T., Huynh-Le, P., & Miyazono, M. (2004). Trigeminal neuralgia caused by venous compression. *Neurosurgery, 55*(2), 334–337, discussion 338–339. doi:10.1227/01.NEU.0000129552.87291.87 PMID:15271239

Matsushima, T., Yamaguchi, T., Inoue, T. K., Matsukado, K., & Fukui, M. (2000). Recurrent trigeminal neuralgia after microvascular decompression using an interposing technique. Teflon felt adhesion and the sling retraction technique. *Acta Neurochirurgica, 142*(5), 557–561. doi:10.1007007010050469 PMID:10898363

Morita, A., Fukushima, T., Miyazaki, S., Shimizu, T., & Atsuchi, M. (1989). Tic douloureux caused by primitive trigeminal artery or its variant. *Journal of Neurosurgery, 70*(3), 415–419. doi:10.3171/jns.1989.70.3.0415 PMID:2915249

Motoyama, Y., Nakagawa, I., Takatani, T., Park, H. S., Kotani, Y., Tanaka, Y., ... Nakase, H. (2016). Microvascular decompression for glossopharyngeal neuralgia using intraoperative neurophysiological monitoring: Technical case report. *Surgical Neurology International, 7*(3Suppl 2), S28–S35. doi:10.4103/2152-7806.173565 PMID:26862458

Park, C. K., Choi, H. J., Lee, S. H., & Rhee, B. A. (2014). Trigeminal neuralgia caused by persistent primitive trigeminal artery. *Journal of Korean Neurosurgical Society, 56*(3), 278–280. doi:10.3340/jkns.2014.56.3.278 PMID:25368776

Polo, G., Fischer, C., Sindou, M. P., & Marneffe, V. (2004). Brainstem auditory evoked potential monitoring during microvascular decompression for hemifacial spasm: Intraoperative brainstem auditory evoked potential changes and warning values to prevent hearing loss--prospective study in a consecutive series of 84 patients. *Neurosurgery, 54*(1), 97–104, discussion 104–106. doi:10.1227/01.NEU.0000097268.90620.07 PMID:14683545

Premsagar, I. C., Moss, T., & Coakham, H. B. (1997). Teflon-induced granuloma following treatment of trigeminal neuralgia by microvascular decompression. Report of two cases. *Journal of Neurosurgery, 87*(3), 454–457. doi:10.3171/jns.1997.87.3.0454 PMID:9285615

Sato, O., Kanazawa, I., & Kokunai, T. (1979). Trigeminal neuralgia caused by compression of trigeminal nerve by pontine vein. *Surgical Neurology, 11*(4), 285–286. PMID:441914

Steinberg, J., Sack, J., Wilson, B., Weingarten, D., Carter, B., Khalessi, A., ... Alksne, J. (2017). (In Press). Tentorial sling for microvascular decompression in patients with trigeminal neuralgia: A description of operative technique and clinical outcomes. *Journal of Neurosurgery*.

Thirumala, P., Meigh, K., Dasyam, N., Shankar, P., Sarma, K. R., Sarma, D. R., ... Balzer, J. (2015). The incidence of high-frequency hearing loss after microvascular decompression for trigeminal neuralgia, glossopharyngeal neuralgia, or geniculate neuralgia. *Journal of Neurosurgery, 123*(6), 1500–1506. doi:10.3171/2014.10.JNS141101 PMID:25932612

Toda, H., Goto, M., & Iwasaki, K. (2015). Patterns and variations in microvascular decompression for trigeminal neuralgia. *Neurologia Medico-Chirurgica, 55*(5), 432–441. doi:10.2176/nmc.ra.2014-0393 PMID:25925756

Wang, D. D., Raygor, K. P., Cage, T. A., Ward, M. M., Westcott, S., Barbaro, N. M., & Chang, E. F. (2017). Prospective comparison of long-term pain relief rates after first-time microvascular decompression and stereotactic radiosurgery for trigeminal neuralgia. *Journal of Neurosurgery*, 1–10. doi:10.3171/2016.9.JNS16149 PMID:28298026

Yamada, Y., Kondo, A., & Tanabe, H. (2006). Trigeminal neuralgia associated with an anomalous artery originating from the persistent primitive trigeminal artery. *Neurologia Medico-Chirurgica, 46*(4), 194–197. doi:10.2176/nmc.46.194 PMID:16636511

Yang, D. B., Jiang, D. Y., Chen, H. C., & Wang, Z. M. (2015). Second microvascular decompression for trigeminal neuralgia in recurrent cases after microvascular decompression. *The Journal of Craniofacial Surgery, 26*(2), 491–494. doi:10.1097/SCS.0000000000001523 PMID:25759921

Zhao, H., Zhang, X., Tang, D., & Li, S. (2017). Nerve Combing for Trigeminal Neuralgia Without Vascular Compression. *The Journal of Craniofacial Surgery, 28*(1), e15–e16. doi:10.1097/SCS.0000000000003161 PMID:27875506

Zheng, X., Feng, B., Hong, W., Zhang, W., Yang, M., Tang, Y., ... Li, S. (2012). Management of intraneural vessels during microvascular decompression surgery for trigeminal neuralgia. *World Neurosurgery, 77*(5-6), 771–774. doi:10.1016/j.wneu.2011.08.031 PMID:22120295

Zhou, X., Liu, Y., Yue, Z., Luan, D., Zhang, H., & Han, J. (2016). Comparison of nerve combing and percutaneous radiofrequency thermocoagulation in the treatment for idiopathic trigeminal neuralgia. *Revista Brasileira de Otorrinolaringologia (English Ed.), 82*(5), 574–579. doi:10.1016/j.bjorl.2015.11.006 PMID:26832635

KEY TERMS AND DEFINITIONS

Internal Neurolysis: The selective surgical disruption of nerve axons to dampen but not destroy their electrical excitability; can be used for the treatment of TN pain in the absence of a compressive artery on the nerve root.

Intraoperative Neuromonitoring (IONM): A system for the real-time assessment of neurologic function in the operating room. Cranial nerve function, in addition to gross motor and sensory functions traversing the spinal cord are commonly assessed.

Microvascular Decompression (MVD): A surgical procedure for the removal of a decompressive artery off of a cranial nerve root entry zone. Separation of these structures during a MVD procedure is often achieved by the placement of an intervening piece of Teflon or other inert material.

Superior Cerebellar Artery (SCA): An artery arising off the superior portion of the basilar trunk that supplies the superior cerebellum, and is the most common compressive artery in cases of TN.

Tentorial Sling for TN: Creation of a sling from a split thickness pedicle of the inferior surface of the tentorium for transposition of a compressive artery away from the trigeminal nerve.

Trigeminal Neuralgia (TN): A rare type of facial pain, characterized by paroxysmal, shock-like pain along the unilateral trigeminal nerve distribution, often triggered by benign stimuli.

Chapter 6 Novel Techniques for Trigeminal Neuralgia Including Trigeminal Neurostimulators

Arvin R. Wali
University of California – San Diego, USA

Jeffrey A. Steinberg
University of California – San Diego, USA

Christian Lopez
University of California – San Diego, USA

Robert C. Rennert
University of California – San Diego, USA

Peter Abraham
University of California – San Diego, USA

Jeffrey Scott Pannell
University of California – San Diego, USA

Michael G. Brandel
University of California – San Diego, USA

John F. Alksne
University of California – San Diego, USA

David R. Santiago-Dieppa
University of California – San Diego, USA

Alexander A. Khalessi
University of California – San Diego, USA

ABSTRACT

Several innovative surgical options for the management of trigeminal neuralgia have emerged over the past 40 years. In addition to microvascular decompression, other techniques have been introduced for the treatment of trigeminal neuralgia and facial nerve pain. This chapter describes the following novel therapeutic modalities: endoscopic microvascular decompression, radiosurgery, radiofrequency, thermocoagulation, glycerol rhizotomoy, balloon compression, Gasserian ganglion stimulation, and subcutaneous trigeminal nerve stimulation. For each of these techniques, this chapter provides a description of the procedure, criteria for patient selection, and discusses published data regarding patient outcomes.

DOI: 10.4018/978-1-5225-5349-6.ch006

INTRODUCTION

Patients with trigeminal neuropathic pain refractory to medical management can be treated with a variety of minimally invasive surgical approaches that either augment or differ from standard microvascular decompression (MVD). For example, endoscopy is increasingly being used to augment traditional microvascular decompressions due to improvements in visualization of the source of vascular or structural compression and ability to intra-operatively confirm an adequate decompression (Artz et al., 2008; C. H. Halpern, S. S. Lang, & J. Y. Lee, 2013; Lang, Chen, & Lee, 2012; Sandell, Ringstad, & Eide, 2014). Other minimally invasive techniques that differ from microvascular decompression include stereotactic radiosurgery surgery (SRS), percutaneous radiofrequency nerve ablation, rhizotomy, balloon compression, and neurostimulation, all of which rely on nerve root lesioning or manipulation to alleviate painful symptoms. Specifically, SRS utilizes radiation, while radiofrequency thermocoagulation and glycerol rhizotomy use percutaneously delivered heat currents and chemicals to achieve nerve root destruction (Hakanson, 1981; Kanpolat, Savas, Bekar, & Berk, 2001; J. K. Lee, Choi, Ko, Choi, & Lim, 2012; William H. Sweet & James G. Wepsic, 1974). Balloon compression similarly utilizes percutaneous placement of an inflatable balloon to cause physical compression of the trigeminal ganglia (Mullan & Lichtor, 1983). Percutaneously delivered neurostimulators can also be used to modulate nerve signals within the trigeminal nerve and distal branches (Holsheimer, 2001). This chapter will discuss the operative nuances of each of these techniques and the published data regarding their comparative efficacy to treat trigeminal nerve pain.

NOVEL NEUROSURGICAL TECHNIQUES

Endoscopic MVD

Brief Description of Procedure

Similarl to the traditional open MVD (O-MVD), endoscopic microvascular decompression (E-MVD) is also approached via a small retrosigmoid craniectomy to expose the borders of the transverse and sigmoid sinuses (Artz et al., 2008; C. H. Halpern et al., 2013; Lang et al., 2012; Sandell et al., 2014). A 1-2 cm dural opening is made and the dural flap is retracted. An endoscope is then inserted through the dural opening. A 0-degree endoscope is typically used, although angled endoscopes may expedite identification of root entry zone vascular anatomy and enhance visualization of the neurovascular conflict in the case of a prominent petrous ridge

(C. H. Halpern et al., 2013). Alternatively, visualization may be improved by the use of small mirrors or drilling the bony ridge (Sandell et al., 2014). Cerebellopontine angle (CPA) structures are exposed after opening the arachnoid plane for drainage of cerebrospinal fluid (C. H. Halpern, S.-S. Lang, & J. Y. Lee, 2013). Upon exposure of the trigeminal nerve, the vasculature is examined utilizing the endoscope and any compressive vessel is mobilized. Decompression is then completed through the placement of Teflon between the offending vessel and the trigeminal nerve. In addition to E-MVD, endoscopy may assist traditional microsurgical technique (endoscopic-assisted MVD (EA-MVD)) to help the operating surgeon visualize the offending vessel and achieve excellent vascular decompression (Casey H Halpern et al., 2013; Teo, Nakaji, & Mobbs, 2006).

Patient Selection

Candidates for E-MVD include patients with clinical exam findings consistent with trigeminal neuralgia with possible MRI evidence of a vascular structure compressing on the dorsal root entry zone of the trigeminal nerve (Brisman, Khandji, & Mooij, 2002; Haines, Jannetta, & Zorub, 1980).

Patient Outcomes

Halpern et al. completed fully endoscopic MVDs in 35 patients with trigeminal neuralgia and completed EA-MVDs in seven trigeminal neuralgia patients (C. H. Halpern et al., 2013). All seven patients that underwent EA-MVD achieved adequate to excellent pain control and 31 of 35 (89%) of patients that underwent E-MVD achieved adequate to excellent pain control via the Barrow Neurologic Institute (BNI) pain (scores 1-2). One patient had the complication of csf-otorrhea, but the authors report that this complication was not directly related to the endoscopic technique. This complication rate (2.4%) among E-MVD patients was comparable to that of patients treated with microsurgical MVD.

Broggi et al. retrospectively reviewed 89 O-MVD, 12 E-MVD, and 40 EA-MVD cases for patients with trigeminal neuralgia, hemifacial spasm, or glossopharyngeal neuralgia (Broggi et al., 2013). Fully endoscopic MVD had a similar rate of excellent pain control (BNI pain scores 1-2) compared to microscopic cases (70% vs. 76%, respectively).

Sandell et al. completed E-MVDs in a 97 trigeminal neuralgia patients (Sandell et al., 2014), finding that endoscopy was essential to identification of the neurovascular conflict in 27.8% of the cases. The overall perioperative complication rate was 5.2%, with no complications directly related to use of the endoscope, and a rate of lasting neurologic deficit of 5.3%. Significant pain relief was achieved in approximately

90% of patients with 100% episodic pain and approximately 80% of patients with a constant pain component.

Bohman et al. reported their experience with E-MVD in 47 patients with trigeminal neuralgia (Bohman, Pierce, Stephen, Sandhu, & Lee, 2014). The most common complication was dizziness/unsteadiness without focal neurological signs, which occurred in 6% of patients. The rate of permanent neurological morbidity was only 2%. 83% of patients reported significant improvements in their preoperative facial pain, with 94% having at least some improvement. Self-rated pain intensity was reduced by an average of 84%.

Lee et al. compared outcomes for 93 trigeminal neuralgia patients that underwent O-MVD and 74 patients that underwent E-MVD (J. Y. K. Lee, Pierce, Sandhu, Petrov, & Yang, 2017). There was a very low rate of overall complications, which did not differ between groups. However, E-MVD patients had a significantly lower rate of headaches at 1-month follow-up (p=0.01).

E-MVD appears to be equally effective as O-MVD to decompress the trigeminal nerve and reduce trigeminal facial pain based a small body of literature evaluating this newer technique. Benefits include improved visualization of the nerve root entry zone afforded by the varied angles of endoscopy. Moreover, one study argues that the endoscope is critical for visualization of neurovascular conflict. As with any new operative technique, there is a learning curve for utilization of the endoscope within the CP angle.

Radiosurgery

Brief Description of Procedure

While the majority of evidence for SRS for the treatment of trigeminal neuralgia derives from publications using the Gamma Knife (GK) system (Singh, Davis, & Sharma, 2016), there has been increased utilization and reporting of outcomes for linear accelerator (LINAC)-based SRS (Varela-Lema, Lopez-Garcia, Maceira-Rozas, & Munoz-Garzon, 2015) and the CyberKnife (CK) system (Singh et al., 2016) in recent years. For SRS using the GK system, treatment planning involves a multispecialty team including neurosurgeons, radiation oncologists, and medical physicists. Local anesthesia is used before attaching a stereotactic coordinate frame to the patient's head. A contrast enhanced thin-slice MRI sequence is then used to visualize the trigeminal nerve root entry zone, where a single isocenter is placed (Alberico, Fenstermaker, & Lobel, 2001). The prescription dose for the treatment typically ranges from 70 to 90 gray (Gy) delivered to the trigeminal nerve root entry zone (J. K. Lee et al., 2012). Some authors argue that higher doses of radiation are associated with greater rates of complications and thus try to limit maximum radiation to less than 90 gray (Bruce E Pollock, Phuong, Foote, Stafford, & Gorman, 2001). Moreover, with SRS alternative targets may also be used, including the brainstem trigeminal nuclei or the centromedian nucleus of the thalamus (Hodaie & Coello, 2013).

Patient Selection (Over MVD)

Results from several studies have suggested that MVD is superior to GK for long-term outcomes (Montano et al., 2015; A. Nanda, V. Javalkar, S. Zhang, & O. Ahmed, 2015). However, some patients may be averse to invasive surgery, have medical contraindications to MVD or have already undergone MVD. Moreover, there is evidence suggesting patients with neuralgia spanning all three trigeminal divisions, minimal amount of nerve compression, and/or focal arachnoiditis have worse MVD outcomes(Sindou, Leston, Decullier, & Chapuis, 2007) and may be better suited for SRS. Additionally, SRS patients avoid the operative risk of MVD and can be discharged on the same day (Anil Nanda, Vijayakumar Javalkar, Shihao Zhang, & Osama Ahmed, 2015). However, patients should be counseled that performing MVD after radiation-based therapy can be significantly more challenging.

Outcomes

Han et al. treated 43 trigeminal neuralgia patients with GK. 7% of patients experienced new facial numbness (Han et al., 1999). 77% of patients were treated successfully, although only 35% of all patients achieved a total reduction in pain and no longer required medications. The average time to initial relief was 31 days.

Lim et al. reported outcomes for 41 idiopathic trigeminal neuralgia patients treated with CK SRS (Lim et al., 2005). 87.8% of patients achieved excellent pain control, with initial pain relief at a median of seven days. 78% of patients experienced long-term relief. 51.2% of patients experienced new-onset numbness after treatment. However, the new onset numbness was only bothersome to a minority of the patients.

Dhople et al. reported their experience using GK to treat 112 patients with classical trigeminal neuralgia (Dhople et al., 2009). The initial response rate was 81%, with a median time to pain relief of two weeks. Seventy percent of patients decreased or discontinued the use of medications for their trigeminal neuralgia symptoms. The rate of new bothersome facial numbness after initial GK was only 6%, and there were no major complications.

Régis et al. analyzed the long-term outcomes of GK in 497 patients with classical trigeminal neuralgia (Regis et al., 2016). Of the treated patients 20.4% experienced hypesthesia at the 5-year mark, although this was very bothersome in only three patients (0.6%). In a median time of 10 days, 91.75% of patients were initially pain free. However, only 71.8% were pain free at three years and 45.3% at 10 years.

These studies demonstrate that radiosurgery is an effective, non-invasive, outpatient treatment to reduce pain associated with trigeminal neuralgia that typically takes effect in one to two weeks. Patients should be counseled that facial numbness is a common side effect from radiosurgery, although not overly bothersome to most patients, and there is a substantial rate of pain recurrence over the ensuing years.

Radiofrequency Thermocoagulation

Brief Description of Procedure

Radiofrequency thermocoagulation (RFT) rhizotomy utilizes heat to lesion the trigeminal nerve to provide pain relief (William H. Sweet & James G. Wepsic, 1974). This technique relies on patient cooperation during portions of the procedure to guide optimal lesioning position based on clinical symptomatology and requires the administration of short-acting anesthetics (William H. Sweet & James G. Wepsic, 1974). A needle is inserted 2-3 cm lateral to the angle of the mouth on the affected side and is advanced toward the base of the skull, aiming for a point at the intersection of a vertical line drawn at the medial ipsilateral pupil and a horizontal line drawn at a point 2-3 cm anterior to the external acoustic meatus (Sebastião Gusmão, Marcelo Oliveira, Uedson Tazinaffo, & Christopher R. Honey, 2003; William H. Sweet & James G. Wepsic, 1974). Penetration of the foramen ovale may result in a vasovagal response, potentially requiring the administration of an anticholinergic medication. The patient is awakened after accurate needle position is confirmed with fluoroscopy. With the patient's input, dermatomal mapping of the trigeminal nerve is performed for optimal lesioning and reduction of sensorimotor complications. An electrode delivers a heating current (55-80° C) for about one minute to the target branches until adequate pain relief is achieved (Kanpolat et al., 2001; William H. Sweet & James G. Wepsic, 1974).

Patient Selection

Candidates for RFT include elderly patients with significant comorbidities, patients unable to tolerate general anesthesia, patients who have failed microvascular decompression, or patient preference for RFT (William H. Sweet & James G. Wepsic, 1974). An important consideration when choosing RFT is the capacity of the patient to communicate the distribution of pain and associated symptoms during the simulation portion of the procedure. Radiofrequency ablation also provides greater division selectivity and may confer a greater benefit for patients presenting with an isolated division neuralgia (Lopez, Hamlyn, & Zakrzewska, 2004).

Patient Outcomes

In a systematic review comparing RFT, glycerol rhizotomy, balloon compression, and stereotactic radiosurgery for trigeminal neuralgia, complete pain relief at 6-months was highest (74-94%) with RFT (Lopez et al., 2004). In a 25-year study of 1,600 patients, RFT provided acute pain relief in 97.6% of patients and more than half of patients at 60- and 120-months (Kanpolat et al., 2001). Similar rates of initial pain relief (94-99%) are reported elsewhere (Mittal & Thomas, 1986; Sweet, 1988; Taha, Tew, & Buncher, 1995). Latchaw et al reported a recurrence free rate of 52% at five years after a single RFT procedure (Latchaw, Hardy, Forsythe, & Cook, 1983). After a 15-year follow up, 95% of patients remained pain-free after one or two RFT procedures.(Taha et al., 1995) Long term recurrence rates have been reported at 25% and 31% for follow-up periods of 5.7- and 14-years, respectively (Kanpolat et al., 2001; Taha et al., 1995). While effective for relieving pain associated with trigeminal neuralgia, RFT is associated with the highest total complication rate (29.2%) among ablative procedures (Lopez et al., 2004). Commonly observed complications include masseter weakness (4-11.9%), corneal numbness (5.7-9.6%) and dysesthesias (4-22%) (Lopez et al., 2004; Sweet, 1988; Taha et al., 1995). Less common complications include cranial nerve palsies, anesthesia dolorosa, and corneal numbness. Previous studies have also noted an inverse correlation between recurrence of pain and the degree of sensory loss after RFT, with lower recurrence rates observed in patients with analgesia after surgery (Latchaw et al., 1983; Taha et al., 1995).

RFT provides excellent, long-term pain relief for patients though this technique may be associated with the highest complication rate compared to other ablative techniques.

Glycerol Rhizotomy

Brief Description of Procedure

Glycerol rhizotomy (GR) remains a commonly performed percutaneous chemical ablative treatment for trigeminal neuralgia that does not require patient cooperation and can thus allow for deeper sedation (Hakanson, 1981). As with RFT, surface landmarks and fluoroscopy guide needle placement through the foramen ovale into the trigeminal cistern. CSF egress may confirm placement. Although not always performed, a contrast cisternography can aid in assessing the volume of the trigeminal cistern (typically 0.3-0.4 mL) to assist in identifying the volume of glycerol required for injection (Kondziolka & Lunsford, 2005; North, Kidd, Piantadosi, & Carson, 1990; B. E. Pollock, 2005). Administration of the full volume of the trigeminal cistern is utilized to treat multi-division neuralgia (Kondziolka & Lunsford, 2005). However, for pain in the V1 distribution, only one-third of the cisternal volume is injected prior to contrast drainage. The less dense glycerol will rise above the contrast agent and selectively lesion the ophthalmic branch. The patient remains in the sitting position 2-3 hours post-glycerol injection and is generally discharged on the same or following day.

Patient Selection

Indications for GR are similar to those previously described for RFT. These include patients who are elderly with significant comorbidities, have failed microvascular decompression or other surgical options, prefer glycerol rhizotomy, or have trigeminal neuralgia secondary to multiple sclerosis (Asplund, Blomstedt, & Bergenheim, 2016; Bender et al., 2012).

Patient Outcomes

Rates of initial complete pain relief after GR have been reported in the range of 85-93% (Kondziolka & Lunsford, 2005; K. Kouzounias, G. Lind, G. Schechtmann, J. Winter, & B. Linderoth, 2010; Slettebo, Hirschberg, & Lindegaard, 1993; Young, 1988). However, recurrence rates are generally higher compared to other ablative techniques and many patients require multiple treatments (Lopez et al., 2004). The median time to recurrence is reported at 21-48 months with subsequent procedures demonstrating decreased median time to recurrence of symptoms (Asplund et al., 2016; Bender et al., 2012; K. Kouzounias et al., 2010; North et al., 1990; Slettebo et al., 1993; Young, 1988). In one study of 101 patients, the median time to recurrence after a single and second GR procedure was 24 months and 8 months, respectively (Konstantinos Kouzounias, Göran Lind, Gastón Schechtmann, Jaleh Winter, & Bengt Linderoth, 2010). Facial pain during glycerol injection and hypesthesias after procedure are associated with favorable pain outcomes and decreased rates of failure (Bender et al., 2012; B. E. Pollock, 2005). New trigeminal deficits are common after GR, with rates of persistent hypesthesias as high as 45% (K. Kouzounias et al., 2010).

In a systematic review, GR was found to have a slightly lower total complication rate (24.8%) compared to RFT (29.2%), but higher than mechanical balloon compression (16.1%) (Lopez et al., 2004). Common complications observed after GR include dystesthesias (8%), corneal numbness (2-8%), masseter weakness (3%), and development of cold sores due to reactivation of the herpes simplex virus (3-

7%) (Asplund et al., 2016; Bender et al., 2012; K. Kouzounias et al., 2010; Lopez et al., 2004; B. E. Pollock, 2005; Young, 1988).

GR, like other ablative techniques, can be efficacious in reducing painful symptoms associated with trigeminal neuralgia. While many patients find initial relief, many patients however have a recurrence of symptoms.

Balloon Compression

Brief Description of Procedure

Mechanical balloon compression is an effective percutaneous treatment of trigeminal neuralgia. Performed on the patient under general anesthesia, surface anatomic landmarks and fluoroscopy guided needle placement into Meckel's cave (Mullan & Lichtor, 1983). Placement of the guiding stylet is dependent on the affected trigeminal branch. Medial, central, and lateral placement targets first-division, third-division, and second- and multi-division neuralgia, respectively(Brown & Pilitsis, 2005). A 4-Fogarty balloon catheter is placed into Meckel's cave and the balloon is inflated with 0.7 mL of contrast material to a pressure in the range of 1000-1200 mm Hg (Brown & Pilitsis, 2005). Average balloon compression times range from 1-3 minutes, but durations up to 7-10 minutes have been reported (Brown, McDaniel, & Weaver, 1993; Brown & Pilitsis, 2005; K. Kouzounias et al., 2010; Lichtor & Mullan, 1990; Mullan & Lichtor, 1983; Skirving & Dan, 2001). Patients treated with mechanical balloon compression are generally discharged on the same day or on post-operative day 1.

Patient Selection

Indications for mechanical balloon compression are similar to RFT and GR, as previously described. Balloon compression minimizes the risk of corneal complications due to its sparing of small nerve fibers and should be considered for patients with first-division neuralgia (Brown & Pilitsis, 2005). Poor candidates include patients who are unable to tolerate general anesthesia.

Patient Outcomes

Numerous studies have reported initial complete pain relief rates in 82-100% of patients (Asplund et al., 2016; Asplund, Linderoth, & Bergenheim, 2010; Brown et al., 1993; Brown & Pilitsis, 2005; Kanpolat et al., 2001; K. Kouzounias et al., 2010; Mullan & Lichtor, 1983; Skirving & Dan, 2001). The median time to recurrence ranges from 20-28 months (Asplund et al., 2016; Brown et al., 1993; K. Kouzounias et al., 2010). The two-year actuarial rates of pain relief reported in one study were 44% and 40%, following a single and repeat balloon compression, respectively (K. Kouzounias et al., 2010). Adequate balloon shape has been shown to significantly correlate with median time to recurrence of symptoms.

Asplund et al found that the median pain free time was greater among patients treated with a "pear-shaped" balloon compared to a "non-pear shaped" balloon (46 months vs 5 months, respectively) (Asplund et al., 2010). Complications related to corneal numbness and keratitis are uncommon compared to RFT and GR (Brown et al., 1993; K. Kouzounias et al., 2010; Lopez et al., 2004). Similarly, anesthesia dolorosa occurs less commonly after balloon compression compared to other percutaneous procedures (Asplund et al., 2010; Lopez et al., 2004; Skirving & Dan, 2001). Rates of dysesthesias and masseter weakness are both reported in the range of 4-20% (Asplund et al., 2016; Brown et al., 1993; Brown & Pilitsis, 2005; K. Kouzounias et al., 2010; Lichtor & Mullan, 1990; Lobato, Rivas, Sarabia, & Lamas, 1990; Lopez et al., 2004; Martin, Teo, & Suttner, 2015; Skirving & Dan, 2001).

These studies demonstrate that balloon decompression may provide excellent pain relief for patients, however the duration of pain relief needs to be further studied.

NEUROMODULATION

Gasserian Ganglion Stimulation

Brief Description of Procedure

Stimulation of the Gasserian ganglion, or trigeminal ganglion, is achieved via a percutaneous approach with fluoroscopic guidance under monitored anesthesia care. A monopolar electrode mounted at the tip of a flexible lead is inserted into the foramen ovale through a 16-gauge needle aimed lateral to the pterygoid. Once the Gasserian ganglion is accessed, the patient is awakened and a test-stimulation is performed until paresthesias are evoked, at which point the needle is removed under fluoroscopic guidance (J. P. Van Buyten, 2015). A trial period of 1-5 days of percutaneous stimulation is performed to identify if there is significant reduction in pain to determine which patients will undergo internalization of the stimulator. Internalization involves the placement of a tunneled pulse generator under the skin typically in the infraclavicular pocket (Holsheimer, 2001; Mehrkens & Steude, 2007). More recent protocols call for a 4-week trial period and many authors report utilizing intraoperative 3D CT scans and electromagnetic neuronavigational systems to maneuver the tip to the clivus (Jean-Pierre Van Buyten et al., 2017).

Patient Selection

Patients that are suitable for Gasserian ganglion nerve stimulation have refractory pain despite medical and other forms of surgical treatment (Taub, Munz, & Tasker, 1997). Moreover, these patients may lack a focal anatomical structural abnormality or have failed prior ablative or decompressive interventions and thus find benefit through modulation of nociceptive signaling. As will be discussed in the outcomes section below, patients that experience the greatest benefit have a positive trial while initially testing the nerve stimulator.

Patient Outcomes

Meyerson and Hakansson were among the first to demonstrate the efficacy of this procedure. In 1986 (Meyerson & Hakanson, 1986), they reported their experience with 14 patients over more than 4 years of follow-up. In this small cohort, 11 of 14 patients (79%) reported significant reduction in pain. In 2001, Holsheimer attempted to more clearly define the efficacy of this intervention by pooling eight cohorts treated between 1980 and 2005 (Holsheimer, 2001). Among 233 patients, 48% reported more than a 50% reduction in symptoms. Efficacy improved to 83% if patients reported relief during the four-week trial period reported. 79% of patients that reported a positive trial test reported a greater than 75% reduction in symptoms. In an attempt to assess the prediction capacity of the trial period, Holsheimer also reported the positive trial percentage for the eight trials but found these results more difficult to extrapolate given high variation (47-80%). Similarly, Mehrkens and Steude reported their results with a cohort of 235 patients followed over 5 years in 2007 (Mehrkens & Steude, 2007). They report 52% of patients had at least a 50% reduction in symptoms, but this efficacy increased to 82% when only looking at the patients with positive trial periods. A recent study by Kustermans et al looked at 22 patients treated between 2010 and 2015 (Kustermans, Van Buyten, Smet, Coucke, & Politis, 2017). They found that 88% of patients with a positive trial stimulation reported a reduction of at least 50% following intervention however, this value declined to 44% at 24 months.

These studies demonstrate that the Gasserian ganglion stimulator is especially efficacious in patients that demonstrate a reduction in painful symptoms during the initial trial period. While Gasserian ganglion stimulator reduces pain levels, this technique may not provide complete pain relief.

Subcutaneous Trigeminal Nerve Stimulation

Brief Description of Procedure

Subcutaneous trigeminal nerve stimulation utilizes peripheral stimulation of the infraorbital and supraorbital nerves by electrodes inserted percutaneously to reduce the sensation of pain returning to the central nervous system (Konstantin V. Slavin, Department of Neurosurgery, Wess, & Department of Neurosurgery, 2005). The procedure is similar to spinal cord stimulation: a trial stage lasting several days precedes the full surgical procedure. During the trial, a temporary electrode placed near the desired nerve branch is stimulated externally. Fluoroscopy (C-arm) provides an anteroposterior view of the head while inserting the electrode. A quadripolar electrode (as is used in spinal cord stimulation) is inserted several centimeters lateral to the eye, directed by a Tuohy needle. The needle is removed once it is 1 cm above the supraorbital ridge and the electrode is advanced under fluoroscopy. Since the supraorbital nerve has a consistent location and the electrode will cross the nerve's course as it exits the foramen, direct visualization of the nerve is not required. Similarly, the infraorbital nerve is accessed by inserting the electrode near the zygoma and placing the electrode across the nerve's path exiting the infraorbital foramen. The device is trialed for five to seven days, recording the painful paresthesias. If stimulation confers more than 50% pain relief, the trial is followed by the surgical insertion of a permanent electrode connected to a pulse generator. Here, an incision behind the ear allows surgeons to anchor the electrode. An incision is made below the clavicle and the pulse generator is placed in a subcutaneous pocket and anchored to the thoracic fascia.

Patient Selection

Similarly to patients suitable for Gasserian ganglion nerve stimulation, patients amenable for subcutaneous trigeminal nerve stimulation have refractory pain despite medical or other surgical interventions (Feletti et al., 2013). Moreover, patients that experience the greatest benefit with trigeminal nerve stimulators have a positive trial during the initial testing.

Patient Outcomes

Johnson and Burchiel reported their experience with 10 patients with implanted subcutaneous pulse generators and quadripolar electrodes in the V1 or V2 distributions for post-traumatic and post-herpetic trigeminal neuropathic pain (Johnson & Burchiel, 2004). 70% of patients reported at least 50% pain relief and a reduction in medication use. In the post-herpetic group, though, 50% (2/4) of patients did not experience a 50% reduction in pain. Overall complication rate requiring reoperation was 30%. Slavin and Wess reported their preliminary efficacy results with eight patients after describing their technique in 2005 (Konstantin V. Slavin et al., 2005). Seven out of eight patients (88%) demonstrated at least a 50% reduction in pain during the trial, prompting a permanent system. Two patients required reoperation: one patient required reoperation to remove the system due to loss of benefit which occurred gradually over 26 months and another required revision due to hardware erosion.

Slavin et al later reported prospective data on 30 patients treated with peripheral nerve stimulation for craniofacial pain (K. V. Slavin, Colpan, Munawar, Wess, & Nersesyan, 2006). Of the 30 patients who underwent trial stimulation, three went on to have infraorbital nerve stimulation and six went on to have supraorbital nerve stimulation (four unilateral and two bilateral). Overall, 73% (16/22) of the patients who received implanted devices experienced at least a 50% reduction in symptoms. Three patients experienced complications such as device failure or infection and had to return to the operating room for removal of the device.

Jakobs et al. reported their experience with eight patients with trigeminal neuralgia (Jakobs, Unterberg, Treede, Schuh-Hofer, & Ahmadi, 2016). Three patients had TN without facial pain, three patients had TN with persistent facial pain, and two patients had post-herpetic neuralgia. Seven out of eight of the patients (88%) reported at least a 50% reduction in symptoms and five out of six patients (83%) were able to stop or reduce their medication use. Two patients (25%) had stimulation-related side effects, though the authors argued simple reprogramming was sufficient to overcome these side effects.

Klein et al published their experience with 10 patients with intractable facial pain due to trigeminal neuralgia due to several factors (classical TN, multiple sclerosis, post-herpetic, and post-radiation therapy, idiopathic facial pain) (Klein, Sandi-Gahun, Schackert, & Juratli, 2016). Using the visual analogue scale, these investigators demonstrated that, among the eight patients who had permanent device placement, the average pain intensity decreased from 9.3 preoperatively to 0.75 post-operatively. Six patients even reported no pain with stimulation.

These small studies demonstrate that subcutaneous trigeminal nerve stimulation may offer select patients relief from trigeminal nerve pain and possible reduction in pain medication use. As with Gasserian ganglion nerve stimulation this method involves typically at least two surgeries and permanent implantation of a battery powered stimulator system.

CONCLUSION

Surgical options for the treatment of trigeminal neuralgia involve diverse mechanisms of action ranging from open surgical decompression with possible endoscopic assistance, to percutaneous lesioning, placement of neurostimulators, or non-invasive radiotherapy. Patients that are not suitable candidates for open microsurgical decompression or seek other forms of therapy have numerous options available to either lesion or modulate painful symptoms stemming from the trigeminal nerve. Future studies will allow for greater delineation of patient subtypes and disease pathogenesis to optimally match therapeutic strategy to a patient's symptoms and preferences for treatment.

REFERENCES

Alberico, R. A., Fenstermaker, R. A., & Lobel, J. (2001). Focal enhancement of cranial nerve V after radiosurgery with the Leksell gamma knife: Experience in 15 patients with medically refractory trigeminal neuralgia. *AJNR. American Journal of Neuroradiology*, *22*(10), 1944–1948. PMID:11733329

Artz, G. J., Hux, F. J., Larouere, M. J., Bojrab, D. I., Babu, S., & Pieper, D. R. (2008). Endoscopic vascular decompression. *Otology & Neurotology*, *29*(7), 995–1000. doi:10.1097/MAO.0b013e318184601a PMID:18698270

Asplund, P., Blomstedt, P., & Bergenheim, A. T. (2016). Percutaneous Balloon Compression vs Percutaneous Retrogasserian Glycerol Rhizotomy for the Primary Treatment of Trigeminal Neuralgia. *Neurosurgery*, *78*(3), 421–428, discussion 428. doi:10.1227/NEU.0000000000001059 PMID:26465639

Asplund, P., Linderoth, B., & Bergenheim, A. T. (2010). The predictive power of balloon shape and change of sensory functions on outcome of percutaneous balloon compression for trigeminal neuralgia. *Journal of Neurosurgery*, *113*(3), 498–507. doi:10.3171/2010.2.JNS091466 PMID:20345223

Bender, M., Pradilla, G., Batra, S., See, A., Bhutiani, N., James, C., . . . Lim, M. (2012). Effectiveness of repeat glycerol rhizotomy in treating recurrent trigeminal neuralgia. *Neurosurgery, 70*(5), 1125-1133.

Bohman, L. E., Pierce, J., Stephen, J. H., Sandhu, S., & Lee, J. Y. (2014). Fully endoscopic microvascular decompression for trigeminal neuralgia: Technique review and early outcomes. *Neurosurgical Focus*, *37*(4), E18. doi:10.3171/2014.7.FOCUS14318 PMID:25270137

Brisman, R., Khandji, A. G., & Mooij, R. B. (2002). Trigeminal nerve-blood vessel relationship as revealed by high-resolution magnetic resonance imaging and its effect on pain relief after gamma knife radiosurgery for trigeminal neuralgia. *Neurosurgery*, *50*(6), 1261–1267. PMID:12015844

Broggi, M., Acerbi, F., Ferroli, P., Tringali, G., Schiariti, M., & Broggi, G. (2013). Microvascular decompression for neurovascular conflicts in the cerebello-pontine angle: Which role for endoscopy? *Acta Neurochirurgica*, *155*(9), 1709–1716. doi:10.100700701-013-1824-8 PMID:23884611

Brown, J. A., McDaniel, M. D., & Weaver, M. T. (1993). Percutaneous trigeminal nerve compression for treatment of trigeminal neuralgia: Results in 50 patients. *Neurosurgery*, *32*(4), 570–573. doi:10.1227/00006123-199304000-00012 PMID:7682678

Brown, J. A., & Pilitsis, J. G. (2005). Percutaneous balloon compression for the treatment of trigeminal neuralgia: Results in 56 patients based on balloon compression pressure monitoring. *Neurosurgical Focus*, *18*(5), E10. doi:10.3171/foc.2005.18.5.11 PMID:15913277

Dhople, A. A., Adams, J. R., Maggio, W. W., Naqvi, S. A., Regine, W. F., & Kwok, Y. (2009). Long-term outcomes of Gamma Knife radiosurgery for classic trigeminal neuralgia: Implications of treatment and critical review of the literature. Clinical article. *Journal of Neurosurgery*, *111*(2), 351–358. doi:10.3171/2009.2.JNS08977 PMID:19326987

Feletti, A., Santi, G. Z., Sammartino, F., Bevilacqua, M., Cisotto, P., & Longatti, P. (2013). Peripheral trigeminal nerve field stimulation: Report of 6 cases. *Neurosurgical Focus*, *35*(3), E10. doi:10.3171/2013.7.FOCUS13228 PMID:23991813

Gusmão, S., Oliveira, M., Tazinaffo, U., & Honey, C. R. (2003). Percutaneous trigeminal nerve radiofrequency rhizotomy guided by computerized tomography fluoroscopy. *Journal of Neurosurgery*, *99*(4), 785–786. doi:10.3171/jns.2003.99.4.0785 PMID:14567619

Haines, S. J., Jannetta, P. J., & Zorub, D. S. (1980). Microvascular relations of the trigeminal nerve: An anatomical study with clinical correlation. *Journal of Neurosurgery*, *52*(3), 381–386. doi:10.3171/jns.1980.52.3.0381 PMID:7359193

Hakanson, S. (1981). Trigeminal neuralgia treated by the injection of glycerol into the trigeminal cistern. *Neurosurgery*, *9*(6), 638–646. doi:10.1227/00006123-198112000-00005 PMID:7322329

Halpern, C. H., Lang, S.-S., & Lee, J. Y. (2013). Fully endoscopic microvascular decompression: Our early experience. *Minimally Invasive Surgery*. PMID:24083024

Halpern, C. H., Lang, S. S., & Lee, J. Y. (2013). Fully endoscopic microvascular decompression: Our early experience. *Minimally Invasive Surgery, 739432*. doi:10.1155/2013/739432 PMID:24083024

Han, P. P., Shetter, A. G., Smith, K. A., Fiedler, J. A., Rogers, C. L., Speiser, B., & Feiz-Erfan, I. (1999). Gamma knife radiosurgery for trigeminal neuralgia: Experience at the Barrow Neurological Institute. *Stereotactic and Functional Neurosurgery, 73*(1-4), 131–133. doi:10.1159/000029771 PMID:10853118

Hodaie, M., & Coello, A. F. (2013). Advances in the management of trigeminal neuralgia. *Journal of Neurosurgical Sciences, 57*(1), 13–21. PMID:23584217

Holsheimer, J. (2001). Electrical stimulation of the trigeminal tract in chronic, intractable facial neuralgia. *Archives of Physiology and Biochemistry, 109*(4), 304–308. doi:10.1076/apab.109.4.304.4246 PMID:11935364

Jakobs, M., Unterberg, A., Treede, R. D., Schuh-Hofer, S., & Ahmadi, R. (2016). Subcutaneous trigeminal nerve field stimulation for refractory trigeminal pain: A cohort analysis. *Acta Neurochirurgica, 158*(9), 1767–1774. doi:10.100700701-016-2881-6 PMID:27372299

Johnson, M. D., & Burchiel, K. J. (2004). Peripheral stimulation for treatment of trigeminal postherpetic neuralgia and trigeminal posttraumatic neuropathic pain: a pilot study. *Neurosurgery, 55*(1), 135-141.

Kanpolat, Y., Savas, A., Bekar, A., & Berk, C. (2001). Percutaneous controlled radiofrequency trigeminal rhizotomy for the treatment of idiopathic trigeminal neuralgia: 25-year experience with 1,600 patients. *Neurosurgery, 48*(3), 524-532.

Klein, J., Sandi-Gahun, S., Schackert, G., & Juratli, T. A. (2016). Peripheral nerve field stimulation for trigeminal neuralgia, trigeminal neuropathic pain, and persistent idiopathic facial pain. *Cephalalgia, 36*(5), 445–453. doi:10.1177/0333102415597526 PMID:26209705

Kondziolka, D., & Lunsford, L. D. (2005). Percutaneous retrogasserian glycerol rhizotomy for trigeminal neuralgia: Technique and expectations. *Neurosurgical Focus, 18*(5), E7. doi:10.3171/foc.2005.18.5.8 PMID:15913283

Kouzounias, K., Lind, G., Schechtmann, G., Winter, J., & Linderoth, B. (2010). Comparison of percutaneous balloon compression and glycerol rhizotomy for the treatment of trigeminal neuralgia. *Journal of Neurosurgery*, *113*(3), 486–492. doi:10.3171/2010.1.JNS091106 PMID:20187700

Kouzounias, K., Lind, G., Schechtmann, G., Winter, J., & Linderoth, B. (2010). Comparison of percutaneous balloon compression and glycerol rhizotomy for the treatment of trigeminal neuralgia. *Journal of Neurosurgery*, *113*(3), 486–492. doi:10.3171/2010.1.JNS091106 PMID:20187700

Kustermans, L., Van Buyten, J. P., Smet, I., Coucke, W., & Politis, C. (2017). Stimulation of the Gasserian ganglion in the treatment of refractory trigeminal neuropathy. *Journal of Cranio-Maxillo-Facial Surgery*, *45*(1), 39–46. doi:10.1016/j.jcms.2016.10.014 PMID:27919593

Lang, S. S., Chen, H. I., & Lee, J. Y. (2012). Endoscopic microvascular decompression: A stepwise operative technique. *ORL; Journal for Oto-Rhino-Laryngology and Its Related Specialties*, *74*(6), 293–298. doi:10.1159/000342795 PMID:23235502

Latchaw, J. P. Jr, Hardy, R. W. Jr, Forsythe, S. B., & Cook, A. F. (1983). Trigeminal neuralgia treated by radiofrequency coagulation. *Journal of Neurosurgery*, *59*(3), 479–484. doi:10.3171/jns.1983.59.3.0479 PMID:6886761

Lee, J. K., Choi, H. J., Ko, H. C., Choi, S. K., & Lim, Y. J. (2012). Long term outcomes of gamma knife radiosurgery for typical trigeminal neuralgia-minimum 5-year follow-up. *Journal of Korean Neurosurgical Society*, *51*(5), 276–280. doi:10.3340/jkns.2012.51.5.276 PMID:22792424

Lee, J. Y. K., Pierce, J. T., Sandhu, S. K., Petrov, D., & Yang, A. I. (2017). Endoscopic versus microscopic microvascular decompression for trigeminal neuralgia: Equivalent pain outcomes with possibly decreased postoperative headache after endoscopic surgery. *Journal of Neurosurgery*, *126*(5), 1676–1684. doi:10.3171/2016.5.JNS1621 PMID:27471895

Lichtor, T., & Mullan, J. F. (1990). A 10-year follow-up review of percutaneous microcompression of the trigeminal ganglion. *Journal of Neurosurgery*, *72*(1), 49–54. doi:10.3171/jns.1990.72.1.0049 PMID:2294184

Lim, M., Villavicencio, A. T., Burneikiene, S., Chang, S. D., Romanelli, P., McNeely, L., ... Adler, J. R. (2005). CyberKnife radiosurgery for idiopathic trigeminal neuralgia. *Neurosurgical Focus*, *18*(5), E9. doi:10.3171/foc.2005.18.5.10 PMID:15913285

Lobato, R. D., Rivas, J. J., Sarabia, R., & Lamas, E. (1990). Percutaneous microcompression of the gasserian ganglion for trigeminal neuralgia. *Journal of Neurosurgery*, *72*(4), 546–553. doi:10.3171/jns.1990.72.4.0546 PMID:2319312

Lopez, B. C., Hamlyn, P. J., & Zakrzewska, J. M. (2004). Systematic review of ablative neurosurgical techniques for the treatment of trigeminal neuralgia. *Neurosurgery*, *54*(4), 973-982.

Martin, S., Teo, M., & Suttner, N. (2015). The effectiveness of percutaneous balloon compression in the treatment of trigeminal neuralgia in patients with multiple sclerosis. *Journal of Neurosurgery*, *123*(6), 1507–1511. doi:10.3171/2014.11.JNS14736 PMID:26067615

Mehrkens, J. H., & Steude, U. (2007). Chronic electrostimulation of the trigeminal ganglion in trigeminal neuropathy: Current state and future prospects. *Acta Neurochirurgica. Supplementum*, *97*(Pt 2), 91–97. PMID:17691294

Meyerson, B. A., & Hakanson, S. (1986). Suppression of pain in trigeminal neuropathy by electric stimulation of the gasserian ganglion. *Neurosurgery*, *18*(1), 59–66. doi:10.1227/00006123-198601000-00010 PMID:2418383

Mittal, B., & Thomas, D. G. (1986). Controlled thermocoagulation in trigeminal neuralgia. *Journal of Neurology, Neurosurgery, and Psychiatry*, *49*(8), 932–936. doi:10.1136/jnnp.49.8.932 PMID:3746327

Montano, N., Conforti, G., Di Bonaventura, R., Meglio, M., Fernandez, E., & Papacci, F. (2015). Advances in diagnosis and treatment of trigeminal neuralgia. *Therapeutics and Clinical Risk Management*, *11*, 289–299. doi:10.2147/TCRM.S37592 PMID:25750533

Mullan, S., & Lichtor, T. (1983). Percutaneous microcompression of the trigeminal ganglion for trigeminal neuralgia. *Journal of Neurosurgery*, *59*(6), 1007–1012. doi:10.3171/jns.1983.59.6.1007 PMID:6631493

Nanda, A., Javalkar, V., Zhang, S., & Ahmed, O. (2015). Long term efficacy and patient satisfaction of microvascular decompression and gamma knife radiosurgery for trigeminal neuralgia. *Journal of Clinical Neuroscience*, *22*(5), 818–822. doi:10.1016/j.jocn.2014.11.028 PMID:25769254

Nanda, A., Javalkar, V., Zhang, S., & Ahmed, O. (2015). Long term efficacy and patient satisfaction of microvascular decompression and gamma knife radiosurgery for trigeminal neuralgia. *Journal of Clinical Neuroscience*, *22*(5), 818–822. doi:10.1016/j.jocn.2014.11.028 PMID:25769254

North, R. B., Kidd, D. H., Piantadosi, S., & Carson, B. S. (1990). Percutaneous retrogasserian glycerol rhizotomy. Predictors of success and failure in treatment of trigeminal neuralgia. *Journal of Neurosurgery, 72*(6), 851–856. doi:10.3171/jns.1990.72.6.0851 PMID:2338568

Pollock, B. E. (2005). Percutaneous retrogasserian glycerol rhizotomy for patients with idiopathic trigeminal neuralgia: A prospective analysis of factors related to pain relief. *Journal of Neurosurgery, 102*(2), 223–228. doi:10.3171/jns.2005.102.2.0223 PMID:15739548

Pollock, B. E., Phuong, L. K., Foote, R. L., Stafford, S. L., & Gorman, D. A. (2001). High-dose trigeminal neuralgia radiosurgery associated with increased risk of trigeminal nerve dysfunction. *Neurosurgery, 49*(1), 58–64. PMID:11440460

Regis, J., Tuleasca, C., Resseguier, N., Carron, R., Donnet, A., Gaudart, J., & Levivier, M. (2016). Long-term safety and efficacy of Gamma Knife surgery in classical trigeminal neuralgia: A 497-patient historical cohort study. *Journal of Neurosurgery, 124*(4), 1079–1087. doi:10.3171/2015.2.JNS142144 PMID:26339857

Sandell, T., Ringstad, G. A., & Eide, P. K. (2014). Usefulness of the endoscope in microvascular decompression for trigeminal neuralgia and MRI-based prediction of the need for endoscopy. *Acta Neurochir (Wien), 156*(10), 1901-1909. doi:10.1007/s00701-014-2171-0

Sindou, M., Leston, J., Decullier, E., & Chapuis, F. (2007). *Microvascular decompression for primary trigeminal neuralgia: long-term effectiveness and prognostic factors in a series of 362 consecutive patients with clear-cut neurovascular conflicts who underwent pure decompression*. Academic Press.

Singh, R., Davis, J., & Sharma, S. (2016). Stereotactic Radiosurgery for Trigeminal Neuralgia: A Retrospective Multi-Institutional Examination of Treatment Outcomes. *Cureus, 8*(4), e554. doi:10.7759/cureus.554 PMID:27182468

Skirving, D. J., & Dan, N. G. (2001). A 20-year review of percutaneous balloon compression of the trigeminal ganglion. *Journal of Neurosurgery, 94*(6), 913–917. doi:10.3171/jns.2001.94.6.0913 PMID:11409519

Slavin, K. V., Colpan, M. E., Munawar, N., Wess, C., & Nersesyan, H. (2006). Trigeminal and occipital peripheral nerve stimulation for craniofacial pain: A single-institution experience and review of the literature. *Neurosurgical Focus, 21*(6), E5. doi:10.3171/foc.2006.21.6.8 PMID:17341049

Slavin, K. V., & Wess, C. (2005). Trigeminal Branch Stimulation for Intractable Neuropathic Pain: Technical Note. *Neuromodulation: Technology at the Neural Interface*, *8*(1), 7–13. doi:10.1111/j.1094-7159.2005.05215.x PMID:22151378

Slettebo, H., Hirschberg, H., & Lindegaard, K. F. (1993). Long-term results after percutaneous retrogasserian glycerol rhizotomy in patients with trigeminal neuralgia. *Acta Neurochirurgica*, *122*(3-4), 231–235. doi:10.1007/BF01405534 PMID:8372713

Sweet, W. H. (1988). Percutaneous methods for the treatment of trigeminal neuralgia and other faciocephalic pain; comparison with microvascular decompression. *Seminars in Neurology*, *8*(4), 272–279. doi:10.1055-2008-1041389 PMID:3074421

Sweet, W. H., & Wepsic, J. G. (1974). Controlled thermocoagulation of trigeminal ganglion and rootlets for differential destruction of pain fibers. *Journal of Neurosurgery*, *40*(2), 143–156. doi:10.3171/jns.1974.40.2.0143 PMID:4587949

Taha, J. M., Tew, J. M. Jr, & Buncher, C. R. (1995). A prospective 15-year follow up of 154 consecutive patients with trigeminal neuralgia treated by percutaneous stereotactic radiofrequency thermal rhizotomy. *Journal of Neurosurgery*, *83*(6), 989–993. doi:10.3171/jns.1995.83.6.0989 PMID:7490643

Taub, E., Munz, M., & Tasker, R. R. (1997). Chronic electrical stimulation of the gasserian ganglion for the relief of pain in a series of 34 patients. *Journal of Neurosurgery*, *86*(2), 197–202. doi:10.3171/jns.1997.86.2.0197 PMID:9010419

Teo, C., Nakaji, P., & Mobbs, R. J. (2006). Endoscope-assisted microvascular decompression for trigeminal neuralgia: technical case report. *Operative Neurosurgery, 59*(suppl_4).

Van Buyten, J. P. (2015). Trigeminal Ganglion Stimulation. *Progress in Neurological Surgery*, *29*, 76–82. doi:10.1159/000434658 PMID:26394074

Van Buyten, J. P., Smet, I., & Van de Kelft, E. (2017). Electromagnetic Navigation Technology for More Precise Electrode Placement in the Foramen Ovale: A Technical Report. *Neuromodulation: Technology at the Neural Interface*, *12*(3), 244–249. doi:10.1111/j.1525-1403.2009.00222.x PMID:22151368

Varela-Lema, L., Lopez-Garcia, M., Maceira-Rozas, M., & Munoz-Garzon, V. (2015). Linear accelerator stereotactic radiosurgery for trigeminal neuralgia. *Pain Physician*, *18*(1), 15–27. PMID:25675056

Young, R. F. (1988). Glycerol rhizolysis for treatment of trigeminal neuralgia. *Journal of Neurosurgery*, *69*(1), 39–45. doi:10.3171/jns.1988.69.1.0039 PMID:2454304

KEY TERMS AND DEFINITIONS

Balloon Compression: The subcutaneous placement and utilization of an inflatable balloon to cause physical compression of trigeminal nerve, thereby lesioning the nerve to treat painful symptoms.

Endoscopic Microvascular Decompression: The microsurgical approach of decompressing the trigeminal nerve from vascular or structural compression while also using endoscopy to better visualize the trigeminal nerve and confirm sufficient decompression.

Gasserian Ganglion Stimulation: The percutaneous placement of a nerve stimulator to modulate nociceptive signaling through the Gasserian ganglion to alleviate painful symptoms.

Glycerol Rhizotomy: The subcutaneous injection of chemical agents to lesion the trigeminal nerve and alleviate painful symptoms.

Radiofrequency Thermocoagulation: The subcutaneous placement of an electrode that uses thermal energy to lesion the trigeminal nerve to treat painful symptoms.

Stereotactic Radiosurgery: The utilization of non-invasive radiation to lesion the trigeminal nerve and provide relief from painful symptoms.

Subcutaneous Trigeminal Nerve Stimulation: Similar to the Gasserian ganglion stimulator, subcutaneous trigeminal nerve stimulation targets distal nerves such as the supraorbital or infraorbital branch of the trigeminal nerve and sends electrical signals to modify nociception to mitigate painful symptoms.

Chapter 7
Endoscopic-Assisted Microvascular Decompression

M. Yashar S. Kalani
Barrow Neurological Institute, USA

Michael R. Levitt
Barrow Neurological Institute, USA

Celene B. Mulholland
Barrow Neurological Institute, USA

Charles Teo
Prince of Wales Private Hospital, Australia

Peter Nakaji
Barrow Neurological Institute, USA

ABSTRACT

Diseases of ephaptic transmission are commonly caused by vascular compression of cranial nerves. The advent of microvascular decompression has allowed for surgical intervention for this patient population. This chapter highlights the technique of endoscopic-assisted microvascular decompression for trigeminal neuralgia and hemifacial spasm. Endoscopy and keyhole techniques have resulted in a minimally invasive and effective treatment of symptoms for patients with neuralgia.

BACKGROUND

Diseases of ephaptic transmission are most frequently caused by contact between a cerebral blood vessel and an adjacent cranial nerve; this contact allows repetitive blood vessel pulsations to stimulate and demyelinate the nerve. In trigeminal neuralgia, abnormal stimulation of the fifth cranial nerve (CN V) results in unilateral

DOI: 10.4018/978-1-5225-5349-6.ch007

paroxysmal, lancinating pain, commonly in the second or third division. Similarly, glossopharyngeal neuralgia is characterized by paroxysmal tongue, palate, and throat pain from stimulation of CN IX. In hemifacial spasm, unilateral spasm of the facial muscles is caused by repetitive stimulation of the facial nerve. Rare disorders of ephaptic transmission include geniculate neuralgia (episodic ear pain due to compression of the nervus intermedius) and combination disorders such as *tic convulsif* (vascular compression of CNs V and VII, resulting in both trigeminal neuralgia and hemifacial spasm). Long-standing hypertension is thought to contribute to the formation of redundant cerebrovascular loops or vascular ectasia that cause cranial nerve compression and result in ephaptic transmission and its associated symptoms.

Cranial nerve compression syndromes have a debilitating effect on a patient's quality of life. Treatment options include medical management (typically with anticonvulsant medications), percutaneous procedures (chemical or electrical rhizotomy, peripheral neurotomy, and radiofrequency ablation), stereotactic radiosurgery, and microvascular decompression (Henson, Goldman et al. 2005, Linskey, Ratanatharathorn et al. 2008, Toda 2008, Dhople, Adams et al. 2009, Dvorak, Finn et al. 2009). Microvascular decompression, in which the vessel causing cranial nerve compression is surgically separated from the nerve using a pledget, is the most effective and durable method of treatment (Fujimaki, Fukushima et al. 1990, Sindou, Leston et al. 2006, Tatli, Satici et al. 2008, Sekula, Frederickson et al. 2011). In this chapter, we review the technique of endoscopic-assisted microvascular decompression.

MAIN FOCUS OF THE CHAPTER

Diagnostic Evaluation

Vascular compression syndromes are best diagnosed by careful history-taking and physical examination. High-resolution magnetic resonance imaging (MRI) with thin-slice T2-weighted sequences (Figure 1A-C), fast imaging employing steady-state acquisition (FIESTA), or constructive interference in steady-state (CISS) techniques may assist in the diagnosis by visualizing vascular compression in the cerebellopontine angle (CPA), but should only be used as an adjunct to clinical suspicion and to rule out uncommon etiologies such as tumors, multiple sclerosis, and arteriovenous malformations.

Figure 1. (A) Axial T2-weighted fast imaging employing steady-state acquisition (FIESTA) magnetic resonance imaging (MRI) demonstrating a vascular loop of the right superior cerebellar artery compressing the right trigeminal nerve. (B) Axial T1- and (C) T2-weighted MRI demonstrating a vascular loop of the vertebral artery compressing the left facial nerve in a case of hemifacial spasm.

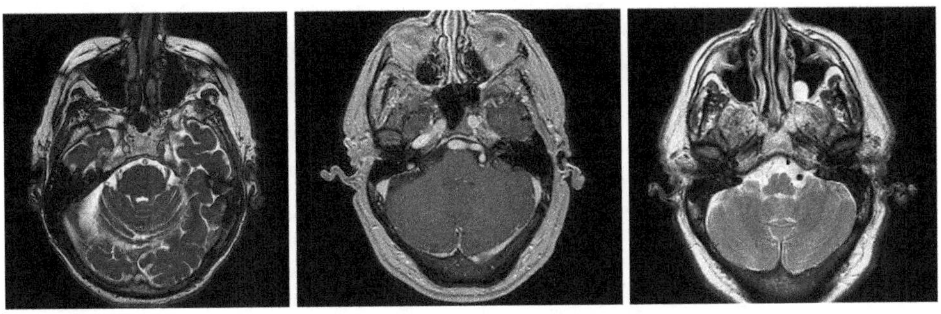

Endoscopic-Assisted Microvascular Decompression Technique

Preoperative Preparation

As with any neurosurgical procedure, careful preoperative assessment of patient risk factors is essential. Patients most commonly present in the fourth or greater decade of life and may require cardiovascular clearance prior to surgery. High-resolution MRI is obtained to identify vascular loops, corroborate patient history, and facilitate intraoperative navigation, which permits a smaller, more targeted incision and craniotomy.

Patient Positioning

After induction of general anesthesia and endotracheal intubation, the patient is placed supine with the head turned contralateral to the side of the craniotomy. We do not favor the use of a shoulder bump because doing so elevates the shoulder into the operative field and limits the anterior angle of approach needed to perform the operation (Figure 2). In patients whose body habitus prevents adequate head turning, the three-quarters prone or park-bench position is used. The patient's head is immobilized using a Mayfield clamp and secured to the operative table. When optimally positioned, the dependent position of the cerebellum obviates the need for rigid retractors.

Figure 2. Patient positioning, site of craniotomy (green dashed line), and incision (red line) for retrosigmoid access to the cerebellopontine angle

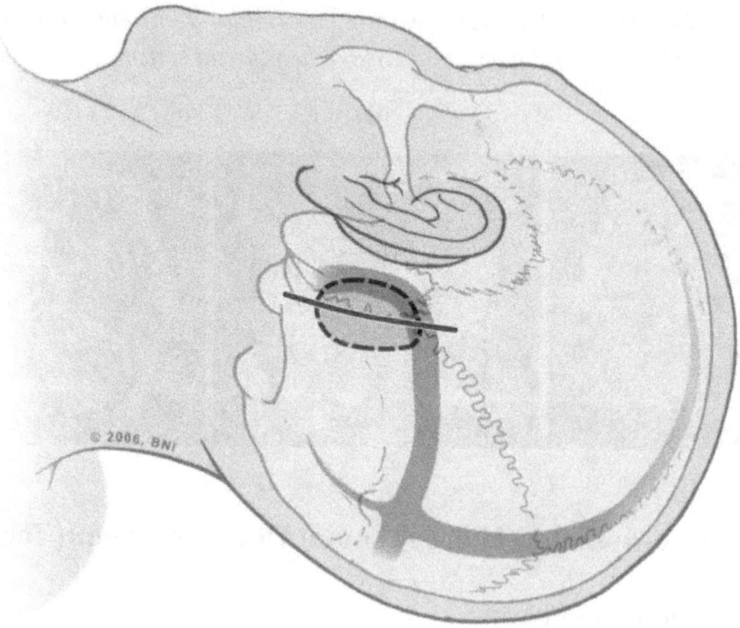

We routinely use intraoperative monitoring of somatosensory and motor-evoked potentials as well as intrafield stimulation of the involved and adjacent cranial nerves. For microvascular decompression of CN V, CNs V, VII and VIII are monitored; for hemifacial spasm and glossopharyngeal neuralgia, CNs V and VII-XI are monitored (Fernandez-Conejero, Ulkatan et al. 2012). Although preoperative lumbar drain placement can facilitate cerebrospinal fluid (CSF) drainage and brain relaxation, brain relaxation is usually accomplished without lumbar drainage by opening the cerebellopontine cistern after craniotomy.

Skin Incision

A 3-cm to 4-cm linear incision is centered on the retromastoid area using neuronavigational guidance (Figure 3). The incision should be roughly one-third above and two-thirds below the transverse sinus to provide the optimal trajectory for the craniotomy. The subcutaneous tissue is then undermined with minimal electrocautery and retracted with fishhooks to minimize ischemic injury. During superficial dissection, the occipital artery should be preserved as it emerges from the digastric groove and courses posterosuperiorly. The mastoid emissary vein, which

Figure 3. Intraoperative photograph demonstrating the size of a right keyhole retrosigmoid craniectomy used for standard microvascular decompression procedures

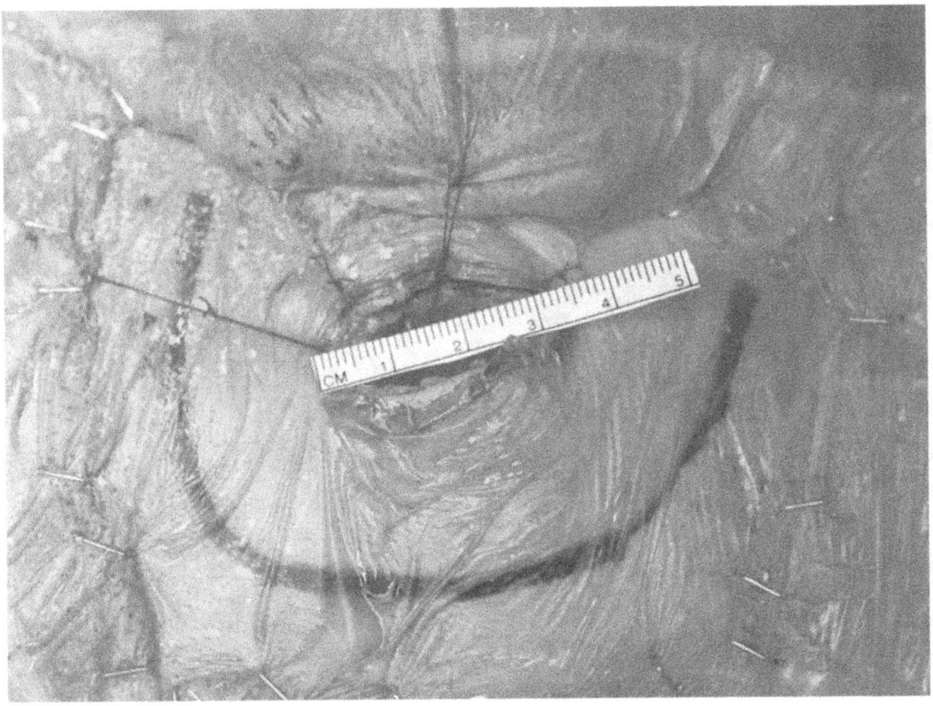

aids in the localization of the superior aspect of the sigmoid sinus, is frequently encountered upon elevation of the suboccipital muscles and periosteum, and it is coagulated and occluded with bone wax and gentle compression.

Keyhole Craniotomy

The ideal location for the craniotomy for microvascular decompression of CN V is at the junction of the transverse and sigmoid sinuses through which both supracerebellar and anterior cerebellar surgical corridors are possible (Figure 4). The craniotomy for lower cranial nerve compression may be centered slightly inferior to the transverse-sigmoid junction. Although the traditional retrosigmoid craniotomy permits visualization of structures from the tentorium to the foramen magnum (Figure 5A), the addition of the endoscope greatly increases the area of visualization (Figure 5B) while reducing the size of the required bony opening. The minimum diameter of the craniotomy is approximately 1.2 cm (enough to fit both an opened bipolar cautery and suction), although 1.5 cm to 2 cm is typical. The bone is thinned using a high-speed drill with a 4-mm or 5-mm drill bit, and the residual

Figure 4. Anatomical dissection demonstrating the anatomy visible via a retrosigmoid craniotomy. For actual surgery, we do not use retractors for this procedure and depend instead on dynamic retraction using a suction and bipolar cautery.

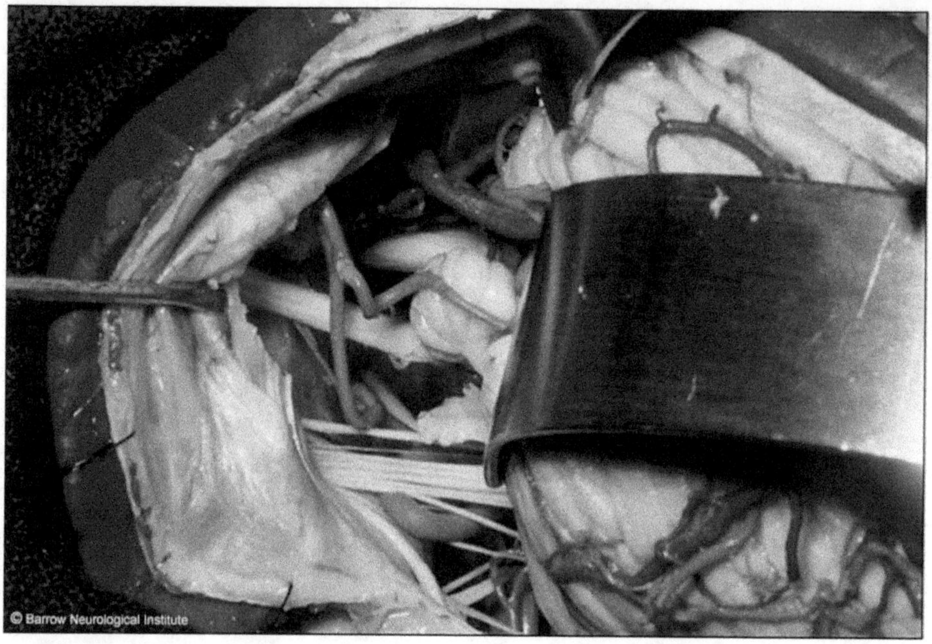

shelf of bone is removed using Kerrison rongeurs or a diamond drill bit. Mastoid air cells are usually exposed and should be thoroughly waxed upon opening and closure to minimize CSF leakage.

Dural Incision and Initial Exposure

The dura is opened sharply in a cruciate fashion with a pedicle based on both the transverse and sigmoid sinuses. Care is taken to avoid coagulating the dura, which shrinks it and prevents watertight closure. The dura is tacked away from the opening and covered with wet sponges to minimize shrinkage and desiccation. Although preoperative lumbar drainage, transient hyperventilation, or intravenous mannitol can be used when needed, cerebellar relaxation and CPA exposure can usually be achieved by draining CSF from the cerebellopontine cistern (Figure 6). Once relaxed, the cerebellar surface can be lined with nonadhesive patties and dynamically retracted with suction and bipolar instruments.

Using the operating microscope, a lateral supracerebellar, infratentorial dissection is performed to expose the petrosal vein (Dandy's vein). The arachnoid membrane

Figure 5. (A) The keyhole retrosigmoid craniotomy allows visualization from the tentorium to the foramen magnum. (B) The addition of the endoscope enhances visualization of the root entry zones of the cranial nerves as well as the exit of cranial nerves into their foramina.

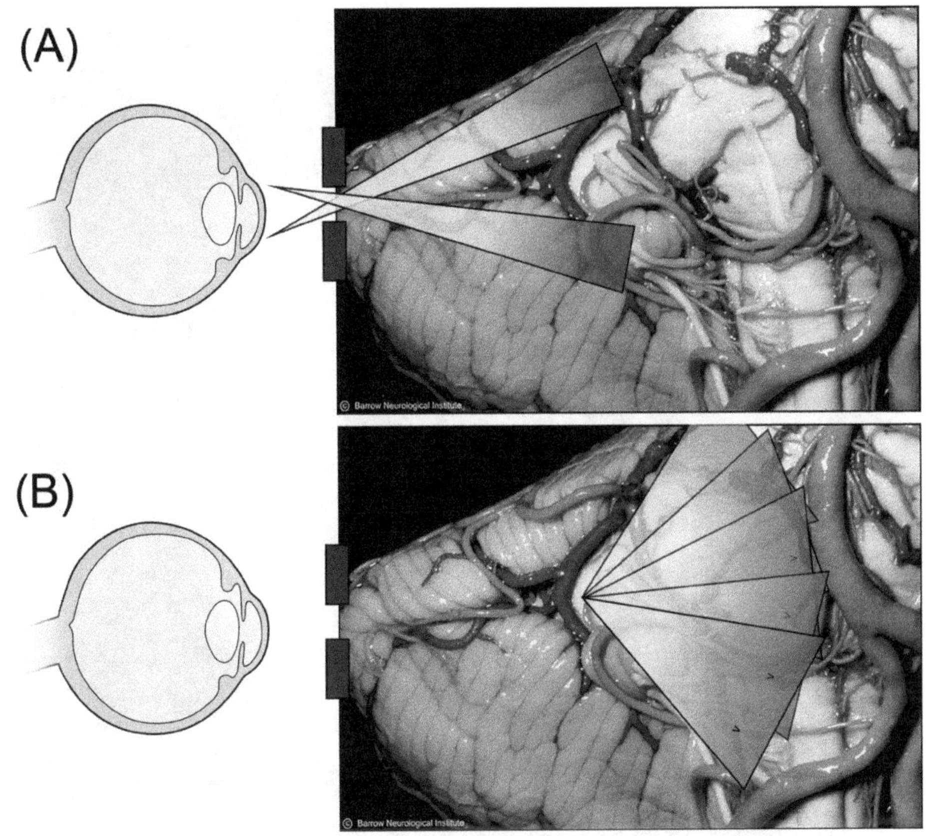

over this vein is sharply dissected, and the vein is mobilized to obtain the operative corridor. Sacrifice of this vein is rarely necessary, but care should be taken to prevent its avulsion as this results in rapid bleeding and greatly reduces visualization. In such cases, an angled bipolar cautery can be used to coagulate the vein at its connection with the tentorium and superior petrosal sinus.

The trigeminal nerve lies deep to the petrosal vein. The nerve is mobilized by sharply dissecting the overlying arachnoid. To avoid inadvertent hearing loss in cases of trigeminal neuralgia, the arachnoid over the internal acoustic canal (IAC) and CNs VII-VIII should not be dissected or manipulated. The trigeminal nerve root can be dissected and exposed in a supracerebellar or precerebellar fashion, depending on the site and vessel causing compression. In hemifacial spasm and

Figure 6. Axial computed tomography demonstrates the steps of sequential cerebrospinal fluid egress, cerebellar relaxation, and access to the cerebellopontine angle. The numbered arrows show the sequential gain in the surgical view and trajectory that is achieved by release of cerebrospinal fluid.

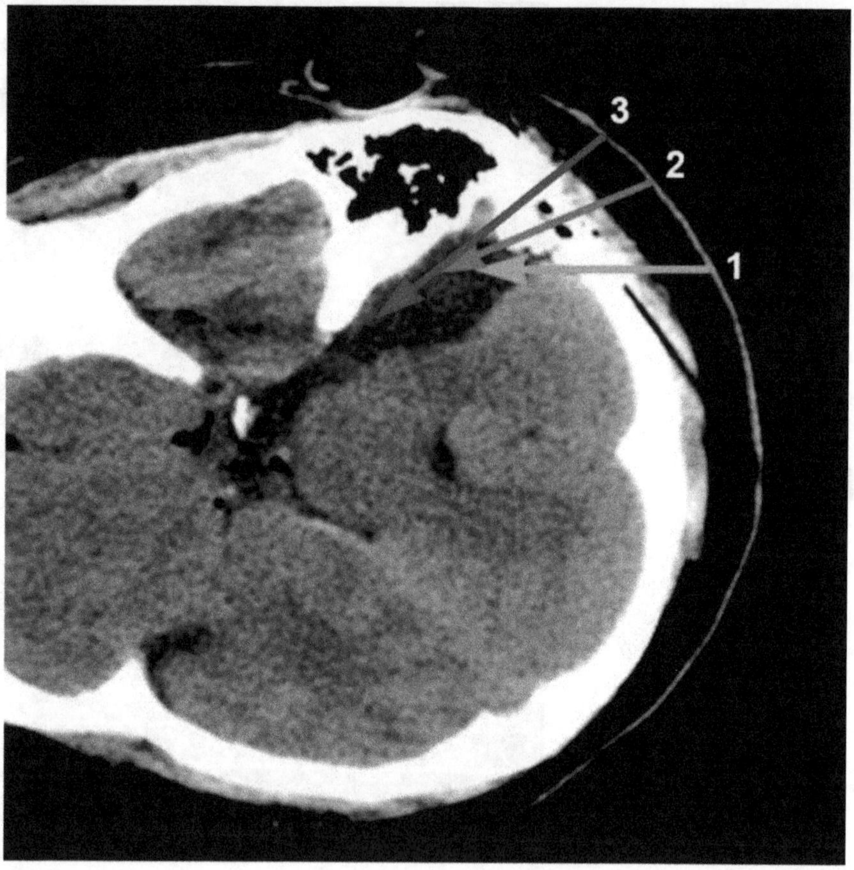

glossopharyngeal neuralgia, exposure requires opening the arachnoid overlying the IAC or lower cranial nerves (IX-XI), respectively. In general, exposure of the lower nerves should be from a more inferior-to-superior trajectory, as the impinging vessels generally come from medially and underneath.

Identification and Transposition of the Compressing Vascular Structures

After the nerve in question has been dissected and mobilized, vascular structures impinging upon it and its root entry zone at the brainstem should be inspected. It is important to be familiar with the native course of vessels and common alterations in their native course associated with disease states (Figure 7). The superior cerebellar artery (SCA) generally runs medial to the trigeminal nerve root, and the anterior inferior cerebellar artery (AICA) runs laterally. The SCA is the most common offending vessel in patients with trigeminal neuralgia; the AICA is the second most common culprit (Lovely and Jannetta 1997, Sekula, Marchan et al. 2008). Occasionally both the SCA and AICA may compress the fifth nerve, effectively sandwiching it. Hemifacial spasm, on the other hand, is usually the result of a loop of the AICA, or less commonly, the posterior inferior cerebellar artery (PICA) or an ectatic vertebral artery, impinging on the root entry zone of CN VII, which is inferior and medial to the CN VII-VIII complex. Vascular compression rarely results in glossopharyngeal neuralgia and is usually the result of a loop of the PICA or vertebral artery. Less commonly, vascular compression syndromes are caused by aberrant veins, a tumor in the CPA, or vascular malformations such as arteriovenous malformations or cavernous malformations (Karibe, Shirane et al. 2004, Deshmukh, Hott et al. 2005, Ferroli, Acerbi et al. 2010, Jayasekera, Vergani et al. 2014). Rarely, an ectatic vertebral or basilar artery may compress one or more cranial nerves. In some patients, the offending vessel may not be identified at the time of surgery (Lee, McCartney et al. 2014).

Although microscopy has been the gold standard for visualization of offending vessels, the development of endoscopic-assisted surgery has improved visualization of the nerve, its root entry zone, and any interaction with vascular structures. Wide-angled (30° and 70°) endoscopic lenses also permit visualization of the posterior aspect of the nerve, which may harbor the site of vascular compression. Endoscopic inspection of the brain stem and nerves, which extends above and below the area that can usually be inspected with a larger retrosigmoid craniotomy, also improves decompression (Figure 8A and 8B). It is critical to utilize proper and meticulous endoscopic technique when operating in the confines of the posterior fossa. Linear placement of instruments under direct and constant endoscopic visualization, and minimal lateral movement of instruments, decreases the likelihood of injury to structures in the CPA.

The introduction of the endoscope into the posterior fossa allows one to visualize structures ventral to the brainstem as well as vascular loops medial to cranial nerves that may impinge upon them (Figure 9A and 9B). Once the offending vessel has been identified, it is mobilized and separated from the nerve. Minimal nerve manipulation is extremely important, especially in the case of hemifacial spasm as traction of the eighth nerve may result in hearing loss. The site of compression is padded with a Teflon pledget, minimizing the transmission of arterial pulsation to the nerve (Figure 9C and 9D). In patients with an ectatic vertebral or basilar artery in which pledget insertion is not feasible, a sling technique may be applied to the artery to

Figure 7. Illustrations show the various vascular relationships and sites of compression noted in cases of trigeminal neuralgia. AICA, anterior inferior cerebellar artery; SCA, superior cerebellar artery; SPV, superior petrosal vein.

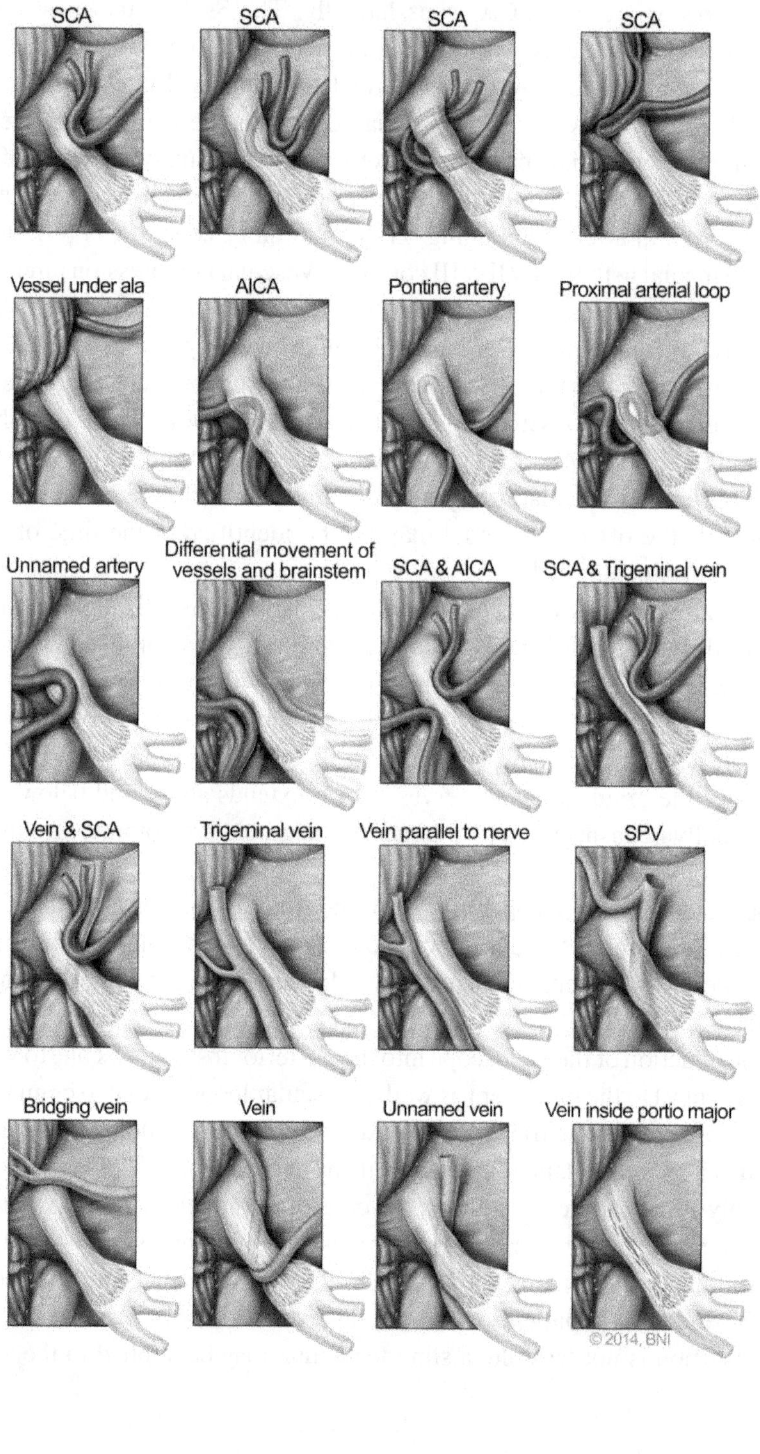

Figure 8. (A and B) Endoscopic views of the trigeminal nerve compressed by branches of the superior cerebellar artery

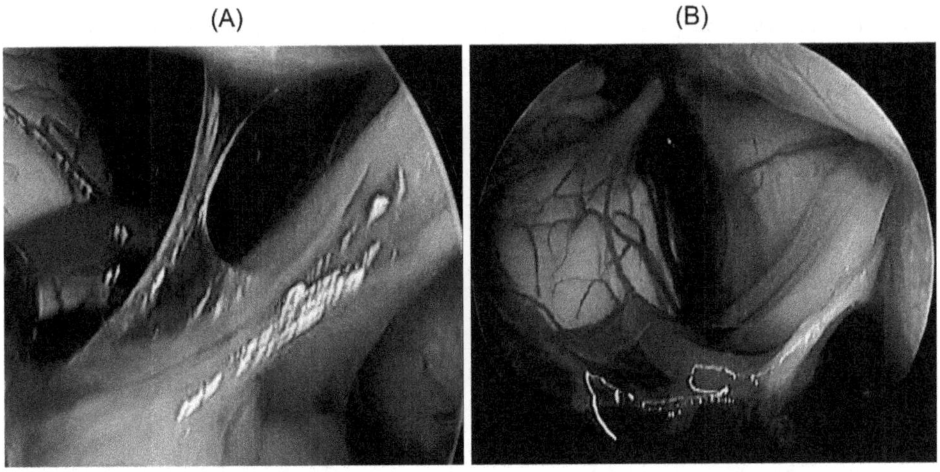

effectively separate the offending vessel from the nerve (Masuoka, Matsushima et al. 2011, Lin, Chen et al. 2012). In patients with glossopharyngeal neuralgia, for which an offending vessel is rarely found, complete transection of CN IX and the upper fascicles of CN X are required to provide symptomatic relief.

Dural and Soft Tissue Closure

Once hemostasis is obtained, the dura is closed in a watertight fashion (Figure 10A), which is essential to prevent CSF leakage in the posterior fossa. If the dura is inadvertently coagulated, a small piece of muscle, fascia, or dural substitute may be used as a patch. A cranioplasty (using methyl methacrylate or simply a burr hole cover) should be performed to prevent direct contact between muscle and dura, which may cause postoperative headache. The soft tissues are closed in layers (Figure 10B).

Postoperative Care

Patients are watched in the intensive care unit overnight. Routine postoperative imaging is not usually necessary. In the rare cases in which a lumbar drain is placed, the patient remains in the intensive care unit until the drain is removed. Most patients are discharged home on the first postoperative day. We do not routinely administer postoperative antibiotics or steroids.

Figure 9. (A and B) Introduction of the endoscope into the cerebellopontine angle for visualization of the contents of the posterior fossa. Note that rotation of the endoscope allows for visualization of the nerve and site of vascular compression from different angles. (C and D) Endoscopic views of the trigeminal nerve after decompression and placement of a pledget.

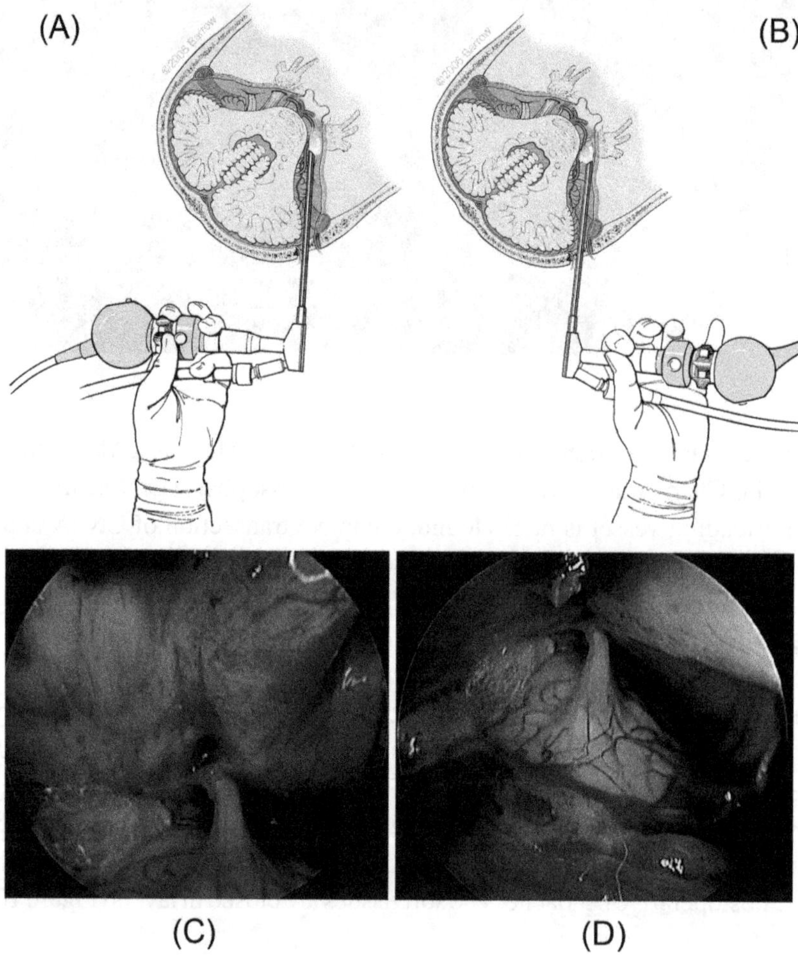

Operative Results

Several studies have examined the safety and efficacy of endoscopic-assisted microvascular decompression. The largest series, by Teo, Nakaji et al. (2006) reviewed 113 patients (65 male and 48 female) undergoing endoscopic-assisted microvascular decompression of the trigeminal nerve. Patients' mean age was 54 years (range, 34-76 y), and the mean duration of symptoms was 2.8 years. Vascular

Figure 10. (A) Intraoperative photo demonstrating watertight closure of the dura. It is critical to obtain watertight closure to minimize the risk of cerebrospinal fluid leakage, especially if a cranioplasty is not performed. (B) Intraoperative photo demonstrating skin closure.

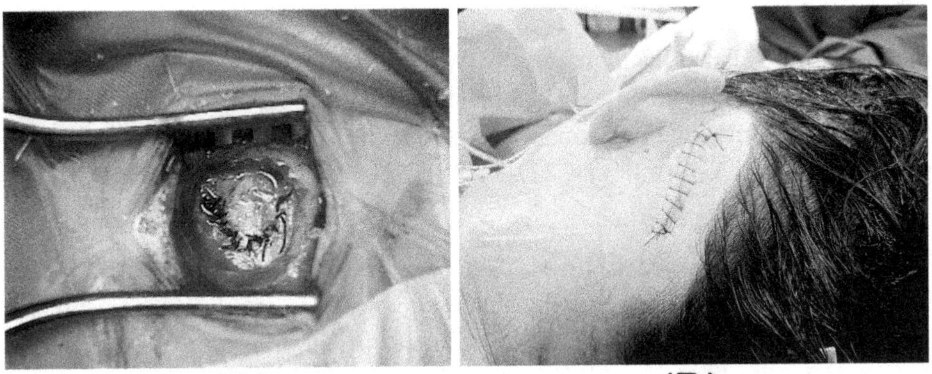

(A) (B)

compression was found in all patients. In 38 of 113 patients (33%), the endoscope improved a suboptimal microscopic view.

In 9 of 113 patients (8%), the endoscope was the sole means of accurately identifying the compressing vessel. In 17 of 113 patients (15%), initial microscopic decompression was found to be inadequate when examined with endoscopy. All suboptimal decompressions were improved with the use of the endoscope. At a mean follow-up of 29 months (range, 9-72 mo), pain relief off medication was noted in 99.1% of patients. Overall operative outcomes were excellent in 91.1% of patients (103/113), good in 7.1% (8/113), and fair in 1.8% (2/113). Complications included 1 patient each who suffered temporary or permanent hearing loss (0.9%) and 7 patients who suffered temporary trigeminal dysesthesia (6.2%). Other series of fully-endoscopic microvascular decompression without the use of a microscope have shown promise, though long-term results are lacking.

CONCLUSION

Endoscopic-assisted microvascular decompression is a safe, minimally invasive, and effective technique for decompression of cranial nerves in the CPA. Improved visualization of cranial nerves and vascular structures using this technique may improve the efficacy of microvascular decompression while reducing the necessary size of the incision and craniotomy.

REFERENCES

Deshmukh, Hott, Tabrizi, Nakaji, Feiz-Erfan, & Spetzler. (2005). Cavernous malformation of the trigeminal nerve manifesting with trigeminal neuralgia: case report. *Neurosurgery, 56*(3).

Dhople, A. A., Adams, J. R., Maggio, W. W., Naqvi, S. A., Regine, W. F., & Kwok, Y. (2009). Long-term outcomes of Gamma Knife radiosurgery for classic trigeminal neuralgia: Implications of treatment and critical review of the literature. Clinical article. *Journal of Neurosurgery, 111*(2), 351–358. doi:10.3171/2009.2.JNS08977 PMID:19326987

Dvorak, T., Finn, A., Price, L. L., Mignano, J. E., Fitzek, M. M., Wu, J. K., & Yao, K. C. (2009). Retreatment of trigeminal neuralgia with Gamma Knife radiosurgery: Is there an appropriate cumulative dose? Clinical article. *Journal of Neurosurgery, 111*(2), 359–364. doi:10.3171/2008.11.JNS08770 PMID:19326978

Fernandez-Conejero, I., Ulkatan, S., Sen, C., & Deletis, V. (2012). Intra-operative neurophysiology during microvascular decompression for hemifacial spasm. *Clinical Neurophysiology, 123*(1), 78–83. doi:10.1016/j.clinph.2011.10.007 PMID:22136736

Ferroli, Acerbi, Broggi, & Broggi. (2010). Arteriovenous micromalformation of the trigeminal root: intraoperative diagnosis with indocyanine green videoangiography: case report. *Neurosurgery, 67*(3 Suppl).

Fujimaki, T., Fukushima, T., & Miyazaki, S. (1990). Percutaneous retrogasserian glycerol injection in the management of trigeminal neuralgia: Long-term follow-up results. *Journal of Neurosurgery, 73*(2), 212–216. doi:10.3171/jns.1990.73.2.0212 PMID:2195139

Henson, C. F., Goldman, H. W., Rosenwasser, R. H., Downes, M. B., Bednarz, G., Pequignot, E. C., ... Andrews, D. W. (2005). Glycerol rhizotomy versus gamma knife radiosurgery for the treatment of trigeminal neuralgia: An analysis of patients treated at one institution. *International Journal of Radiation Oncology, Biology, Physics, 63*(1), 82–90. doi:10.1016/j.ijrobp.2005.01.033 PMID:16111575

Jayasekera, B. A., Vergani, F., Gholkar, A., & Jenkins, A. J. (2014). Trigeminal neuralgia from an Arteriovenous malformation: An intra-operative diagnosis. *British Journal of Neurosurgery*, 1–2. PMID:25222749

Karibe, H., Shirane, R., Jokura, H., & Yoshimoto, T. (2004). Intrinsic arteriovenous malformation of the trigeminal nerve in a patient with trigeminal neuralgia: Case report. *Neurosurgery, 55*(6), 1433. doi:10.1227/01.NEU.0000143147.57383.AA PMID:15574228

Lee, A., McCartney, S., Burbidge, C., Raslan, A. M., & Burchiel, K. J. (2014). Trigeminal neuralgia occurs and recurs in the absence of neurovascular compression. *Journal of Neurosurgery*, *120*(5), 1048–1054. doi:10.3171/2014.1.JNS131410 PMID:24506241

Lin, C. F., Chen, H. H., Hernesniemi, J., Lee, C. C., Liao, C. H., Chen, S. C., ... Hsu, S. P. (2012). An easy adjustable method of ectatic vertebrobasilar artery transposition for microvascular decompression. *Clinical Neurology and Neurosurgery*, *114*(7), 951–956. doi:10.1016/j.clineuro.2012.02.021 PMID:22390889

Linskey, M. E., Ratanatharathorn, V., & Penagaricano, J. (2008). A prospective cohort study of microvascular decompression and Gamma Knife surgery in patients with trigeminal neuralgia. *Journal of Neurosurgery*, *109*(Suppl), 160–172. PMID:19123904

Lovely, T. J., & Jannetta, P. J. (1997). Microvascular decompression for trigeminal neuralgia. Surgical technique and long-term results. *Neurosurgery Clinics of North America*, *8*(1), 11–29. PMID:9018702

Masuoka, J., Matsushima, T., Kawashima, M., Nakahara, Y., Funaki, T., & Mineta, T. (2011). Stitched sling retraction technique for microvascular decompression: Procedures and techniques based on an anatomical viewpoint. *Neurosurgical Review*, *34*(3), 373–379, discussion 379–380. doi:10.100710143-011-0310-0 PMID:21347661

Sekula, R. F. Jr, Frederickson, A. M., Jannetta, P. J., Quigley, M. R., Aziz, K. M., & Arnone, G. D. (2011). Microvascular decompression for elderly patients with trigeminal neuralgia: A prospective study and systematic review with meta-analysis. *Journal of Neurosurgery*, *114*(1), 172–179. doi:10.3171/2010.6.JNS10142 PMID:20653393

Sekula, R. F. Jr, Marchan, E. M., Fletcher, L. H., Casey, K. F., & Jannetta, P. J. (2008). Microvascular decompression for trigeminal neuralgia in elderly patients. *Journal of Neurosurgery*, *108*(4), 689–691. doi:10.3171/JNS/2008/108/4/0689 PMID:18377247

Sindou, M., Leston, J., Howeidy, T., Decullier, E., & Chapuis, F. (2006). Microvascular decompression for primary Trigeminal Neuralgia (typical or atypical). Long-term effectiveness on pain; prospective study with survival analysis in a consecutive series of 362 patients. *Acta Neurochirurgica*, *148*(12), 1235–1245, discussion 1245. doi:10.100700701-006-0809-2 PMID:16804643

Tatli, M., Satici, O., Kanpolat, Y., & Sindou, M. (2008). Various surgical modalities for trigeminal neuralgia: Literature study of respective long-term outcomes. *Acta Neurochirurgica, 150*(3), 243–255. doi:10.100700701-007-1488-3 PMID:18193149

Teo, Nakaji, & Mobbs. (2006). Endoscope-assisted microvascular decompression for trigeminal neuralgia: technical case report. *Neurosurgery, 59*(4 Suppl 2).

Toda, K. (2008). Operative treatment of trigeminal neuralgia: review of current techniques. *Oral Surg Oral Med Oral Pathol Oral Radiol Endod, 106*(6), 788-805.

KEY TERMS AND DEFINITIONS

Endoscopic-Assisted Surgery: Use of the endoscope to assist with an operation primarily performed with an operative microscope.

Keyhole Surgery: Techniques of surgery whereby craniotomies are garnished at appropriate locations and sizes to address pathologies without undue exposure of adjacent brain. Keyhole surgery does not exclusively refer to addressing lesions with small craniotomies that hinder the completion of the operation; but rather, to craniotomies that are of adequate size to perform the operation while minimizing unnecessary exposure or trauma to the brain.

Microvascular Decompression: Technique of separating an offending vessel from an adjacent neural structure.

Chapter 8
Glycerol Rhizotomy as a Treatment Modality for Trigeminal Neuralgia

Alexander B. Dru
University of Arizona College of Medicine – Tucson, USA

Hasan A. Zaidi
Barrow Neurological Institute, USA

Andrew G. Shetter
Barrow Neurological Institute, USA

ABSTRACT

In this chapter, the authors discuss the use of glycerol rhizotomy (GR) as a treatment modality for trigeminal neuralgia. GR was first described by Håkanson and has been used for more than 40 years as a minimally invasive, safe option for the management of facial pain. Here, the authors discuss the history behind the discovery of GR, relevant biochemical mechanisms of neurolysis, indications, a step-by-step procedural outline for GR and intraoperative cisternography, potential side effects, efficacy of treatment, and new applications for the imaging technique. GR has stood the test of time in neurosurgery, and this chapter demonstrates its utility in patients who are poor surgical candidates for microvascular decompression and for whom medical treatment has failed to manage their intractable pain.

INTRODUCTION

Trigeminal neuralgia (TN) has the highest incidence in elderly patients, many of whom also have comorbid medical conditions that preclude long, invasive surgical procedures under anesthesia to treat their facial pain. Glycerol rhizotomy (GR), as described in this chapter, is an appropriate procedure for these individuals.

DOI: 10.4018/978-1-5225-5349-6.ch008

Percutaneous GR poses little surgical risk, may be performed under local anesthesia, and carries a favorable side-effect profile; thus, it is well suited for many patients with trigeminal neuralgia who would not be able to tolerate either the invasiveness of direct decompression or potential adverse effects of anticonvulsants, such as carbamazepine, traditionally used for this condition.

BACKGROUND

History of Glycerol Rhizotomy

Like many paramount medical treatments, the discovery of glycerol's neurolytic effects and potential therapeutic application in TN was made by chance. During the 1970s in Stockholm, stereotactic gamma knife radiation was used in an attempt to ablate the trigeminal (gasserian) ganglion and dull pain signals in TN patients. Both glycerol and metrizamide were trialed as carriers of tantalum dust—a radiopaque material—that was injected to the trigeminal cistern as a visual waypoint for stereotactic calculations (Håkanson & Leksell, 1979). Glycerol became the medium of choice because of its documented role in human triglyceride synthesis, favorable viscosity, and prior use as a vehicle for phenol neurolysis, which was the predominant percutaneous TN treatment of the time (Jefferson, 1963). Håkanson and colleagues began to notice that injection of the medium alone appeared to relieve facial pain before the radio-ablative procedure was set to take place. The group subsequently outlined a method for the direct injection of glycerol into the trigeminal cistern and published the first case series in 1981 (Håkanson, 1981).

Mechanism of Neurolysis by Glycerol

Glycerol ($C_3H_8O_3$) is a colorless, odorless trivalent alcohol that serves as a precursor for phospholipid and triacylglycerol synthesis in the human liver and adipose tissue. Glycerol's three hydroxyl groups and carbon backbone yield a molecule with a versatile solubility profile, allowing it readily dissolve in water as well as easily traverse animal cell membranes. Additionally, glycerol is a relatively benign chemical, with feline studies demonstrating that large quantities of 7.5%–15% solutions injected directly into the lumbosacral subarachnoid space are required before systemic damage occurs in the form of proliferative arachnoiditis and widespread peripheral demyelination (Baxter & Schacherl, 1962).

Glycerol's mechanism of neurolysis is two-part, stemming from the disruption of tight junctions between Schwann cells and the outer axolemma of peripheral nerves, and hypertonicity osmotic shifts resulting in neuron damage. Small-diameter, unmyelinated neurons are traditionally thought to be most vulnerable to hypertonic damage. Animal neurons bathed in hypertonic glycerol will shrink initially before equilibrating their intracellular solute concentration with the external environment. As the glycerol solution dissipates, fibers then swell considerably before reaching a second equilibration. Although the axon proper and conduction properties remain relatively undisturbed in this isolated set of conditions, the hypertonic microenvironment of glycerol solutions cause marked structural changes in both myelinated and unmyelinated neurons (Freeman, Reuben, Brandt, & Grundfest, 1966; King, Jewett, & Sundberg, 1972).

Håkanson and Rengachary et al. in the early 1980s noted neuron swelling and axolysis after intra- and perineural glycerol injection; the most substantial evidence was observed in large myelinated fibers with relative sparing of smaller myelinated and unmyelinated neurons (Håkanson, 1981; Rengachary, Watanabe, Singer, & Bopp, 1983). Pal et al. confirmed this work in 1989 by observing a positive correlation between the extent of myelinated neural tissue damage with fiber diameter and longer exposure to glycerol (Pal, Dinda, Roy, & Banerji, 1989). A more recent study by Isik et al. in 2002 evaluated histopathological changes in dog trigeminal ganglia after glycerol solution injection under electron and light microscopy; they concluded that both myelinated and unmyelinated neurons underwent axolysis (Isik et al., 2002). Glycerol's primary neurolytic effect appears to take place at the site of injection, with little evidence of retrograde transport and subsequent widespread neuronal destruction. Stajcic injected proton-labeled glycerol into distal branches of rat maxillary nerves, which yielded radioactive concentrations $<0.1\%$ in all areas distal to the foramen rotundum as well as in both ipsilateral and contralateral gasserian ganglia (Stajcic, 1990).

Equally important as hypertonicity for neurolysis is the actual rate of alteration of the osmotic microenvironment in causing neural destruction. More damage is likely induced in a neuron subjected to sudden large changes in tonicity than in a neuron exposed to a relatively slow infusion of glycerol, thereby minimizing rapid diameter alterations. Glycerol requires a minimum of 30 minutes to equilibrate across an animal cell. It is postulated that injection followed by evacuation would cause greater physical disturbance to the trigeminal root than a simple glycerol injection allowed to slowly exit the cistern via subarachnoid diffusion (Linderoth & Lind, 2012).

Glycerol-Induced Alterations to Healthy and Damaged Neurons

Long-term suppression of pain signals from the trigeminal ganglion is the key to proper relief for TN patients. Several groups have studied the effects of glycerol on various types of damaged and healthy neurons.

Burchiel and Russell in 1985 observed the effects of glycerol injections on healthy and damaged nerves by generating rat saphenous neuromas. The neuroma model was created by sectioning the saphenous nerve, which was studied 7 days after its formation. At baseline, the neuroma discharged both spontaneously and in response to light mechanical stimulation. The application of anhydrous glycerol on normal nerves showed rapid loss of C-fiber–type conduction within 5 minutes with progression to complete conduction blockade of all fibers by 30 minutes. The authors concluded that after application glycerol rapidly results in a non-specific blockade of both spontaneous and stimulated discharges of large and small fibers (Burchiel & Russell, 1985). Rappaport et al. in 1986 also observed a significant reduction in autotomy in rat sciatic neuromas when injected with glycerol compared with saline and alcohol, which they attributed to the mechanism of decreased chronic neurologic pain from GR (Rappaport, Seltzer, & Zagzag, 1986).

The groups led by Sweet and Hellstrand were some of the first to start experimentation specific to pain modulation with glycerol applied to isolated trigeminal roots and injections into the trigeminal cistern. Sweet's conclusions of decreased trigeminal root potentials from both C and alpha-delta fibers were recorded in the very short term—only minutes after glycerol injection in Meckel's cave (Sweet, Poletti, & Macon, 1981). Unpublished work from Hellstrand's group (Håkanson, 1981), as described by Håkanson, outlines studies on both cat trigeminal roots and frog nerves. They witnessed a decrease in potentials with glycerol application but a recovery of function when the tissues were washed with saline. This called into question the longer-term effects of glycerol application on abolition of nociceptive transmission due to the concern that any neuronal disruption would be short-lived as glycerol would diffuse from the offending neurons.

Studies of longer-term effects of GR on trigeminal roots were carried out by Bennet in two research groups. In 1983, Bennet and Jannetta showed that trigeminal roots continued to exhibit elevated threshold potentials and latency of signal transmission compared with a healthy root 6 weeks post-GR in human patients (Bennett & Jannetta, 1983). In a subsequent study by Bennett and Lunsford, evoked potential N20 peak differences (at the maxillary gum) of the normal and pathologic sides of patients were actually reduced at 6 weeks after GR. This "normalization" of the N20 peaks lead to the conclusion that partially damaged axons are more selectively attacked in GR (Bennett & Lunsford, 1984). Further characterization by various groups demonstrated, within the trigeminal ganglion, that large-diameter myelinated fibers exhibit the most significant conduction changes in the aftermath of GR (Håkanson, 1991; Lunsford, Bennett, & Martinez, 1985).

It is readily apparent that the body of current research points to GR exerting its temporal, hypertonic effects preferentially on large-diameter myelinated fibers. Ultimately the osmotic insult to damaged trigeminal roots results in a normalization of evoked potential firing and pain perception. More work in 1997 by Eide and colleagues additionally suggests that GR leads to additional normalization of centrally mediated temporal summation of pain perception (Eide & Stubhaug, 1997).

MAIN FOCUS OF THE CHAPTER

Indications for Glycerol Rhizotomy

The most frequent indication for GR is idiopathic typical trigeminal neuralgia (TN1 in the Burchiel classification system [Burchiel, 2003]) in patients whose pain is inadequately controlled on medications or those experiencing unacceptable drug side effects. Atypical trigeminal neuralgia (Burchiel's TN2) and trigeminal neuralgia associated with multiple sclerosis may respond to GR as well, although some studies suggest lower response rate for these conditions. GR is not indicated for post-herpetic trigeminal neuralgia or facial pain due to intentional or unintentional injury to the trigeminal nerve (Burchiel's trigeminal differentiation pain and trigeminal neuropathic pain, respectively).

The decision whether to undergo surgical treatment, and, if so, which procedure to choose is highly subjective on the part of the patient. It is important that physicians provide patients with a detailed and honest description of the various options available to them so they can pick the course with which they feel most comfortable.

Preoperative Considerations for Glycerol Rhizotomy

A full medical history and physical examination, with special note of TN symptoms including severity of pain, sensory deficits, and any hearing issues, should be well documented. As with any procedure using radiocontrast dyes, allergies and kidney function should be elucidated in the clinic before the patient undergoes GR. A preoperative MRI is warranted to identify unsuspected structural abnormalities or demyelinating disease.

Procedural Outline for Glycerol Rhizotomy

Various modifications to the original procedure outlined by Håkanson (1981) include variations in depth of anesthesia, patient positioning, imaging modalities to localize the trigeminal cistern and needle tip, glycerol solution mixture and dosing methodology, head position angle, and duration of sustained head position after rhizotomy. The procedure described below is adopted from Schmidek and Sweet's *Operative Neurosurgical Techniques* (6th ed.) (Linderoth & Lind, 2012).

Anesthesia Principles and Patient Positioning

Current anesthesia protocol involves a combination of 0.5% lidocaine solution, intravenous propofol, and low-dose benzodiazepine for anxiolysis approximately 1 hour prior to surgery. Intubation is not required unless concern for airway patency is present; oxygen via nasal cannula is often sufficient. Of note in any procedure that instruments a portion of the trigeminal body is the potential for a trigeminal depressor response. Such incidents have been described in up to 20% of cases specifically during cannulation of the foramen ovale or glycerol injection (Cheng, Lim, Chang, & Barbaro, 2014). Therefore, atropine may be dosed at the first signs of bradycardia if warranted by the surgeon or anesthesiologist.

The patient is placed in the supine position with his or her neck slightly extended and the head rotated approximately 20 degrees away from the affected side. Lateral and oblique C-arm fluoroscope imaging is utilized to identify the location of the foramen ovale.

Anatomical Landmarks and Trigeminal Cisternography

Ideally, the trigeminal cistern is cannulated via an anterior percutaneous route, coursing with the mandibular branch of the trigeminal nerve and passing through the foramen ovale as it approaches the body of the gasserian ganglion. An external landmark for the point of skin puncture is 3–4 cm lateral to the corner of the mouth on the affected side. A 20-gauge lumbar cannula is inserted after local anesthesia. The trajectory of the needle should be directed in a path created by the intersection of two planes with an axial and sagittal orientation. The axially oriented plane is made by three points: the skin puncture site, a point 0.5 cm anterior to the anterior margin of the mandibular joint, and the foramen ovale. The sagittally oriented plane includes the skin puncture site, the medial margin of the pupil in neutral position, and the foramen ovale.

Experienced surgeons suggest that first contacting the boney medial foramen wall and subsequently redirecting the needle laterally helps to ensure proper entry. Fluoroscopy can provide additional feedback to attain ideal passage. As the needle passes the foramen, the patient may experience pain in the V3 distribution and bradycardia with penetration of the gasserian ganglion.

Once the needle enters the trigeminal cistern, there may be spontaneous drainage of cerebrospinal fluid (CSF) as its current location enters the subarachnoid space. CSF drainage is most common during the first GR, but may not be present during subsequent procedures. Additionally, brisk CSF flow has been anecdotally noted if the cannula has erroneously entered the subtemporal space. As a rule, the tip should not pass the clival contour on lateral imaging. If it does, the injection may cause pain to the ipsilateral eye and will not be in the proper area for suitable neurolysis. If the surgeon is not using cisternography, the appearance of spontaneous CSF flow, fluoroscopy, and a glycerol test all can be used together to verify proper needle placement.

Cisternography has changed little since described by Håkanson (1981). The landmark study by Arias in 1986 suggests that similar efficacy of pain relief and nerve branch selectivity may be attained without the use of cisternography (Arias, 1986). In this chapter, both techniques are presented. For cisternography, the contrast medium of choice is iohexol (300 mg iodine/mL) with a typical injected volume ranging from 0.25 to 0.4 mL. With the patient's head flexed to minimize drainage out of the cistern into the posterior fossa, contrast is slowly injected. Fluoroscopy during injection is necessary to confirm the intracisternal positioning of the cannula. Due to the presence of a subdural-extracisternal section of Meckel's cave, contrast may accidentally be injected in this area if prior CSF drainage was not confirmed, or if the needle becomes dislodged during the injection process. Some physicians prefer to use the original cannula as a guide—after its location in the cistern has been confirmed by CSF flow and fluoroscopy—to introduce a second injection needle for iohexol.

To remove contrast from the cistern after cannulation, the patient may be placed in a sitting position and the injecting syringe removed from the cannula to allow passive drainage. The patient may be placed in a Trendelenburg position to allow outflow through the posterior fossa if not all contrast drains through the cannula. Complete evacuation of contrast, which may be confirmed by fluoroscopy, is necessary for the most inferior trigeminal fibers to be infiltrated by glycerol. Additionally, gentle flushing of the cistern with several milliliters of saline will help clear any remaining contrast.

Glycerol Injection and Nerve Branch Selection

The glycerol formulation should be anhydrous and sterile. To prevent spillage from the cistern, the injection should take place with the patient sitting upright. The effective volume of injected glycerol ranges from 0.18 to 0.3 mL; however, larger volumes (>0.35 mL) have been required if all three segments (V1–V3) of the trigeminal ganglion require injection. Injecting glycerol into specific trigeminal branches can be achieved as well using several techniques.

Generally, the trigeminal V1, V2, and V3 branches are oriented superior to inferior within the trigeminal cistern, respectively. Therefore, the glycerol needle tip location should be positioned in the cistern with this basic theme in mind. For V3 neuralgia, the tip should be in the lower cistern whereas V1/V2 neuralgias require injection in the upper portion.

The volume of glycerol injected also plays a role in the specific neurolysis of trigeminal fibers. Within a cistern that has been completely evacuated of contrast, small-volume injections of glycerol (<0.2 mL) will deposit in the bottom of the cistern, preferentially affecting the V3 and lower V2 fibers. This can be augmented by slightly flexing the patient's head so only the lowest area of the cistern fills, with any small excess of glycerol flowing into the posterior fossa. Increasing the volume of injected glycerol will cause rhizolysis of the upper V2 and V1 fibers.

If specific lysis of the V1 and V2 branches with preservation of V3 is desired, leaving a small volume of iohexol in the cistern protects the lower fibers from the glycerol. The densities of standard iohexol, glycerol, and CSF are 1.345 g/L, 1.242 g/L, and 1.007 g/L, respectively. Therefore, within the cistern, the glycerol will layer above the denser iohexol.

Head positioning has a role in the selective neurolysis of trigeminal roots. For enhanced V1 selectivity, it is prudent for the patient to be sitting upright with his or her head maximally flexed (~40 degrees). For V2 treatments, the head should be flexed to 25 degrees. For V3 treatments the head should remain upright in the sagittal plane with a slight lateral tilt toward the pathologic side. Bergenheim et al. studied the efficacy of head positioning and quality of specific branch lysis. They concluded head flexion only played a significant role for ophthalmic branch rhizotomy and was progressively less selective for maxillary and mandibular branches (Bergenheim, Hariz, & Laitinen, 1991, 1993). For patients not undergoing trigeminal cisternography, branch selection is still possible using the glycerol test.

A glycerol test may be used in any patient (with or without cisternography) to not only verify the correct positioning of the needle in Meckel's cave but also aid in selective nerve branch identification (Arias, 1986). The test involves injecting 0.05 mL glycerol with the patient sitting with his or her head flexed to a degree based on the desired lysis of V1–V3 roots noted above. Facial sensation is tested with both pinprick and cotton to test response, which usually occurs within 1–5 minutes of glycerol injection. The test is considered positive if various paresthesias (cold, numbness, tingling, etc) or, more rarely, attacks of neuralgia occur in the desired trigeminal distribution(s). With a positive test, the proper volume of glycerol for neurolysis may be injected: V1: 0.1 mL; V2, V3, and V1–V2: 0.25 mL; V2–V3: 0.3 mL; and V1–V3: 0.40 mL (Arias, 1986).

Immediately before the injection of glycerol, confirmation of CSF flow through the cannula ensures the tip is still in the cistern. As a rule, smaller diameter needles tend to cause less pain to the patient. Needles with an outer diameter of 0.7 mm are generally adequate, cause less pain to the patient, and have a lower risk of mechanical damage to trigeminal cistern contents. Needles up to 0.9 mm may be used if the practitioner requires a more robust tool to penetrate the soft tissues.

Concerns for Patients Undergoing Multiple GRs

For patients who are expected to undergo or have undergone multiple GRs, certain considerations must be addressed. First, these patients may have their trigeminal cistern permanently marked. This procedure is simple, requiring a small-volume injection of glycerol–tantalum slurry into the cisternal space. The suspension is formulated by adding 0.5 g of 0.042-mm tantalum grain into 2 mL of glycerol. Permanent marking will successfully outline the bottom of the cistern, and the patient often no longer requires additional cisternography (unless the iohexol used helps with branch selectivity, see above). In this case, when the cannula tip is confirmed to be in the previously marked cistern by radiography, glycerol may be injected outright. In patients with a marked cistern, there should be CSF flow upon cannulation and if no CSF flow is observed, a new cisternogram is warranted.

For repeat patients with persistent facial pain after the procedure, it is important not to be overzealous with re-doing GRs within 3–4 weeks. The delay will allow a later-responding patient to achieve relief without increasing the likelihood of intracisternal adhesions from the glycerol or contrast (Rappaport & Gomori, 1988). Harries and Mitchell in 2011 looked at the safety and efficacy of repeat GR in 179 patients and found that repeat GR had an overall success rate of 92.1% in curbing facial pain. The average time to repeat treatment was 22.9 months. Although repeat GRs may cause structural changes to the cistern over time, which is evident when initial images are analyzed, Harries and Mitchell did not find a relation between the number of prior rhizotomies and likelihood of a complication ($p=0.87$) (Harries & Mitchell, 2011).

SOLUTIONS AND RECOMMENDATIONS

Postoperative Considerations for Glycerol Rhizotomy

After the glycerol injection, the patient's head must remain in the desired position for at least 1 hour. There is no current evidence suggesting that a particular head position held for more than 1 hour improves the quality of rhizolysis. Around 50% of patients have immediate relief from pain paroxysms. Still, either during or in the immediate aftermath of the procedure, many patients frequently experience paresthesias or pain paroxysms lasting less than 1 minute. These fits usually last between 1 and 5 days, but cases recurring up to 3 weeks post-rhizotomy have been reported (Lunsford, 1985).

For most patients, GR is performed on an outpatient basis. In older patients or those requiring general anesthesia, an overnight stay in the hospital may be prudent.

At 24 hours post-GR, light touch sensation can be examined over the entire trigeminal nerve distribution and can be repeated at a 3-month follow-up visit. Postoperative occurrence of fever, facial rashes, mouth ulcerations, and changes in vision should be immediately reported to the physician. For patients with TN previously controlled by carbamazepine, a drug-tapering schedule may be initiated after GR and continued typically for 1–2 weeks. For patients on higher doses of carbamazepine or multi-drug regimens, specific plans should be tailored to the patient.

Efficacy of Glycerol Rhizotomy

Inter-Series Variability

Outcomes from 22 case series dating from 1983 to 2011 are examined in this section. Variations in surgical expertise and shifts in practice through the years undeniably muddy the waters when trying to compare patient outcomes through the years. During the evolution of GR, there were major changes in practice, such as the routine use of cisternography, with adoption of iohexol in 1986, which impacted efficacy in pain relief and decreased rates of certain complications such as aseptic meningitis (see *Complications* section below).

Variation in technique with regard to visualization of the cistern and injection of glycerol presents the biggest issue in evaluating different studies over the years. For example, the use of cisternography before 1990 was not common. In the published series evaluated by the authors, techniques range from the use of modern cisternography in 16 of the groups (Bergenheim & Hariz, 1995; Blomstedt & Bergenheim, 2002; Burchiel, 1988; Dieckmann, Bockermann, Heyer, Henning, & Roesen, 1987; Febles et al.; Fujimaki, Fukushima, & Miyazaki, 1990; S. Håkanson, 1983; Henson et al., 2005; Ischia, Luzzani, & Polati, 1990; Jho & Lunsford, 1997; Kondziolka & Lunsford, 2005; Lunsford, 1985; Pollock, 2005; Slettebo, Hirschberg, & Lindegaard, 1993; Steiger, 1991; Waltz, Dalessio, Copeland, & Abbott, 1989; Young, 1988) to drop-wise glycerol injection with observation of regional anesthesia by patient feedback in four of the groups (Jagia et al., 2004; North, Kidd, Piantadosi, & Carson, 1990; Saini, 1987; Xu-Hui et al., 2011).

In addition to the non-standardized use of cisternography, which many groups would agree positively correlates with proper needle placement and quality of neurolysis, other variables within these 22-case series include the volume of glycerol injected and patient treatment history. With respect to glycerol injection, which is always presented as a range of volumes in these series, five of the groups reported an upper volume limit >0.5 mL with the maximum being 0.7 mL (more than double the recommended 0.18–0.30 mL glycerol volume) (Fujimaki et al., 1990; Ischia et al., 1990; Jho & Lunsford, 1997; Slettebo et al., 1993; Waltz et al., 1989). Prior patient treatment by GR or another lytic procedure is an additional factor that was impossible to standardize among the 22 studies. This complicates comparisons with not only reporting levels of pain control and sensory disturbance before and after the procedure, but also would impact the volume of glycerol injected if only specific branches of the trigeminal nerve were targeted.

Early and Late Outcomes

Of the 22 studies, 67–97% of patients reported being "pain free" within 2 weeks of their first injection (Beck, Olson, & Urig, 1986; Bergenheim & Hariz, 1995). Interestingly, Beck's group in 1986 (Beck et al., 1986) had the lowest initial pain-free percentage of patients, yet reported using cisternography in only 31% of their patients. Time to first follow-up as well as total follow-up range was widely different among the 22 case series, the longest of which was by Xu-Hui's group with an average of 13.1 years and maximum of 23 years (Xu-Hui et al., 2011). As a result of this variability, it seems more reasonable to observe the result of GR by examining how early patients' pain recurs. The rates of "early" pain recurrence (<2 years from injection) were between 2 and 47%, with an average of approximately 20% (Arias, 1986; Burchiel, 1988). The rates of "late" pain recurrence (≥2 years from injection) ranged from 10% to 92%, with an average of approximately 50% (Arias, 1986; Saini, 1987).

Interestingly, the use of cisternography does not appear to be associated with lower rates of early or late pain recurrence (Arias, 1986). In the 16 groups that used cisternography in all patients, the range of pain recurrence before and after 2 years was 11–47% and 25–75%, respectively. For three groups (Arias, 1986; Young, 1988; Beck et al., 1986) who used cisternography intermittently, the range of pain recurrence before and after 2 years was 2–11% and 10–34%, respectively (Beck did not report pain recurrence after 2 years). For two groups (Saini, 1987; North et al., 1990) who did not use cisternography in any of their patients, the range of pain recurrence before and after 2 years was 40–41% and 55–92% respectively. Xu-Hui et al. in 2011 (Xu-Hui et al., 2011) published results from a cohort of 3,370 GR-treated TN patients (of whom 2,750 completed full follow-up) and did not use cisternography. They reported that 2,469 patients (74%) had complete pain relief with one GR procedure. Patients' pain recurrence rates were <0.3%, 21%, 7%, 4%, and 3% at < 1, 1–5, >5–10, >10–15, and >15–23 years, respectively.

Outcomes in Trigeminal Neuralgia Patients With Multiple Sclerosis

A history of MS can be found in approximately 2–8% of all patients suffering from TN, a 20-fold increase compared with the general population (Mohammad-Mohammadi,

Recinos, Lee, Elson, & Barnett, 2013; O'Connor, Schwid, Herrmann, Markman, & Dworkin, 2008). The symptoms of TN in MS patients are very similar to idiopathic trigeminal neuralgia (ITN), with paroxysmal electric shock-like sensation in one or more trigeminal nerve distributions; however, a key difference is that bilateral pathology occurs more frequently in MS patients. A recent series by Mohammad-Mohammadi et al. in 2013 showed 4% of the MS group presenting with bilateral TN (Mohammad-Mohammadi et al., 2013).

All surgical interventions for TN can reasonably be attempted on patients with MS-associated TN (other than microvascular decompression), with GR being no exception. As alluded to earlier in this chapter, the initial rates of pain control after GR are similar between individuals suffering from TN and those with MS-TN. A retrospective review by Bender et al. in 2013 looked at GR results in ITN and MS-TN patients. Their cohort had a total of 822 patients treated between 1998 and 2010, with 759 suffering from ITN and 63 with MS-TN. After GR, 67% of the ITN patients and 68% of MS-TN patients reported having no facial pain (BNI score I) at 1-month follow-up (Bender et al., 2013).

In the past, reports suggested statistically significantly higher long-term recurrence rates of pain in MS-TN patients than ITN patients undergoing GR. In 1987, Dieckmann et al. reported a pain recurrence rate of 40% vs. 10% at 2 years in 34 patients with MS-TN and 252 individuals with ITN, respectively (Dieckmann et al., 1987). This idea received additional validation by Linderoth and Håkanson in 1989, who published rates of 61% and 38% for pain recurrence at 8–79 months in 23 MS-TN patients and nearly 300 ITN patients, respectively (Linderoth & Håkanson, 1989). More recently, data from Kondziolka et al. in 1994 and Bender et al. in 2013 have potentially ousted this finding. Kondziolka and colleagues showed an identical 75% rate of pain recurrence at 3 years in the 480 patients observed with MS-TN and ITN (Kondziolka, Lunsford, & Bissonette, 1994). Similarly, Bender's cohort did not find a statistically significant difference ($p=0.40$) in median time to recurrence of pain post-GR between the MS-TN (20 months) and ITN (25 months) patient populations (Bender et al., 2013).

Complications of Glycerol Rhizotomy

Various sensory, motor, vascular, and infectious disturbances are known to complicate GR; however, the procedure is generally well tolerated compared with other surgical treatments for TN. Due to the trigeminocardiac reflex, severe bradycardia or even asystole are known potential complications from GR during the manipulation of the trigeminal nerve. This is an extremely rare complication, and only a single case of cardiopulmonary arrest after rhizolysis with subsequent death in the postoperative stage has been published (Jho & Lunsford, 1997).

Facial Sensory Disturbance

The most common, relatively mild, adverse effect of GR is a transitory facial hypesthesia reported to occur in up to 98% of patients in the 2011 study by Xu-Hui. The mildly impaired sensation usually subsided after 6 months (4% of patients had persistent hypesthesia) (Xu-Hui et al., 2011).

The most feared complication of GR—severe postoperative facial sensory disturbance (anesthesia dolorosa)—is quite rare. In the earlier days of the procedure, before cisternography or other techniques were used to localize the cannula, severe anesthesia dolorosa occurred in 26 patients in a series of 469 cases published by Saini (5.5%) (Saini, 1987). The more recent series of Pollock in 2005 (98 patients) and Xu-Hui et al. (Pollock, 2005; Xu-Hui et al., 2011) in 2011 did not report a single case of anesthesia dolorosa. Corneal anesthesia after GR occurs in 0.9–7% of patients (Ischia et al., 1990; Lunsford, 1985; Saini, 1987).

Facial dysesthesia, or an abnormal unpleasant sensation when touched, typically occurs in <4% of patients (Jho & Lunsford, 1997), but it was reported by Jagia et al. to occur in 40% of their group of 115 patients (Jagia et al., 2004). According to the Jagia study, dysesthesia was defined as "altered facial sensations," so it is not clear how many of these were painful or how to view their result compared with other authors' results. A known cause of facial dysesthesia is chronic inflammatory change to the trigeminal root from repeated neurolysis. Herpetic eruptions post-GR are another cause of dysesthesia, which is discussed below (see *Infectious Processes*). Suffice it to say that in patients undergoing initial GR, dysesthesia does not occur frequently.

Facial Motor Disturbance

Trigeminal motor weakness may occur secondarily to GR in 0–3.4% of patients (Jho & Lunsford, 1997; Saini, 1987; Xu-Hui et al., 2011). The mandibular division of the trigeminal nerve contains the motor neurons responsible for innervating the muscles of mastication: the masseter, temporalis, and medial and lateral pterygoid muscles. Both mechanical damage and chemical damage as the cannula passes through the foramen ovale and from glycerol, respectively, are thought to be responsible for this complication, which results in isolated masseter weakness. The paresis is short lived and usually resolves in less than 4 weeks.

Hemorrhage

Hemorrhage has been documented as a short-term complication of GR in 0.15% of patients (Xu-Hui et al., 2011). Most bleeding is from the buccinator muscles, the foramen ovale veniplex, or branches of the external artery. Some amount of venous bleeding is inevitable, but serious arterial sources of bleeding—such as the middle meningeal or internal carotid artery—can be avoided or minimized with intraoperative fluoroscopic imaging.

Infectious Processes

Infectious complications after GR fall under the following categories: herpes simplex activation, aseptic meningitis, and bacterial meningitis. Of those, activation of latent herpes simplex is the most common, and least worrisome. Case series describe extremely wide rates of this complication, from 3% to 77% (Dieckmann et al., 1987; Saini, 1987). The most recent large case series of 1,174 patients by Kondziolka and Lunsford in 2005 recorded this complication simply as "common" (Kondziolka & Lunsford, 2005). The most frequent manifestation of herpes simplex is ulceration of the mouth and gums with no therapy required.

Aseptic meningitis is the second most common infectious sequelae of GR, occurring in in 0–7% of patients (Håkanson, 1983; Waltz et al., 1989). Negative CSF cultures with pleocytosis, nuchal rigidity, fever, and malaise should raise suspicion. Although antibiotics should be started for patients with meningeal signs, antibiotics can be discontinued after negative bacterial cultures and patients can be transitioned to steroids. Patients typically improve in several days with no long-term issues. One of the suspected culprits of aseptic meningitis was the use of metrizamide as a contrast agent before 1986. With the adoption of iohexol, case reports of this complication have significantly dropped. In a series of 100 patients by Arias in 1986, half of the patients were given metrizamide contrast injection, and 4% of these patients developed aseptic meningitis; in contrast, none of the non-contrast patients developed the condition.(Arias, 1986)

Bacterial meningitis is the most infrequent infection resulting from GR and occurs in 0–2% of patients (Burchiel, 1988; Håkanson, 1983). A study by Henson et al. in 2005 reported bacterial infections in 8% of their patients (79 in the series) (Henson et al., 2005), but generally speaking the rate is quite low. The infecting bacteria originate from oral mucosa and the upper respiratory tract (Aspevall, Hillebrant, Linderoth, & Rylander, 1991). There are no reports in the literature to date of serious complications or death from bacterial meningitis post-GR.

Comparison of Glycerol Rhizotomy to Other Surgical Procedures

There are no randomized controlled trials comparing any of the various surgical procedures available for TN to one another. Evaluating the relative risks and benefits reported in non-randomized trials is problematic because of the often significant differences in diagnostic criteria, surgical techniques, outcome measures, and length of the follow-up. There is a general observational consensus that the non-ablative procedure of trigeminal microvascular decompression results in the best chance of long-term pain cessation in patients who are able and willing to undergo posterior fossa craniotomy. Of the less invasive ablative procedures—GR, percutaneous thermal rhizotomy (TR), percutaneous balloon compression (BC), and stereotactic radiosurgery (SRS)—there is no agreement about the best approach. It is clear that SRS usually requires weeks to months to provide pain relief, while the percutaneous procedures have a much more immediate effect. It is also apparent that BC requires a general anesthetic and may not be appropriate for patients with serious medical comorbidities.

Lopez et al. (Lopez, Hamlyn, & Zakrzewska, 2004) identified 175 studies referencing these 4 ablative procedures and evaluated them using predefined quality criteria. There were 22 studies that met their criteria for determining complications and 9 studies that could be used to assess pain relief. They concluded that TR had a higher rate of complete pain relief than GR or SRS, but it also resulted in a greater incidence of complications related to facial numbness. There was not sufficient data on BC to make a statement on this procedure. In 2011, Zakrzewska and Akram (Zakrzewska & Akram, 2011) updated those findings using a similar methodology (review of a large database to extract the few studies that met their rigid selection criteria). Their conclusions: "There is little evidence to help comparative decision making about the best surgical procedure. Well-designed studies are urgently needed." Given the lack of definitive evidence, individual surgeons may or may not prefer GR over the other ablative procedures based on their personal experience and the availability of resources at their institution.

FUTURE RESEARCH DIRECTIONS

Adjunct Therapy to Retrosigmoid Microvascular Decompression

Although preoperative imaging or surgery may localize a vessel (commonly the superior cerebellar artery) compressing the trigeminal nerve as the culprit for TN, in 3–17% of reported cases, the surgeon does not visualize an offending vessel during open decompression (Ammori, King, Siripurapu, Herwadkar, & Rutherford, 2013; Revuelta-Gutierrez, Lopez-Gonzalez, & Soto-Hernandez, 2006; Revuelta-Gutierrez, Martinez-Anda, Coll, Campos-Romo, & Perez-Pena, 2013; Sindou, Chiha, & Mertens, 1994). In 2013, Goodwin and colleagues at Johns Hopkins and University of Pennsylvania published a novel use of GR as a complement to these operations. They documented 14 patients, 7 of whom did not have operative evidence of vascular compression of the trigeminal nerve (only 2 patients had preoperative MRI evidence of trigeminal compression). For the 7 with either no or minimal compression from a small artery, they injected 0.1–0.2 mL of glycerol via a 25-gauge needle into the inferior third of the cisternal portion of the trigeminal nerve. All patients (including those with microvascular decompression) subjectively reported significant improvement in their pain. No systematic pain scale (e.g., BNI scale) was used to describe pain levels, but at 3 months, 79% of patients were "pain free." The authors agree that further work to increase the case number and quantify pain levels needs to occur in the future, but that glycerol injection into an operated cistern via retrosigmoid approach is a reasonable strategy for this subset of patients (Goodwin et al., 2013).

CONCLUSION

Glycerol rhizotomy for the treatment of idiopathic trigeminal neuralgia is a minimally invasive option for elderly and young patients who are poor surgical candidates due to preexisting health conditions or who are adverse to the notion of general anesthesia and open craniotomy. The procedure is generally well tolerated and can be performed under local anesthesia sedation. There is a low risk of adverse side effects, such as sensory derangements, hemorrhage, or infection. Although the longer-term recurrence of TN symptoms is more common than with microvascular decompression, the efficacy of GR is in line with procedures in its class and belongs in the repertoire of practicing neurosurgeons.

REFERENCES

Ammori, M. B., King, A. T., Siripurapu, R., Herwadkar, A. V., & Rutherford, S. A. (2013). Factors Influencing Decision-making and Outcome in the Surgical Management of Trigeminal Neuralgia. *Journal of Neurological Surgery. Part B, Skull Base*, *74*(2), 75–81. doi:10.1055-0033-1333617 PMID:24436892

Arias, M. J. (1986). Percutaneous retrogasserian glycerol rhizotomy for trigeminal neuralgia. A prospective study of 100 cases. *Journal of Neurosurgery*, *65*(1), 32–36. doi:10.3171/jns.1986.65.1.0032 PMID:3712027

Aspevall, O., Hillebrant, E., Linderoth, B., & Rylander, M. (1991). Meningitis due to Gemella haemolysans after neurosurgical treatment of trigeminal neuralgia. *Scandinavian Journal of Infectious Diseases*, *23*(4), 503–505. doi:10.3109/00365549109075101 PMID:1957134

Baxter, D. W., & Schacherl, U. (1962). Experimental studies on the morphological changes produced by intrathecal phenol. *Canadian Medical Association Journal*, *86*, 1200–1205. PMID:13866009

Beck, D. W., Olson, J. J., & Urig, E. J. (1986). Percutaneous retrogasserian glycerol rhizotomy for treatment of trigeminal neuralgia. *Journal of Neurosurgery*, *65*(1), 28–31. doi:10.3171/jns.1986.65.1.0028 PMID:3712026

Bender, M. T., Pradilla, G., Batra, S., See, A. P., James, C., Pardo, C. A., ... Lim, M. (2013). Glycerol rhizotomy and radiofrequency thermocoagulation for trigeminal neuralgia in multiple sclerosis. *Journal of Neurosurgery*, *118*(2), 329–336. doi:10.3171/2012.9.JNS1226 PMID:23121430

Bennett, M. H., & Jannetta, P. J. (1983). Evoked potentials in trigeminal neuralgia. *Neurosurgery*, *13*(3), 242–247. doi:10.1227/00006123-198309000-00005 PMID:6312364

Bennett, M. H., & Lunsford, L. D. (1984). Percutaneous retrogasserian glycerol rhizotomy for tic douloureux: Part 2. Results nd implications of trigeminal evoked potential studies. *Neurosurgery*, *14*(4), 431–435. doi:10.1227/00006123-198404000-00007 PMID:6728145

Bergenheim, A. T., & Hariz, M. I. (1995). Influence of previous treatment on outcome after glycerol rhizotomy for trigeminal neuralgia. *Neurosurgery*, *36*(2), 303–309, discussion 309–310. doi:10.1227/00006123-199502000-00009 PMID:7731510

Bergenheim, A. T., Hariz, M. I., & Laitinen, L. V. (1991). Selectivity of retrogasserian glycerol rhizotomy in the treatment of trigeminal neuralgia. *Stereotactic and Functional Neurosurgery*, *56*(3), 159–165. doi:10.1159/000099402 PMID:1796220

Bergenheim, A. T., Hariz, M. I., & Laitinen, L. V. (1993). Retrogasserian glycerol rhizotomy and its selectivity in the treatment of trigeminal neuralgia. *Acta Neurochirurgica. Supplementum*, *58*, 174–177. PMID:8109286

Blomstedt, P. C., & Bergenheim, A. T. (2002). Technical difficulties and perioperative complications of retrogasserian glycerol rhizotomy for trigeminal neuralgia. *Stereotact Funct Neurosurg, 79*(3-4), 168-181. doi: 7083070830

Burchiel, K. J. (1988). Percutaneous retrogasserian glycerol rhizolysis in the management of trigeminal neuralgia. *Journal of Neurosurgery*, *69*(3), 361–366. doi:10.3171/jns.1988.69.3.0361 PMID:3404233

Burchiel, K. J. (2003). A new classification for facial pain [Review]. *Neurosurgery*, *53*(5), 1164–1166, discussion 1166–1167. doi:10.1227/01.NEU.0000088806.11659.D8 PMID:14580284

Burchiel, K. J., & Russell, L. C. (1985). Glycerol neurolysis: Neurophysiological effects of topical glycerol application on rat saphenous nerve. *Journal of Neurosurgery*, *63*(5), 784–788. doi:10.3171/jns.1985.63.5.0784 PMID:4056882

Cheng, J. S., Lim, D. A., Chang, E. F., & Barbaro, N. M. (2014). A review of percutaneous treatments for trigeminal neuralgia. *Neurosurgery*, *10*(Suppl 1), 25–33, discussion 33. doi:10.1227/NEU.0000000000000168700006123-201403001-00003 PMID:24509496

Dieckmann, G., Bockermann, V., Heyer, C., Henning, J., & Roesen, M. (1987). Five-and-a-half years' experience with percutaneous retrogasserian glycerol rhizotomy in treatment of trigeminal neuralgia. *Applied Neurophysiology*, *50*(1-6), 401–413. PMID:3502439

Eide, P. K., & Stubhaug, A. (1997). Sensory perception in patients with trigeminal neuralgia: Effects of percutaneous retrogasserian glycerol rhizotomy. *Stereotactic and Functional Neurosurgery*, *68*(1-4 Pt 1), 207–211. doi:10.1159/000099925 PMID:9711718

Febles, C., Werner-Wasik, M., Rosenwasser, R. H., Goldman, W. H., Curran, W. J., & Andrews, D. W. (n.d.). A comparison of treatment outcomes with Gamma Knife radiosurgery versus Glycerol Rhizotomy in the management of trigeminal neuralgia. *International Journal of Radiation Oncology, Biology, Physics, 57*(2), S253. doi: 10.1016/s0360-3016(03)01087-3

Freeman, A. R., Reuben, J. P., Brandt, P. W., & Grundfest, H. (1966). Osmometrically determined characteristics of the cell membrane of squid and lobster giant axons. *The Journal of General Physiology*, *50*(2), 423–445. doi:10.1085/jgp.50.2.423 PMID:11526838

Fujimaki, T., Fukushima, T., & Miyazaki, S. (1990). Percutaneous retrogasserian glycerol injection in the management of trigeminal neuralgia: Long-term follow-up results. *Journal of Neurosurgery*, *73*(2), 212–216. doi:10.3171/jns.1990.73.2.0212 PMID:2195139

Goodwin, C. R., Yang, J. X., Bettegowda, C., Hwang, B., James, C., Biser, A., ... Lim, M. (2013). Glycerol rhizotomy via a retrosigmoid approach as an alternative treatment for trigeminal neuralgia. [pii]. *Clinical Neurology and Neurosurgery, 115*(12), 2454–2456. doi:10.1016/j.clineuro.2013.09.009 PMID:24161889

Håkanson, S. (1981). Trigeminal neuralgia treated by the injection of glycerol into the trigeminal cistern. *Neurosurgery, 9*(6), 638–646. doi:10.1227/00006123-198112000-00005 PMID:7322329

Håkanson, S. (1983). Retrogasserian glycerol injection as treatment of tic douloureux. *Advances in Pain Research and Therapy, 5*, 927–933.

Håkanson, S. (1991). In G. H. Fromm (Ed.), *Surgical treatment: retrogasserian glycerol injection.* Boston: ButterworthHeinemann.

Håkanson, S., & Leksell, L. (1979). Stereotactic radiosurgery in trigeminal neuralgia. In G. F. Pauser G., Gross D. (Ed.), Gesichtsschmerz: Schmerzstudien (pp. 231-237). New York: Gustav Fischer Verlag.

Harries, A. M., & Mitchell, R. D. (2011). Percutaneous glycerol rhizotomy for trigeminal neuralgia: Safety and efficacy of repeat procedures. *British Journal of Neurosurgery, 25*(2), 268–272. doi:10.3109/02688697.2011.558946 PMID:21545328

Henson, C. F., Goldman, H. W., Rosenwasser, R. H., Downes, M. B., Bednarz, G., Pequignot, E. C., . . . Andrews, D. W. (2005). Glycerol rhizotomy versus gamma knife radiosurgery for the treatment of trigeminal neuralgia: an analysis of patients treated at one institution. *Int J Radiat Oncol Biol Phys, 63*(1), 82-90. doi: 10.1016/j.ijrobp.2005.01.033

Ischia, S., Luzzani, A., & Polati, E. (1990). Retrogasserian glycerol injection: A retrospective study of 112 patients. *The Clinical Journal of Pain, 6*(4), 291–296. doi:10.1097/00002508-199012000-00006 PMID:2135029

Isik, N., Pamir, M. N., Benli, K., Erbengi, A., Erbengi, T., & Ruacan, S. (2002). Experimental trigeminal glycerol injection in dogs: histopathological evaluation by light and electron microscopy. *Stereotact Funct Neurosurg, 79*(2), 94-106. doi: 7010570105

Jagia, M., Bithal, P. K., Dash, H. H., Prabhakar, H., Chaturvedi, A., & Chouhan, R. S. (2004). Effect of cerebrospinal fluid return on success rate of percutaneous retrogasserian glycerol rhizotomy. *Reg Anesth Pain Med, 29*(6), 592-595. doi: S1098733904005206

Jefferson, A. (1963). Trigeminal Root and Ganglion Injections Using Phenol in Glycerine for the Relief of Trigeminal Neuralgia. *Journal of Neurology, Neurosurgery, and Psychiatry*, *26*(4), 345–352. doi:10.1136/jnnp.26.4.345 PMID:14043050

Jho, H. D., & Lunsford, L. D. (1997). Percutaneous retrogasserian glycerol rhizotomy. Current technique and results. *Neurosurgery Clinics of North America*, *8*(1), 63–74. PMID:9018706

King, J. S., Jewett, D. L., & Sundberg, H. R. (1972). Differential blockade of cat dorsal root C fibers by various chloride solutions. *Journal of Neurosurgery*, *36*(5), 569–583. doi:10.3171/jns.1972.36.5.0569 PMID:5067506

Kondziolka, D., & Lunsford, L. D. (2005). Percutaneous retrogasserian glycerol rhizotomy for trigeminal neuralgia: technique and expectations. *Neurosurg Focus, 18*(5), E7. doi: 180507

Kondziolka, D., Lunsford, L. D., & Bissonette, D. J. (1994). Long-term results after glycerol rhizotomy for multiple sclerosis-related trigeminal neuralgia. *The Canadian Journal of Neurological Sciences*, *21*(2), 137–140. doi:10.1017/S0317167100049076 PMID:8087740

Linderoth, B., & Håkanson, S. (1989). Paroxysmal facial pain in disseminated sclerosis treated by retrogasserian glycerol injection. *Acta Neurologica Scandinavica*, *80*(4), 341–346. doi:10.1111/j.1600-0404.1989.tb03890.x PMID:2816292

Linderoth, B., & Lind, G. (2012). Retrogasserian Glycerol Rhizolysis in Trigeminal Neuralgia. In A. Quinones-Hinojosa (Ed.), Schmidek and Sweet: Operative Neurosurgical Techniques (6th ed.; Vol. 2, pp. 1393-1408). Philadelphia: Elsevier.

Lopez, B. C., Hamlyn, P. J., & Zakrzewska, J. M. (2004). Systematic review of ablative neurosurgical techniques for the treatment of trigeminal neuralgia. *Neurosurgery, 54*(4), 973-982; discussion 982-973.

Lunsford, L. D. (1985). *Trigeminal neuralgia: treatment by glycerol rhizotomy*. New York: McGraw-Hill.

Lunsford, L. D., Bennett, M. H., & Martinez, A. J. (1985). Experimental trigeminal glycerol injection. Electrophysiologic and morphologic effects. *Archives of Neurology*, *42*(2), 146–149. doi:10.1001/archneur.1985.04060020060016 PMID:3977642

Mohammad-Mohammadi, A., Recinos, P. F., Lee, J. H., Elson, P., & Barnett, G. H. (2013). Surgical outcomes of trigeminal neuralgia in patients with multiple sclerosis. *Neurosurgery*, *73*(6), 941–950, discussion 950. doi:10.1227/NEU.0000000000000128 PMID:23921703

North, R. B., Kidd, D. H., Piantadosi, S., & Carson, B. S. (1990). Percutaneous retrogasserian glycerol rhizotomy. Predictors of success and failure in treatment of trigeminal neuralgia. *Journal of Neurosurgery*, *72*(6), 851–856. doi:10.3171/jns.1990.72.6.0851 PMID:2338568

O'Connor, A. B., Schwid, S. R., Herrmann, D. N., Markman, J. D., & Dworkin, R. H. (2008). Pain associated with multiple sclerosis: systematic review and proposed classification. *Pain, 137*(1), 96-111. doi: 10.1016/j.pain.2007.08.024

Pal, H. K., Dinda, A. K., Roy, S., & Banerji, A. K. (1989). Acute effect of anhydrous glycerol on peripheral nerve: An experimental study. *British Journal of Neurosurgery*, *3*(4), 463–469. doi:10.3109/02688698909002832 PMID:2803594

Pollock, B. E. (2005). Percutaneous retrogasserian glycerol rhizotomy for patients with idiopathic trigeminal neuralgia: A prospective analysis of factors related to pain relief. *Journal of Neurosurgery*, *102*(2), 223–228. doi:10.3171/jns.2005.102.2.0223 PMID:15739548

Rappaport, Z. H., & Gomori, J. M. (1988). Recurrent trigeminal cistern glycerol injections for tic douloureux. *Acta Neurochirurgica*, *90*(1-2), 31–34. doi:10.1007/BF01541263 PMID:2449803

Rappaport, Z. H., Seltzer, Z., & Zagzag, D. (1986). The effect of glycerol on autotomy. An experimental model of neuralgia pain. *Pain*, *26*(1), 85–91. doi:10.1016/0304-3959(86)90175-2 PMID:3737232

Rengachary, S. S., Watanabe, I. S., Singer, P., & Bopp, W. J. (1983). Effect of glycerol on peripheral nerve: An experimental study. *Neurosurgery*, *13*(6), 681–688. doi:10.1227/00006123-198312000-00012 PMID:6318149

Revuelta-Gutierrez, R., Lopez-Gonzalez, M. A., & Soto-Hernandez, J. L. (2006). Surgical treatment of trigeminal neuralgia without vascular compression: 20 years of experience. *Surg Neurol, 66*(1), 32-36; discussion 36. doi: 10.1016/j.surneu.2005.10.018

Revuelta-Gutierrez, R., Martinez-Anda, J. J., Coll, J. B., Campos-Romo, A., & Perez-Pena, N. (2013). Efficacy and safety of root compression of trigeminal nerve for trigeminal neuralgia without evidence of vascular compression. *World Neurosurgery*, *80*(3-4), 385–389. doi:10.1016/j.wneu.2012.07.030 PMID:22889619

Saini, S. S. (1987). Reterogasserian anhydrous glycerol injection therapy in trigeminal neuralgia: Observations in 552 patients. *Journal of Neurology, Neurosurgery, and Psychiatry*, *50*(11), 1536–1538. doi:10.1136/jnnp.50.11.1536 PMID:3501000

Sindou, M. P., Chiha, M., & Mertens, P. (1994). Anatomical findings observed during microsurgical approaches of the cerebellopontine angle for vascular decompression in trigeminal neuralgia (350 cases). *Stereotactic and Functional Neurosurgery*, *63*(1-4), 203–207. doi:10.1159/000100316 PMID:7624636

Slettebo, H., Hirschberg, H., & Lindegaard, K. F. (1993). Long-term results after percutaneous retrogasserian glycerol rhizotomy in patients with trigeminal neuralgia. *Acta Neurochirurgica*, *122*(3-4), 231–235. doi:10.1007/BF01405534 PMID:8372713

Stajcic, Z. (1990). Evidence that the site of action of glycerol in relieving tic douloureux is its actual site of application. *Deutsche Zahnarztliche Zeitschrift*, *45*(1), 44–46. PMID:1701698

Steiger, H. J. (1991). Prognostic factors in the treatment of trigeminal neuralgia. Analysis of a differential therapeutic approach. *Acta Neurochirurgica*, *113*(1-2), 11–17. doi:10.1007/BF01402108 PMID:1799138

Sweet, W. H., Poletti, C. E., & Macon, J. B. (1981). Treatment of trigeminal neuralgia and other facial pains by retrogasserian injection of glycerol. *Neurosurgery*, *9*(6), 647–653. doi:10.1227/00006123-198112000-00006 PMID:6976524

Waltz, T. A., Dalessio, D. J., Copeland, B., & Abbott, G. (1989). Percutaneous injection of glycerol for the treatment of trigeminal neuralgia. *The Clinical Journal of Pain*, *5*(2), 195–198. doi:10.1097/00002508-198906000-00011 PMID:2520403

Xu-Hui, W., Chun, Z., Guang-Jian, S., Min-Hui, X., Guang-Xin, C., Yong-Wen, Z., & Lun-Shan, X. (2011). Long-term outcomes of percutaneous retrogasserian glycerol rhizotomy in 3370 patients with trigeminal neuralgia. *Turkish Neurosurgery*, *21*(1), 48–52. PMID:21294091

Young, R. F. (1988). Glycerol rhizolysis for treatment of trigeminal neuralgia. *Journal of Neurosurgery*, *69*(1), 39–45. doi:10.3171/jns.1988.69.1.0039 PMID:2454304

Zakrzewska, J. M., & Akram, H. (2011). Neurosurgical interventions for the treatment of classical trigeminal neuralgia [Review]. *Cochrane Database of Systematic Reviews*, (9). doi:10.1002/14651858.CD007312.pub2 PMID:21901707

KEY TERMS AND DEFINITIONS

Anesthesia Dolorosa: Painful sensation in an area of the face that is normally numb to tactile stimulation.

Foramen Ovale: An opening in the greater wing of the sphenoid bone that allows the passage of five anatomical structures: the V3 branch of the trigeminal nerve, the lesser petrosal nerve, the otic ganglion, the accessory branch of the middle meningeal artery, and the emissary veins connecting the cavernous sinus and pterygoid plexus.

Hypesthesia: Decreased tactile sensation of the skin.

Trigeminal Cistern (Meckel's Cave): A cerebrospinal fluid-filled dural pouch created by a fold in the tentorium cerebelli overlying the apex of the petrous part of the temporal bone. It is bound superolaterally by the cerebellar tentorium, superomedially by the lateral cavernous sinus, medially by the clivus, and inferiorly by the skull base.

Trigeminal Cisternography: An imaging technique involving injecting a radiopaque contrast solution into the trigeminal cistern, then visualizing the cavity under fluoroscopy to provide real-time anatomical information on Meckel's cave and structures within its confine.

Trigeminal (Gasserian) Ganglion: The sensory root of the trigeminal nerve housed in Meckel's cave, which gives off three major branches: the ophthalmic (V1) branch, maxillary (V2) branch, and mandibular (V3) branch for sensation over the face. It lies just laterally to the internal carotid artery and posterolaterally to the cavernous sinus.

Trigeminocardiac Reflex: The rapid onset of hypotension, dysrhythmia, or respiratory depression after the stimulation of any sensory branch(es) of the trigeminal nerve.

Chapter 9
Balloon Rhizotomy Treatment for Trigeminal Neuralgia

Stephen Haines
University of Minnesota, USA

ABSTRACT

No single surgical procedure can achieve lasting pain relief in all patients with trigeminal neuralgia. Percutaneous balloon compression trigeminal rhizotomy is an alternative outpatient procedure for patients in whom open operation or other percutaneous procedures are infeasible or have failed. The instrumentation required and a stepwise description of the procedure are given. Limited information on results is available, but suggest that approximately 95% of patients will get immediate relief of their pain with a median duration of pain estimated between 20 and 28 months. As many as 20% of patients may remain pain free and off medication at 5 years. Serious complications are rare but include meningitis, hemorrhage, extensive facial dysesthesia or analgesia and cranial nerve dysfunction.

INTRODUCTION

Balloon compression rhizotomy has become an important part of the surgeon's armamentarium for the management of trigeminal neuralgia. Based on the initial ganglion decompression operation of Taarnhoj (Taarnhoj, 1952) and subsequent interpretation by Shelden (Shelden, Pudenz, Freshwater, & Crue, 1955) and others (cited in Mullan & Lichtor (Mullan & Lichtor, 1983)) that ganglion compression was more effective than decompression, Mullan & Lichtor (1983) introduced it as a percutaneous alternative to open trigeminal ganglion compression. The procedure was repopularized by Mullan & Brown (Mullan & Brown, 1996) and Brown and

DOI: 10.4018/978-1-5225-5349-6.ch009

Pilitsis (Brown & Pilitsis, 2005). It has replaced glycerol injection in the author's practice because it is quicker and easier on patient and surgeon. The author still regards radiofrequency rhizotomy as the preferred percutaneous technique, but in certain circumstances balloon rhizotomy has advantages over radiofrequency rhizotomy and provides outcomes that appear to be better than those obtained with stereotactic radiosurgery.

SURGICAL PROCEDURE

We originally performed the procedure using the Mullan Trigeminal Ganglion Microcompression Set (Cook Medical LLC., P.O. Box 4195 Bloomington, IN 47402-4195). This set is no longer commercially available. We have combined a number of commercially available instruments and supplies to make a usable kit for the procedure (Lim, Ladd, Grande, & Haines, 2017).

The operation is done under general anesthesia. The patient is positioned supine with the neck extended to facilitate modified submento-vertex fluoroscopic views to identify the foramen ovale. Brown and Pilitsis (2005) recommend placing an external pacemaker prior to starting the procedure in the event that trigeminal compression produces asystole. In our experience, with appropriate cholinergic blockade we have never had to use the pacemaker.

The procedure can be done in an operating room, procedure room or imaging facility so long as biplane fluoroscopy is available for guiding the placement of the needle and monitoring balloon inflation shape. We have preferred to use the operating room. One c-arm fluoroscope is positioned for a true lateral image of the skull base (planum spenoidale, sella turcica and clivus) and one for a modified submento-vertex view of the foramen ovale. The surgeon stands on the side of the patient's pain (and therefore the side of needle placement). The base of the lateral fluoroscope should be opposite the surgeon.

The balloon catheter is prepared by filling it with contrast that is approved for intrathecal use (in case the balloon ruptures). The appropriate depth of passage of the balloon catheter through the cannula is determined visually, fixed by a friction adapter and measurements made so that depth can be confirmed after the passage of the balloon catheter.

Various external landmarks are used to guide the initial placement of cannula and should be marked before draping. The needle puncture site is generally 2.5 cm lateral to the oral fissure. The landmarks of 3 cm anterior to the external auditory meatus along the inferior edge of the zygomatic process and the midpupillary line are generally attributed to Hartel (Abdennebi & Guenane, 2014). With good success, we have used the "upside-down ventriculostomy" landmarks of half the distance from the external auditory canal to the lateral canthus of the eye and the midpupillary line.

In either case, the skin is sterilely prepped and the insertion site puncture with a large gauge needle or fine blade. The 11 gauge cannula is passed through the entry point toward the foramen ovale. The surgeon places one finger in the oral cavity during the initial passage to be alerted to penetration of the oral cavity which should result in discarding the contaminated cannula and starting over. After the initial placement to the skull base, gloves are changed and AP and lateral fluoroscopic images obtained. The trajectory is adjusted to place the tip of the cannula in the foramen ovale.

A stylet is passed through the cannula to make pathway for the balloon catheter. Depth and position of the stylet penetration is monitored fluoroscopically. Once satisfactory position is obtained (the balloon typically rests with its proximal edge at the clival line) the stylet is removed and replaced with the balloon catheter. The inflation syringe is attached.

The balloon is gradually inflated, watching the pressure and checking intermittently with the lateral fluoroscope to see the shape of the inflated balloon. A balloon that is too proximal with demonstrate rapid pressure rise with little visible inflation. A balloon that is too distal will not rise to the desired pressure and will take on a spherical shape distant from the clivus.

Ideal inflation will produce a "pear shaped" balloon with the small extrusion at the distal tip of the balloon thought to be balloon protruding through the opening to Meckel's cave. The balloon should be inflated to 1.4 atmospheres. We typically hold inflation for 90 seconds, although adjustments depending on prior procedures may be done in recurrent trigeminal neuralgia.

Once the inflation is complete, the balloon is deflated to negative pressure, the complete emptying of the balloon is confirmed fluoroscopically and balloon catheter and cannula are removed together. The balloon should not be pulled back with the cannula in place as the currently available cannulae are not designed to prevent shearing of the balloon or catheter.

A bandaid is applied to the puncture site.

EXPECTED OUTCOMES

It is generally acknowledged that "There is either no, or very low quality, evidence for most neurosurgical procedures for the treatment of trigeminal neuralgia because of the poor quality of the trials." (Zakrzewska & Akram, 2011). Therefore, estimates of frequency and duration of pain relief are based on observational (usually case series) reports. The authors have reviewed such reports looking for Kaplan-Meier estimates of the duration of pain relief as a marker of sufficient sample size to allow for meaningful follow-up and appropriate reporting of the time sensitive outcome of pain relief. The non-Kaplan-Meier reports cited by Wang, et. al. (Wang, Bender, & Bettegowda, 2016) have been reviewed for additional estimates of pain relief. Only reports in which the reported outcome of "pain free off medication" can be determined are included.

As can be seen from the Tables 1 and 2, there is limited information and substantial variation between reported series of patients. Initial relief ranges from

Table 1. Pain relief in studies reporting Kaplan-Meier estimates of duration of relief

Author	Initial Pain Relief	Median Duration	N	Endpoint*
(Bergenheim, Asplund, & Linderoth, 2013)	90%	28 months	100	~18% pain free at 8 years
Brown & Pilitsis 2005	92%	Not reached	56	~85% pain free at 28 months
(Chen, Tu, & Lee, 2012)	93.8%	Not reached	122	~60% pain free at 10 years
(Kouzounias, Lind, Schechtmann, Winter, & Linderoth, 2010)	85%	21 months	66	~22% pain free at 4 years
(Teo & Suttner, 2015)	~95%	20 months	83	~18% pain free at 10 years

* Endpoint estimated from Kaplan Meier graphic displays in publication.

Note: in several of these studies the median duration of relief reported in the text did not correspond to the estimated median time to recurrence from the published Kaplan-Meier graph.

Table 2. Pain relief in studies not reporting Kaplan-Meier estimates of duration of relief

Author	Initial Pain Relief	Median Duration	N	Endpoint*
(Fraioli, Esposito, Guidetti, Cruccu, & Manfredi, 1989)	89.9%	Not stated	159	Not available
(Lichtor & Mullan, 1990)	100%	Not stated	100	20% pain free at 5 years
(Lobato, Rivas, Sarabia, & Lamas, 1990)	100%	Not stated	144	Not available
(Brown, Mcdaniel, Weaver, Burchiel, & Young, 1993)	94%	Not stated	50	Not available
(Correa & Teixeira, 1998)	90%	Not stated	158	8.2% pain free at 3 years
(Skirving & Dan, 2001)	99%	Not stated	496	19.2% pain free at 5 years
(Omeis, Smith, Kim, & Murali, 2008)	83%	Not stated	29	Not available
Abdennebi & Guenane 2014	92.7%	Not stated	901	Not available

Note: Studies identified in Table 1 of Wang, et. al. (2016).

83 to 100 percent with most reports near 95 percent. Relief for 5 – 10 years after the procedure ranges from 18 to 60 percent with most reports near 20 percent. The median duration of relief ranges from 20 to 28 months.

The comments of Zakrzewska & Akram (2011) cited above apply and the quality of the published data do not allow more detailed study of the reports to strengthen the reliability of these estimates.

Complications

Complications are well summarized in Bergenheim, et. al. (2013) and Wang, et. al. (2016). A brief catalogue of concerns follows:

- **Bradycardia:** In early reports, some patients experienced severe bradycardia or even cardia arrest at the time of needle insertion or balloon inflation. The authors agree with the recommendation of Bergenheim, et. al. (2013) that appropriate analgesia and anticholinergic premedication (they recommend remifentanil and atropine) reduces the risk of this complication to very low levels.
- **Hemorrhage:**
    - Cheek hematomas are relatively common but rarely significant. Their frequency may be reduced by compression of the puncture site at the end of the procedure.
    - Subdural, subarachnoid and intraparenchymal hemorrhage have been reported. These are thought to be related to improper needle placement.
    - Carotid cavernous fistula has been reported.
- **Nerve Dysfunction:**
    - While facial numbness is expected in most patients, disabling facial dysesthesia or anesthesia should be very unusual. However, the reports in the literature onthis subject are quite varied.
    - Masseter weakness is occasionally seen and usually self-limited.
    - Diplopia is occasionally reported.
- **Infection:** Meningitis is reported in up to 1 percent of patients in large series. Care to avoid puncture of the oral mucosa is an important preventive measure.
- **Death:** Death has been reported but is extremely unusual.

RECOMMENDATIONS

Percutaneous balloon compression trigeminal rhizotomy has a high rate of initial success, provides most patients 1.5 to 2 years of pain relief and can readily be repeated. The results are similar to other percutaneous procedures for trigeminal neuralgia. Appropriate comparative trials do not exist. It is the author's impression that patients are most likely to get long relief from the radiofrequency trigeminal rhizotomy with the balloon rhizotomy the next most effective in producing long duration of relief. In the authors' experience, glycerol rhizotomy appears to give results similar to balloon rhizotomy. Balloon rhizotomy, however, has the advantages of not requiring the assistance of the patient (as is true for radiofrequency rhizotomy) and not having the risk of a toxic agent entering the CSF circulation around the brainstem (as can happen with glycerol rhizotomy) and minimizing patient discomfort by being done under general anesthesia. In addition, the degree of expected facial numbness is low making corneal anesthesia and its attendant risks very unlikely in patients with first division pain.

Reliable reports of patients achieving freedom from pain without requiring medication following stereotactic radiosurgery for trigeminal neuralgia suggest that this goal is achieved in about 55 – 60 percent of patients, a figure which is substantially lower that the author achieves with either balloon or radiofrequency rhizotomy.

For these reasons, for patients in whom microvascular decompression is determined not to be appropriate, the authors first choice of percutaneous procedure is radiofrequency rhizotomy. There are four specific circumstances when balloon compression rhizotomy is chosen:

- **V1 (First Division) Pain:** For these patients the likelihood of corneal anesthesia is less with balloon rhizotomy
- **Inability to Cooperate With the Surgeon During the Procedure:**
    - Patients who do not speak the language of the surgeon
    - Patients with advanced multiple sclerosis and cognitive involvement
    - Patients with dementia
    - Patients on large doses of medication that, when combined with the short acting anesthetics required for radiofrequency or glycerol rhizotomy are judged to be unlikely to participate reliably
- Patients unwilling to undergo the procedure with local anesthesia and transient anesthetics.
- Patients in whom other procedures have failed.

Balloon compression rhizotomy is a useful addition to the armamentarium of physicians who treat patients with trigeminal neuralgia. No single procedure can manage all trigeminal neuralgia patients and the comprehensive trigeminal neuraglia treatment program will offer several different procedures that can be tailored to patient-specific needs. It is a surgical procedure with infrequent serious complications when done carefully, but the serious complications can require urgent neurosurgical intervention and therefore this procedure should be done by neurosurgeons or procedural specialists who are part of a team with immediately available neurosurgical backup.

REFERENCES

Abdennebi, B., & Guenane, L. (2014). Technical considerations and outcome assessment in retrogasserian balloon compression for treatment of trigeminal neuralgia. Series of 901 patients. *Surgical Neurology International*, *5*(1), 118. doi:10.4103/2152-7806.137838 PMID:25101213

Bergenheim, A. T., Asplund, P., & Linderoth, B. (2013). Percutaneous Retrogasserian Balloon Compression for Trigeminal Neuralgia: Review of Critical Technical Details and Outcomes. *World Neurosurgery*, *79*(2), 359–368. doi:10.1016/j.wneu.2012.03.014 PMID:22480980

Brown, J. A., Mcdaniel, M. D., Weaver, M. T., Burchiel, K. J., & Young, R. F. (1993). Percutaneous Trigeminal Nerve Compression for Treatment of Trigeminal Neuralgia - Results in 50 Patients. *Neurosurgery*, *32*(4), 570–573. doi:10.1227/00006123-199304000-00012 PMID:7682678

Brown, J. A., & Pilitsis, J. G. (2005). Percutaneous balloon compression for trigeminal neuralgia: Reduced dysesthesias and masseter weakness using intraluminal compression pressure monitoring in a consecutive series of 56 patients. *Neurosurgery*, *57*(2), 414–414. doi:10.1093/neurosurgery/57.2.414a

Chen, J. F., Tu, P. H., & Lee, S. T. (2012). Repeated Percutaneous Balloon Compression for Recurrent Trigeminal Neuralgia: A Long-Term Study. *World Neurosurgery*, *77*(2), 352–356. doi:10.1016/j.wneu.2011.06.013 PMID:22120364

Correa, C. F., & Teixeira, M. J. (1998). Balloon compression of the Gasserian ganglion for the treatment of trigeminal neuralgia. *Stereotactic and Functional Neurosurgery*, *71*(2), 83–89. doi:10.1159/000029651 PMID:10087472

Fraioli, B., Esposito, V., Guidetti, B., Cruccu, G., & Manfredi, M. (1989). Treatment of Trigeminal Neuralgia by Thermocoagulation, Glycerolization, and Percutaneous Compression of the Gasserian Ganglion and or Retrogasserian Rootlets - Long-Term Results and Therapeutic Protocol. *Neurosurgery*, *24*(2), 239–245. doi:10.1227/00006123-198902000-00014 PMID:2783993

Kouzounias, K., Lind, G., Schechtmann, G., Winter, J., & Linderoth, B. (2010). Comparison of percutaneous balloon compression and glycerol rhizotomy for the treatment of trigeminal neuralgia. *Journal of Neurosurgery*, *113*(3), 486–492. doi:10.3171/2010.1.JNS091106 PMID:20187700

Lichtor, T., & Mullan, J. F. (1990). A 10-Year Follow-up Review of Percutaneous Microcompression of the Trigeminal Ganglion. *Journal of Neurosurgery*, *72*(1), 49–54. doi:10.3171/jns.1990.72.1.0049 PMID:2294184

Lim, J. J., Ladd, B. M., Grande, A. W., & Haines, S. J. (2017). Letter: Prepackaged Instrument Kit for Percutaneous Balloon Compression Rhizotomy for the Treatment of Trigeminal Neuralgia: Improvised Solution for an Unexpected National Supply Shortage. *Operative Neurosurgery*, *13*(4), E19–E20. doi:10.1093/ons/opx061 PMID:28838119

Lobato, R. D., Rivas, J. J., Sarabia, R., & Lamas, E. (1990). Percutaneous Microcompression of the Gasserian Ganglion for Trigeminal Neuralgia. *Journal of Neurosurgery*, *72*(4), 546–553. doi:10.3171/jns.1990.72.4.0546 PMID:2319312

Mullan, S., & Brown, J. A. (1996). Trigeminal neuralgia. *Neurosurgery Quarterly*, *6*(4), 267–288. doi:10.1097/00013414-199612000-00003

Mullan, S., & Lichtor, T. (1983). Percutaneous microcompression of the trigeminal ganglion for trigeminal neuralgia. *Journal of Neurosurgery*, *59*(6), 1007–1012. doi:10.3171/jns.1983.59.6.1007 PMID:6631493

Omeis, I., Smith, D., Kim, S., & Murali, R. (2008). Percutaneous balloon compression for the treatment of recurrent trigeminal neuralgia: Long-term outcome in 29 patients. *Stereotactic and Functional Neurosurgery*, *86*(4), 259–265. doi:10.1159/000138770 PMID:18552523

Shelden, C. H., Pudenz, R. H., Freshwater, D. B., & Crue, B. L. (1955). Compression rather than decompression for trigeminal neuralgia. *Journal of Neurosurgery*, *12*(2), 123–126. doi:10.3171/jns.1955.12.2.0123 PMID:14368343

Skirving, D. J., & Dan, N. G. (2001). A 20-year review of percutaneous balloon compression of the trigeminal ganglion. *Journal of Neurosurgery*, *94*(6), 913–917. doi:10.3171/jns.2001.94.6.0913 PMID:11409519

Taarnhoj, P. (1952). Decompression of the trigeminal root and the posterior part of the ganglion as treatment in trigeminal neuralgia; preliminary communication. *Journal of Neurosurgery*, *9*(3), 288–290. doi:10.3171/jns.1952.9.3.0288 PMID:14939059

Teo, M. K., & Suttner, N. J. (2015). Effective management of lower divisional pain in trigeminal neuralgia using balloon traction. *British Journal of Neurosurgery*, *29*(3), 343–346. doi:10.3109/02688697.2014.990419 PMID:25496298

Wang, J. Y., Bender, M. T., & Bettegowda, C. (2016). Percutaneous Procedures for the Treatment of Trigeminal Neuralgia. *Neurosurgery Clinics of North America*, *27*(3), 277–295. doi:10.1016/j.nec.2016.02.005 PMID:27324995

Zakrzewska, J. M., & Akram, H. (2011). Neurosurgical interventions for the treatment of classical trigeminal neuralgia. *Cochrane Database of Systematic Reviews*, (9): CD007312. doi:10.1002/14651858.CD007312.pub2 PMID:21901707

Chapter 10
Radiosurgery for Trigeminal Neuralgia

Daivik B. Vyas
Stanford School of Medicine, USA

Eric S. Sussman
Stanford School of Medicine, USA

Lily H. Kim
Stanford School of Medicine, USA

Arjun V. Pendharkar
Stanford School of Medicine, USA

Allen Ho
Stanford University, USA

Steven Chang
Stanford University, USA

ABSTRACT

Trigeminal neuralgia is a debilitating neuropathic condition characterized by recurrent paroxysms of shock-like pain across the distribution of the trigeminal nerve, often brought on by innocuous stimuli. Available therapies presently include symptomatic management using anti-convulsant drugs and invasive surgical procedures to target the pathogenic drivers of disease or ablate the trigeminal nerve. Radiosurgery is a treatment modality that offers a minimally invasive, low-risk alternative that has promising clinical utility in the management of refractory trigeminal neuralgia. Radiosurgical approaches like Gamma Knife (GKS) and Cyberknife (CK) utilize image-guided, algorithm-defined dose contouring to disrupt pathogenic pain signaling by delivering targeted amounts of radiation along different points on the trigeminal nerve. This chapter reviews the structure of radiotherapy paradigms, treatment protocol, major outcomes, associated risks, relative clinical utility, and areas of further research that underlie the use of CK and GKS in managing trigeminal neuralgia.

DOI: 10.4018/978-1-5225-5349-6.ch010

INTRODUCTION

Trigeminal neuralgia (TN) is a rare neurological condition characterized by recurrent unilateral paroxysms of electric shock-like pain across the distribution of the trigeminal nerve. The characteristic, stabbing pain of TN presents with maximal intensity at symptom onset and is often brought on by identifiable, innocuous stimuli such as facial touch, brushing, or chewing. Episodes of pain may last up to two minutes, and are followed by a refractory period in which pain symptoms are no longer triggered. Similarly, while the episodes of pain most often occur unilaterally, rare bilateral episodes may occur; however, the pain sensation never crosses to the opposite side. Episodes of trigeminal neuropathic pain occur more frequently along the maxillary (V2) and mandibular (V3) divisions of the trigeminal nerve, though the ophthalmic (V1) division may still be affected.

Epidemiologically, trigeminal neuralgia is a rare disorder. The annual incidence rate is estimated to be between 4-13/100,000/year. (Macdonald, Cockerell, Sander, & Shorvon, 2000; Koopman et al., 2009; Katusic, Beard, Bergstralh, & Kurland, 1990) Incidence rates increase significantly with age in both men and women, with the average of onset being between 50-53 years old. (Maarbjerg, Gozalov, Olesen, & Bendtsen, 2014). Disease rates are found to be significantly higher in women than in men (Katusic et al., 1990). The majority of trigeminal neuralgia cases are found to be idiopathic; however, individual reports of familial trigeminal neuralgia have been reported. (Smyth, Greenough, & Stommel, 2003; Fleetwood, Innes, Hansen, & Steinberg, 2001)

Based on its clinical presentation and the case history, trigeminal neuralgia may be classified as *classical trigeminal neuralgia* or as *classical trigeminal neuralgia with concomitant persistent facial pain* (formerly known as *atypical trigeminal neuralgia*). (Headache Classification Committee of the International Headache Society [IHS], 2013) The presentation of classical TN, as described above, is characterized by bouts of lancinating pain lasting for up to two minutes and occurring along the distributions of V1-V3. However, patients with this form of TN do not feel pain in between their recurrent paroxysms. In contrast, patients with the atypical variant of TN feel a persistent pain along the distribution of V1-V3 in between episodes, albeit of a lesser intensity. In these cases, the pain is qualitatively different and is often characterized as burning or tingling rather than as shock-like. Electrophysiological evidence suggests that while microvascular compression may contribute to the etiology, central sensitization that results in over-activation of nociceptive signaling may produce the characteristic persistent facial pain seen in this atypical form. (Obermann et al., 2007) Diagnostically, however, there remains significant overlap between the typical and atypical variants of classical trigeminal neuralgia. The general criteria for a diagnosis of classical trigeminal neuralgia include a minimum of three episodes of pain occurring without radiation along the distribution of the trigeminal nerve. Characteristically, this pain must fulfill three of the four following criteria: 1) occur in paroxysms; 2) be of severe intensity; 3) be lancinating or stabbing in quality; or, 4) be brought on by innocuous stimuli.

In addition to its symptomatic profile, trigeminal neuralgia may be classified as primary or secondary according to its etiology. For the primary, or classical, form of trigeminal neuralgia, the predominant model of pathogenesis involves compression of the nerve root by an aberrant vascular loop. As first described by the American neurosurgeon Walter Dandy (1934), these anatomic variations in cerebral vasculature can alter the course and integrity of the trigeminal nerve by direct indentation, elevation, bending, or attachment to the nerve root. Persistent mechanical disruption due to pulsatile blood flow at the site of compression may drive damage to nerve fibers at a cellular level. On pathology, vascular compression has been shown to cause focal demyelination and the apposition of adjacent nerve fibers without any astrocytic intervention. (Hilton, Love, Gradidge, & Coakham, 1994) In this process of central demyelination, neighboring axons may interact via ephaptic transmission to generate ectopic potentials along parallel but separate sensory information streams, such as between the ascending tracts that carry signals for tactile sensation and pain. (Smith & McDonald, 1980; 1999) Anatomically, neurovascular compression has found to occur because of aberrance by arteries, veins, or both. This structural abnormality most often occurs in the superior cerebellar artery, though compression has also been shown to occur by way of cerebral veins, as well as the anterior inferior cerebellar, basilar, and posterior cerebellar arteries. (Hamlyn & King, 1992; Yoshino et al., 2003; Barker, Jannetta, Bissonette, Larkins, & Jho, 1996)

In contrast to this mechanism of injury, the etiology of secondary trigeminal neuropathy involves a clinically-discernible disease state. According to IHS criteria, pain along the trigeminal distribution can be attributed to acute infection or post-herpetic injury by Herpes zoster, trauma, multiple sclerosis lesions, or neoplasia at the level of CN V. It is to note that in the most recent IHS criteria, the term "secondary trigeminal neuralgia" is not used; rather, the pain phenotype is described as a painful trigeminal neuropathy to include forms of trigeminal pain resulting from processes like post-herpetic neuralgia. While this scheme encompasses a wide array of possible mechanisms, the broader symptomatic profiles included as part of this category reduce the distinction of secondary trigeminal neuralgia as a unique pain syndrome. To account for this, alternative classification criteria have been proposed by Cruccu et al. (2016) to maintain the distinction of secondary trigeminal neuralgia as phenotypically different from secondary neuropathies, as well as to provide diagnostic grading of TN-related pain for improved management.

At present, trigeminal neuralgia may be managed using a variety of pharmacological and surgical treatment options. The first-line therapy for pain management in trigeminal neuralgia is medical treatment using the anti-convulsant drug carbamazepine because of its high rate of success in achieving pain control (Gronseth et al., 2008). Other drugs that are indicated for pain control include oxcarbazepine, baclofen, lamotrigine, and pimozide. While anti-epileptic drugs such as phenytoin, gabapentin, clonazepam, and valproate are also used in pain management and show therapeutic benefit, their clinical efficacy is not sufficiently known to recommend or refuse their use in treatment guidelines. Generally, while medical therapy has been shown to be efficacious at pain management, its role is restricted by the exclusively symptomatic focus of treatment, as well as by an overall decrease in efficacy over the long-run.

For patients that are refractory to medical treatment, surgical intervention using open and percutaneous neurosurgical procedures is indicated. Microvascular decompression (MVD) is commonly used and, as eponymously suggested, involves the separation of the trigeminal nerve root from a compressive vascular aberrant. In a study of 1185 patients over a 20-year period, MVD demonstrated immediate post-operative relief in 82% of patients, with one-year complete relief rates of 75% and ten-year complete relief in 64% of patients. 16% of patients showed immediate partial relief, with a one-year and ten-year partial relief outcomes of 9% and 4%, respectively. (Barker et al., 1996) Although MVD does offer a robust, long-term pain-free outcome, it has a complication profile that includes CSF leak, cranial neuropathy, infection, DVT, and pulmonary embolism. (Gronseth et al., 2008) While MVD is designed to target the pathogenic drivers of trigeminal neuralgia, percutaneous procedures utilize minimally invasive ablation techniques to lesion the trigeminal nerve. These ablative techniques utilize thermal, chemical, and mechanical mechanisms to damage sensory fibers in the trigeminal nerve, and include techniques such as radiofrequency rhizotomy, glycerol rhizotomy, and percutaneous balloon compression. Collectively, these techniques achieve pain relief in over 90% of cases, however long-term follow-up often shows high rates of recurrence at one-year and five-year follow-ups. (Spina, Mortini, Alemanno, Houdayer, & Iannacone, 2017) Additionally, these percutaneous techniques may result in complications such as corneal disturbance, keratitis, dysesthesia, and anesthesia dolorosa. Additional techniques used for pain management in trigeminal neuralgia include neuromodulation, subdermal analgesia, cryotherapy, and peripheral neurectomy (for review, see Spina et al., 2017).

In addition to medical and invasive procedures, stereotactic radiosurgery has been increasingly studied and applied for pain management in trigeminal neuralgia. Beginning with Hermann Moritz Gocht in the late 19th century, the use of ionizing radiation was increasingly recognized as a potential treatment modality for managing neuropathic pain (Artico, De Caro, Fraioli, & Giuffrè, 1997). Interest in the use of radiosurgery for pain management slowly declined as attention was increasingly paid to the role of pharmacotherapies for managing pain and to the development of safer neurosurgical techniques. Similarly, research into the mechanisms of ionizing radiation began revealing the damage that it could incur (Lettmaier, 2014). The interest in radiosurgery gained traction in the latter half of the 20th century, as new methods of radiosurgery were utilized and their clinical outcomes better defined. In 1951, the Swedish neurosurgeon Lars Lekell utilized an orthovoltage x-ray beam to perform the first radiosurgery on a patient with trigeminal neuralgia (Leksell, 1951). In 1971, Leksell would go on to report that patients who had undergone gamma-wave radiosurgery using a stereotactic external-beam apparatus in 1953 demonstrated pain-free resolution of trigeminal neuralgia nearly two decades later. (Leksell, 1971) The Leksell Gamma Knife began the widespread popularization of using Gamma Knife surgery (GKS) in the management of trigeminal neuralgia. Then, in the 1990s, American neurosurgeon John R. Adler Jr. and his group would report the development and preliminary results of the CyberKnife (CK)–a frameless, image-guided stereotactic apparatus that delivered linear accelerator-derived radiation to targets. (Adler et al., 1997) Since then, radiosurgery has become a mainstay treatment for trigeminal neuralgia, and research at present focuses on refining treatment parameters and characterizing the outcomes of larger and more long-term case series.

In comparison to other therapeutic methods, stereotactic radiosurgery offers a few key advantages. The intended goal of radiosurgical treatment is to address the cause of pain by directly lesioning the nerve target that mediates pain signaling. Compared to medical therapy, whose action and efficacy is directly limited by the amount of drug in circulation at any given time, radiosurgery addresses non-symptomatic factors to offer the possibility of a longer duration of pain-relief. When compared to invasive surgery, radiosurgery offers the advantage of minimally-invasive approach and same-day discharge, reducing the risk of complications. Furthermore, radiosurgery offers an additional treatment modality in cases where trigeminal neuralgia is refractory to medication, surgery, or both. While being the least invasive procedural approach to TN management, radiosurgery also allows the possibility of being repeated in cases where initial treatment does not elicit an effective response. Finally, radiation therapy can provide pain management for candidates where invasive approaches are contraindicated, as in the case of elderly patients and those with significant medical comorbidities.

The general outcomes of radiosurgery demonstrate it is a favorable treatment mechanism, with pain-relief beginning shortly after treatment and remaining at high rates through short-term follow-up. The median latency of pain relief onset has been consistently reported as beginning between 1 to 2 months following treatment. (Kondziolka et al., 2011; Maesawa et al., 2001; Règis et al., 2016; Young, Shivazad, Kryscio, St. Clair, & Bush, 2013; Smith et al., 2011) Clinical outcomes from these studies generally illustrate an increasing rates of pain relief from treatment to first follow-up, with higher radiation doses corresponding to better clinical outcomes. However, the overall pain-free rate begins to decrease over time, with rates of recurrence ranging from 34-45%. (Wolf & Kondziolka, 2016) Side effects typically seen after radiosurgery for trigeminal neuralgia are also dose-dependent, and include sensory dysfunction of the trigeminal nerve, dysesthesia, numbness, reduced corneal reflex masticator weakness, diplopia, and–very rarely–anesthesia dolorosa.

POSSIBLE MECHANISM OF ACTION

At present, the mechanism by which radiosurgery elicits its clinically-evident effects remains largely unknown. Through its controlled lesioning of only sections of the trigeminal nerve root, radiosurgery can induce anatomic changes that are evident on histology. In a study of rhesus monkeys that underwent single- and double-point trigeminal nerve irradiation at clinical dosages (60-100 Gy), examination of the nerve tissue revealed a dose-dependent demyelination, axonal degeneration, fragmentation, and structural derangement. (Zhao, Yang, Jiang, Zheng, & Zhang, 2010) Similarly, in a study examining radiobiological changes in two baboons that underwent single isocenter GKS, histology revealed focal axonal degeneration impacting large and small myelinated and unmyelinated axons. (Kondziolka, et al., 2000) In both studies, dosages of 100 Gy elicited nerve necrosis. From this evidence, it may be theorized that the focal axonal breakdown brought on by dose targeting results in a selective loss of afferent signal transmission. Additionally, while Obermann et al. (2007) have previously described the susceptibility of A-delta nociceptive fibers to demyelination in the context of vascular compression, neither of the present studies reveals fiber-specific radiation effects.

In addition to physical damage, radiosurgery may alter the pain signaling along the trigeminal nerve through changes in cellular electrophysiology. In an in vitro study examining the effects of radiation on ionic conductance, the delivery of ionizing radiation induced significant reductions in peak sodium current after an 800-1000 second post-treatment delay; no such effects were seen on potassium currents. (Schwarz & Fox,1979) Conceptually, this reduction in sodium current is suggested to have stabilized the membrane and reduced the excitability and signal transmission of neurons. However, it is important to note that these experiments took place at dosages higher than the clinical range, and were performed as patch-clamp recordings on dissected sciatic nerve fibers from frogs. Given endogenous nerve composition differences, as well as pathological demyelination from vascular compression, patient trigeminal nerves may be more susceptible to conductance changes at lower doses, though physiological evidence is needed. (Gorgulho,

2012) Additionally, while pain relief onset typically begins one to four months after treatment, the range of latencies has been reported anywhere from between immediately post-treatment (i.e. 1 day) to 6 months later. (Smith et al., 2011; Régis et al., 2016) This range of responses may overlie individual genetic or physiological variations in factors like membrane composition, myelination, or axonal integrity that may contribute to radiation efficacy and response.

DEFINING TARGETS AND DOSE DEFINITION

Target and dose definition in stereotactic radiosurgery can be characterized according to two primary goals: 1) optimization of dose coverage along pathologically-relevant structures (i.e. maximal dose coverage along the trigeminal nerve), and 2) minimization of non-target injury and side effects (i.e. avoiding non-trigeminal brainstem or cerebral structures). To that end, radiosurgery planning utilizes information about structural anatomy, tissue heterogeneity, radiation beam properties, and apparatus parameters to define the ideal target and dose parameters for each patient.

The process of defining the target site that will receive maximum radiation draws upon information from general neuroanatomy and patient-specific, image-guided target delineation. Early studies using GKS to target the Gasserian ganglion did not show consistent results, though inaccuracies in target localization, patient stabilization, and dose volume may have contributed to these poorer outcomes. (Lindquist, Kihlström, & Hellstrand, 1991) In its present state, radiosurgery for trigeminal neuralgia has a reproducible set of radiosurgical parameters that have been consistently shown to elicit clinically significant pain-free states by targeting the proximal trigeminal nerve, with high-dose radiation (70-90 Gy). From a microanatomic perspective, this region of the trigeminal nerve, located an average 2.55 mm from the root entry zone (REZ), is the site of the peripheral-central myelin transition (Peker, Kurtaya, Uzün, & Pamir, 2006). While it is conceptually suggested that this transition zone is the site of greatest radiosensitivity, recent evidence suggests that the distance of dose delivery from REZ is not associated with significant pain relief outcomes (Sharim et al., 2017). Given the variability of target definition methodologies, as well as the dose-dependent nature of pain response, the optimal target-dose relationship for radiosurgery requires further refinement.

GKS and CK both utilize pre-treatment imaging from CT and MRI to best localize portions of the trigeminal nerve that will receive the highest dose of radiation, while minimizing the volume of non-target neural structures that are irradiated. (Figure 1) GKS may utilize CT or T2-weighted fast spin echo MRI for targeting and dose contouring. While evidence regarding the relationship between pre-treatment image quality and clinical outcome is scarce, a study of 112 patients

Figure 1. CyberKnife Planning for Trigeminal Neuralgia. (Above) 3-dimensional treatment plan with collimated radiation beam geometry for CyberKnife therapy for trigeminal neuralgia. (Below) Sample CyberKnife contoured treatment plan for trigeminal neuralgia around trigeminal nerve with sparing of brainstem and optic nerve.

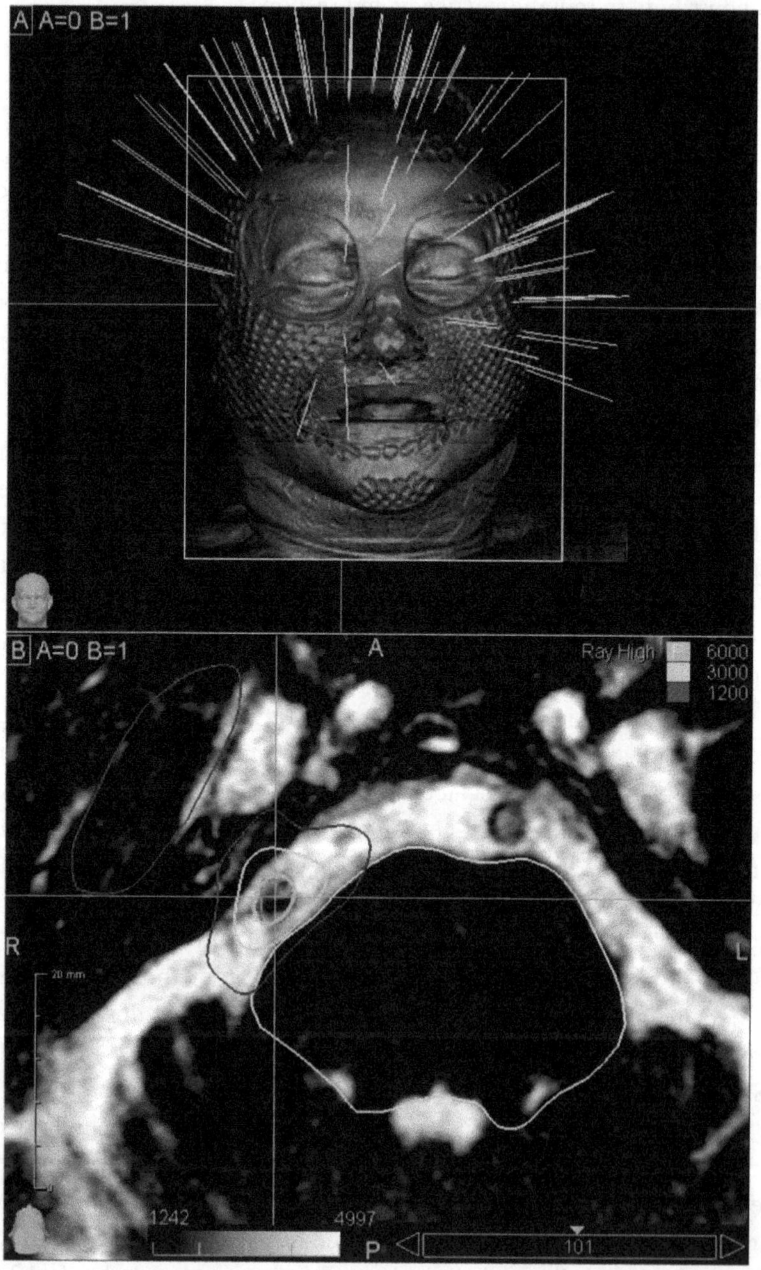

with trigeminal neuralgia undergoing GKS finds no correlation between MRI imaging quality, defined according to the visualization of the pre-pontine trigeminal nerve, and treatment response. (Cheuk et al., 2004) In the case of CK, pre-treatment CT is required, however, the use of fused T2 weighted MRI-CT images for treatment planning has become increasingly common. (Adler et al., 2009; Fariselli et al., 2009) The utilization of three-dimensional Fourier transformations during MR imaging through a methodology known as Constructive Interference in Steady State (CISS) or Fast Imaging Employing Steady State (FIESTA) has been shown to provide robust, high-resolution distinction between cranial nerves and CSF. (Casselman et al., 1993) In the context of trigeminal neuralgia, magnetic resonance FIESTA has shown excellent visualization of the trigeminal root entry zone, surrounding vasculature, and divisions of the trigeminal nerve in Meckel's cave, highlighting its clinical utility in structural mapping. (Chávez et al., 2005)

After obtaining imaging, an apparatus-specific software packages utilizes contouring algorithms to define prescription dose strength for user-defined target and non-target regions. In GKS, a planning platform (GammaPlan) is utilized for defining the treatment isocenter, which is the spatial point through which the central radiation beam passes. Additionally, this provides an opportunity for contouring calculated dose distributions around anatomical structures, and defining the isodose lines that signify the relative percentage strength of radiation dose that will be delivered within each contour. Through this, dose constraints may be placed and dose distribution optimized using a grid-based method of beam placement. Similarly, through this platform, sector blocking and isocenter weighting may be performed to restrict radiation delivery on or near critical structures. For Cyberknife, the treatment platform (Multiplan) operates in a similar fashion, but with the added capability of modulating radiation delivery through non-isocentric beams.

For both radiosurgical modalities, algorithms are utilized for calculation of dose distribution. Traditionally, for GKS, dose calculation has utilized manual, measurement-based skull definition and a tissue maximum ratio (TMR) algorithm that assumes homogeneous density in target tissue equivalent to that of water. Given the inherent error associated with this assumption, though, the most recent version of the GammaPlan software features two new algorithms sets (Rojas-Villabona, Kitchen, & Paddick, 2016). In the first, known as TMR 10, utilized Monte Carlo simulations on input data to refine calculated dosages. Second, the software introduces a convolution algorithm that accounts for tissue heterogeneity by using material densities derived from CT imaging; the CT image-based approach is also utilized for automatic skull definition. Xu et al. (2015) conducted a retrospective comparison of the two treatment algorithms on a sample of 65 patients who underwent radiosurgery for trigeminal neuralgia. While the CT-based skull definition method may provide a more accurate reproduction of the skull surface, on comparison the two methods show a relatively small dosimetric difference of less than 0.3 Gy. However, when comparing the TMR 10 and the convolution dose calculations, when controlling for image-based skull definition, treatment time was on average 8.4% higher for the convolution method. These findings suggest the possibility of underdosing in the TMR 10 algorithm and promotes the clinical utility of the convolution method, especially in cases of radiosurgery near bone-tissue interfaces of heterogeneous density, such as at the level of the pontine brain stem and skull base.

In the case of Cyberknife two primary dose calculation algorithms have been utilized to treat trigeminal neuralgia: Ray-Tracing and Monte Carlo calculation. In the traditional Ray-Tracing method, the algorithm calculates required radiation dosage by determining the possible intersection points for a source ray (e.g. radiation beam) against target volumes, such as heterogeneous tissues, pathological structures, and radiation beam-modifiers. These determined intersection points are then used to calculate the ray depth, dose magnitude, and any attenuation of the dose that may occur along the path of the ray. (Siddon, 1985) Monte Carlo calculations utilize clinically-determined measurement data, including a central axis depth dose curve, dose profile at maximum dosage, and cone output factors, through a dual-source model to determine the radiation dosage. (Deng, Ma, Hai, & Nath, 2003)

A key distinction between the Ray-Tracing and Monte Carlo algorithms is the method of correction for tissue heterogeneity. In the Ray-tracing method, a water phantom is used to pre-measure beam data prior to treatment and tissue heterogeneity corrections are only made along the primary beam path. This method works well for relatively homogeneous structures such as the brain, however heterogeneous tissues may not have as much dose correction, resulting in possible dose overestimation. In contrast, the Monte Carlo algorithm reduces the discrepancy in tissue heterogeneity correction by using stochastic sampling and calculated particle interaction probabilities to determine the effective dose deposition in target tissue. (Sharma, Ott, Williams, & Dickow, 2010) Given these heterogeneous correction differences, the Monte Carlo algorithm is believed to be a more accurate method of dose calculation. In the case of trigeminal neuralgia, preliminary comparison of both calculation algorithms has shown prospective clinical utility for using the Monte Carlo approach. In a study of 10 patients that had dose calculation performed using both algorithms, the Monte Carlo algorithm determined a prescribed isodose line of 76-79%, relative to the 80% of Ray-Tracing. Additionally, the calculated volume of brainstem receiving 12 Gy and the conformity index were reported to be higher in Monte Carlo calculation. (Ho et al., 2012) Although the data suggest greater accuracy in dose delivery and volume calculations using the Monte Carlo approach, the clinical significance of these calculations remains uncertain and warrants further inquiry in larger patient samples.

Variable machine properties, which include factors such as total beam count, source-to-axis distance (SAD), aperture size, and beam weighting also contribute to the dose definition parameters. Depending on the model, Gamma Knife systems employ isocentric radiation delivery that focuses gamma radiation beams at a singular focal point. Isocenter weights may be adjusted to better localize delivery according to each patient's unique anatomy. Conventionally, the proximal trigeminal nerve is irradiated with a single 4-mm isocenter, though methodologies often incorporate methods of source plugging or sector blocking by using additional isocenters and location-specific radiation source plugs to lower the dose delivery to the brainstem by up to 40%. (Descovich et al., 2010; Li & Ma, 2004) Selective blocking at high dosages (90 Gy) has shown significantly higher mean doses delivered to the trigeminal nerve with a higher rate of therapeutic response, though this has been associated with increased incidence of trigeminal nerve dysfunction. (Massager et al., 2006) However, the increased dysfunction rate has not been reported in other experiments that utilized plugging to restrict brain stem dosages to less than 16 Gy. (Pan et al., 2010) Selective plugging approaches must be employed with discretion to restrict dose delivery to critical structures, while avoiding the possible risk of nerve dysfunction.

Unlike GKS, the Cyberknife apparatus allows for dose delivery in an isocentric or non-isocentric manner. Uniquely, the method of non-isocentric dose delivery allows for a more homogenous distribution of radiation dose across the target volume. Optimized parameters for the non-isocentric method of dose delivery have previously shown high rates of pain relief and decreased rates of facial numbness, positing its clinical utility in the treatment of trigeminal neuralgia. (Adler et al., 2009) Additionally, the use of secondary collimators that are composed of tungsten cones allows for further control of beam diameter through variations across 12 possible aperture sizes that range from 5 to 60 mm. The "trigeminal node set" is a frequently utilized set of collimator sizes that yields apertures of 6 and 4 mm for cone sizes of 7.5 and 5 mm, respectively, when set at an SAD of 65 cm. (Descovich et al., 2010) The use of small cones in the context of trigeminal neuralgia allows for radiation be collimated into a pencil beam of minimal width so that it allows for precise, targeted dose delivery without beam overlap across non-target structures.

GAMMA KNIFE

The Gamma Knife (Elekta Instruments, Stockholm, Sweden) treatment process consists of three distinct phases: planning, treatment, and follow-up. On the day of treatment, patients are first given light sedation and a local anesthetic, after which a stereotactic head frame is fixed to the patient's skull with pins that penetrate in about 2 mm. Pre-treatment imaging is undertaken and patients undergo a CT or T2-weighted fast echo MRI that is subsequently uploaded on to GammaPlan for contouring, target definition, isocenter targeting, beam plugging, and dosimetry calculation. The physician team working on dosimetry and the treatment process typically consists of a radiation oncologist, neurosurgeon, and physicist. Once the treatment parameters have been defined, the patient is taken to the treatment room, where they are placed on a Gamma Knife couch and their head is situated in the hemispherical collimator helmet. The collimator helmet is the primary unit of the treatment apparatus, and features 192-source (Perfexion unit) or 201-source (model B, C, and 4C) ports through which ^{60}Co-derived ionizing gamma radiation will be collimated and delivered as beams converging at the contoured isocenters that are defined in the individual treatment plan. As is characteristic of stereotactic radiosurgery, beams of gamma radiation are delivered with submillimeter accuracy to the defined target structure for up to 2 hours, depending on the prescribed dose. Upon completion of the treatment, the couch slides the patient away from the treatment unit, and the treatment team removes the stereotactic frame. Patients are usually discharged the same day after a short observation period, unless any complications require further monitoring. Follow-up is coordinated with the treatment team, and usually occurs monthly up until 6 months, after which it may be annual. Further imaging may be required prior to follow-up to assess the target site and monitor for any edema or post-radiation changes to local tissue.

The extensive body of literature on the use of GKS for trigeminal neuralgia is characterized by key trends associated with pain relief outcomes (Table 1). In the short-term, the latency between treatment and the onset of pain relief lasts approximately one to two months, though reported medians for this latency range from 10 days (Régis et al., 2016) to 3 months (Flickinger et al., 2001). In Cheuk et al. (2004) the median response time was 2 weeks, with a range of 0 to 24 weeks. Remarkably, 27 of the patients 96 patients (31.4% of respondents) in their study had a 0-week latency, suggesting an immediate response to GKS. In Kondziolka et al. (2010) the median pain response time for 449 patients was one month, with the range extending from one day to one year. Factor assessment in this study suggested that classical trigeminal neuralgia, no prior surgical intervention, and pain of ≤ 3 years prior to GKS were associated with a shorter latency period. Similarly, in a study of 250 patients, Young et al. (2013) found that the 29 patients who had a previous history of surgical intervention for trigeminal neuralgia reported an increased latency to pain relief. Thus, while the latency of pain relief onset may approximate to one month, individual variability, including factors such as previous invasive pain interventions, may influence the time at which pain relief begins following treatment.

In the short term, within one year of treatment, GKS demonstrates robust pain-free and pain-relief rates upwards of 75% in the majority of case series. (Guo,

Table 1. Selected outcomes in case series for gamma knife surgery in trigeminal neuralgia

Study	N	Dmax [a] (Range) [Gy]	Follow-Up [b] (Range) [mo]	Latency [c] [mo]	Pain Response [d] [%]	Reccurence [%]	Complications [%]
Kondziolka et al., (1996)	50	70 (60-90)	18 (11-36)	1	2-year: 88 Follow-up: 94	6	6
Flickinger et al., (2001)	87	75	26 (1-36)	3	Follow-up: 83	42	24
Maesawa et al., (2001)	220	80 (60-90)	22 (6-78)	2	6-mo: 82.3 Follow-up: 69.1	13.6	8.1
Cheuk et al., (2004)	96	75 (60-80)	–	2	Follow-up: 89.6	–	13.5
Fountas et al., (2007)	106	80 (70-85)	36 (12-72)	–	Initial: 89.6 1-yr: 76.4 5-yr: 60	–	21.7
Kondziolka et al., (2010)	503	80 (60-90)	24 (3-156)	1	Initial: 89 1-yr: 80 10-yr: 30	43	10.5
Young et al., (2013)	250	90	58.8	0.16	Initial: 85.6 Follow-up: 89.5	14.3	32.9
Lucas et al., (2014)	446	90 (80-97)	21.1	5	1-yr: 84.5 5- yr: 46.9	45.1	42
Kotecha et al., (2016)	870	86 (70-95)	36.5 (0-207.9)	–	Initial: 86 4-yr: 86.7	–	30
Régis et al., (2016)	497	85 (70-90)	43.8 (12-174.4)	10	Initial: 91.75 1-yr: 85.9 10-yr: 45.3	34.4	14.5
Taich et al., (2016)[e]	263	85 (80-97)	24 (6-48)	2.5	6-mo: 79% 3-yr: 70.2%	–	–

– indicates information that is not reported.

[a] Median Dmax reported for all studies except Flickinger et al. (2001) and Young et al. (2013), where single maximum dose was used on all patients.

[b] Median follow-up reported for all studies. No data available from Cheuk et al. (2001), and no range presented in Young et al. (2013) and Lucas et al. (2014).

[c] Median latency reported for all studies except Fountas et al. (2007) and Kotecha et al. (2016), in which information was unavailable.

[d] Defined as complete, partial, or greater than 50% pain relief. "Follow-up" refers to pain response rates at the most recent follow-up.

[e] Individual rates of recurrence and complication not reported; study reports results of multivariate analysis identifying factors associated with each.

Chao, Reuther, Barnett, & Suh, 2008) In Maesawa et al. (2001), 81.4% of the 220 patients reported achieving greater than 50% pain relief, with 85.6% achieving this level at the end of the first year. Similarly, complete pain relief, defined as absence of pain with or without medications, was reported by 64.9% of patients at 6 months and 70.3% of patients at one year. In their study, greater than 50% pain relief was maintained at one year by 75.8% of patients. Notably, a lack of previous surgical history for trigeminal neuralgia was significantly associated with maintenance of complete relief. Similarly, in a retrospective study of 106 patients with medically refractive trigeminal neuralgia 92.9% of patients without a prior history of surgery, and 85.7% of patients with a history of surgery, showed an initial response, which was defined as a decrease in pain severity or frequency. At one year, a pain-free outcome was achieved in 82.5% of patients who had no history of surgery, and in 69.4% of patients who had previous interventions. (Fountas et al., 2007) GKS management of trigeminal neuralgia provides strong initial pain relief in most patients, though the likelihood of initial short-term response may depend on the previous surgical history of the patient.

While the initial short-term responses are high, long-term durability of the pain response in GKS is shown to variably decrease over time, with the largest case series illustrating 5-year pain relief rates of 45-65%. In Maesawa et al. (2001), for instance, pain-free state progressively declined over time, such that at 5 years, only 55.8% of patients showed greater than 50% pain relief, while only 37.7% of patients maintained a complete pain relief response at 5 years. In that case series, patients received 60-65 Gy of radiation, which is comparatively lower than the present clinical standard; however, the decline in pain-free rates over time has been illustrated in studies featuring higher median doses. In Lucas et al. (2014), 446 patients underwent GKS for trigeminal neuralgia, receiving radiation doses ranging from 80-97 Gy); pain-relief state was scored according to the Barrow Neurological Institute pain scale (BNI). The BNI is a common scale present in the assessment of pain following radiosurgery for TN, and has 5 grades: 1 = no pain, no medications; 2 = some pain, no medications; 3 = some pain, adequately controlled with medications; 4 = some pain, not adequately controlled with medications; 5 = severe pain or no relief. (Chen & Lee, 2010) In their study, Lucas et al. found that pain relief (BNI 1 – 3) at 1, 3, and 5 years was 84.5%, 70.4%, and 46.9%, respectively. Moreover, a BNI 1 level of pain relief at 1, 3, and 5 years was achieved in only 62.9%, 43.5%, and 22.0% of patients with classical trigeminal neuralgia. Multivariate regression from Lucas et al. (2014) suggests that factors associated with the durability of a long-term GKS response include post-SRS numbness, BNI score improvement at 6 months, and Burchiel Type 1 pain, defined as pain in which greater than 50% of the symptoms are episodic rather than constant (Burchiel Type 2).

Given patient variability and dosimetry differences across various GKS outcomes studies, a definitive optimal dosage remains uncertain. However, doses in a range of 70-90 Gy have shown the most reproducible pain-relief outcomes. In Kondziolka et al. (1996), for example, 50 patients were treated with radiation doses across a range from 60-90 Gy. In that study, a radiation dose greater than 70 Gy significantly increased the likelihood of achieving and maintaining complete pain relief. However, the caveat to treatment at higher doses is the increased likelihood of developing post-radiation side effects. In Kotecha et al. (2016) 870 patients who underwent GKS for trigeminal neuralgia were divided into 3 tiers of treatment doses: ≤ 82 Gy, 83-86 Gy, and ≥ 90 Gy. The 4-year pain response rate was highest for patients treated with greater than 90 Gy (92%) and lowest for those treated with 82 Gy or less (79%). Moreover, patients treated with ≥ 90 Gy had longer times to pain failure compared to those treated with ≤ 82 Gy. However, patients treated with 83 Gy or greater were at increased risk of developing facial numbness. Similarly, in a study where 94% of the 263-patient sample was treated with greater than 85 Gy of radiation, 79% showed pain relief of BNI pain scores less than 3. However, dose prescription of 90 Gy was associated with development of facial numbness. (Taich et al., 2016). In addition to this dose-dependent efficacy and complication relationship, the length of nerve irradiated has been correlated with an increase in the likelihood of new onset dysesthesia. (Flickinger et al., 2001) Clinical evidence therefore suggests that the optimal range of a GKS radiation dose for managing trigeminal neuralgia is between 70-90 Gy, however this is accompanied by an associated increase in the risk of developing more common post-therapy complications such as cranial nerve dysfunction, numbness, and paresthesias. Although further studies are required, preliminary evidence suggests that radiosurgical treatment of trigeminal neuralgia within 3 years of symptom onset can lead to a shorter latency period, longer interval of non-medication pain relief, and longer duration of adequate pain control. (Mousavi et al., 2015)

Long-term recurrence rates of trigeminal neuralgia following GKS therapy are variable, and can range from as low as 6% (Kondziolka et al., 1996) to as high as 44.2% (Pan et al., 2010) In Kondziolka et al. (2010) 42.9% of the 503 patients had symptom recurrence. Factors determined to be associated with earlier pain recurrence included age, trigeminal neuralgia with additional symptoms (e.g. atypical TN), 3 or more previous surgeries, and the absence of any new facial sensory symptoms. Furthermore, factors associated with earlier pain recurrence in patients that had initial post-GKS pain relief included trigeminal neuralgia with additional symptoms and the absence of new facial symptoms. For patients in whom initial GKS therapy fails, repeat GKS remains a viable treatment option with a median pain cessation rate of 88%, although it may be associated with an increased risk of post-treatment nerve dysfunction and new-onset hypesthesia. (Tuleasca et al., 2014) In Aubuchon et al. (2011), a 37-patient sample received a mean retreatment dose of 84.4 Gy, resulting in greater than 50% pain-relief in 81% of the patients. Notably, however, trigeminal dysfunction was present in 57% of patients after the second GKS. In a larger, 152-patient sample, 84% of patients achieved pain relief of BNI Grade 3 or better following secondary GKS, with a 5-year maintenance rate of 46%. (Helis et al., 2015) The outcomes associated with repeat GKS studies suggest that there is a high possibility of pain relief following secondary treatment, though this must be considered in the context of an increased risk of developing post-treatment complications.

CYBERKNIFE

The Cyberknife (Accuray Inc., Sunnyvale, California) treatment process is like GKS in that it also consists of three phases: planning, treatment, and follow-up. Treatment planning begins with patients undergoing CT and possible T2-weighted MRI imaging prior to their treatment day. During imaging, patients are fitted with a custom-built thermoplastic mask for non-invasive head fixation. Imaging is uploaded onto the MultiPlan platform for target definition, contouring, and dosimetry calculation to develop an individual treatment plan for the patient. The treatment team consists of a radiation oncologist, physicist, and neurosurgeon. On the day of treatment, the patient is taken to the Cyberknife facility and placed onto the treatment couch. As CK does not utilize any stereotactic frame, sedation or anesthesia are not required. In lieu of a stereotactic frame or hemispheric radiation-source helmet, the Cyberknife apparatus achieves targeted dose delivery through an external 6-MV linear accelerator mounted on a robotic arm that can move along 6 distinct axes to deliver photon radiation. During treatment, the patient's head is immobilized using their thermoplastic mask, and the robot arm of the CK unit moves around the patient to deliver radiation doses with submillimeter accuracy. At various points throughout the treatment, the Cyberknife collects x-ray images of patient position using 2 x-ray sources positioned at 45° and 2 flat-paneled silicon detector units; these images allow for active correction of beam targeting for any patient motion to ensure high-fidelity dose delivery. Treatment may last up to 90 minutes, after which patients are typically discharged the same day. Cyberknife therapy may occur in one instance or fractionated over the course of five days, usually during the same week. Follow-up is coordinated at monthly intervals, followed by at 6 months, and then annually. Imaging may be repeated for continued monitoring of anatomical or morphological changes following radiotherapy.

Given the relatively more recent utilization of Cyberknife for treating trigeminal neuralgia, outcomes literature has been largely restricted to single-institution studies. Despite this, the efficacy of Cyberknife therapy largely mimics that of GKS, but with the possibility of a shorter latency of symptom onset that occurs within days to weeks, rather than months (Table 2). In a study of 41 patients that received a median

Table 2. Selected outcomes in case series of Cyberknife therapy for trigeminal neuralgia

Study	N	Dmax [a] (Range) [Gy]	Follow-Up [b] (Range) [mo]	Latency [c] [mo]	Pain Response [d] [%]	Reccurence [%]	Complications [%]
Lim et al., (2005)	41	78 (71.4-86.3)	11 (6-15)	0.23	Initial: 92.7 Follow-up: 78	15.8	51.2
Villavicencio et al., (2008)	95	75 (50-86.4)	22 (12-46)	0.46	Initial: 92 Follow-up: 50	31	18
Adler et al., (2009)	46	73.5 (71.4-86.2)	10.5 (6-29)	1.2	Follow-up: 96	2	17
Borchers et al., (2009)	46	73.5 (71.4-86.2)	10.5 (6.2-31.6)	–	Initial: 97.8 Follow-up: 87	15.6	39.1
Lazzara et al., (2013)	16	73.06 (72.91-73.73)	11.8 (1-27)	1.9	Follow-up: 88	28.6	12.5

– indicates information that is not reported.

[a] Medians reported for Lim et al. (2005) and Villavicencio et al. (2008). Means reported for Adler et al. (2009), Borchers et al. (2009), and Lazzara et al. (2008).

[b] Means reported for Lim et al. (2005) and Lazzara et al. (2013). Medians reported for Villavicencio et al. (2008), Adler et al. (2009), and Borchers et al. (2009).

[c] Medians reported for Lim et al. (2005) and Villavicencio et al. (2008). Means reported for Adler et al. (2009) and Borchers et al. (2009).

[d] Defined as complete, partial, or greater than 50% pain relief. "Follow-up" refers to pain response rates at the most recent follow-up.

maximum dose of 78 Gy, 38 patients (92.7%) reported successful pain relief in a median latency of 7 days, across a range of less than 24 hours to 4 months. (Lim et al., 2005) A larger, multi-center analysis of 95 patients receiving a median maximal dose of 75 Gy similarly reported a median time to pain relief of 14 days, across a range from 0.3 to 180 days. While 92% of patients in this later study reported some initial pain relief, 67% of patients were reported as having successful treatment, defined as a score of 1 on the Boulder-Stanford pain relief scale. (Villavicencio et al., 2008) The Boulder-Stanford pain relief scale, initially defined in Lim et al. (2005), uses patient self-assessment to assign a score along a 4-point scale: 1 = greater than 90% pain relief, no medications; 2 = between 50 and 90% pain relief, reduction in medication use; 3 = less than 50% pain relief, no change in medication use; 4 = no change in symptoms. In a retrospective review of 46 patient cases treated with a median dose of 73.5 Gy, 97.2% of patients reported initial pain relief immediately or within weeks of treatment, while a Boulder-Stanford level 1 degree of pain relief was maintained in 73.9% of patients. (Borchers et al., 2009) In contrast, Lazzara et al. (2013) report an average time of 1.9 months between treatment and achievement of maximum therapeutic response. GKS and CK therefore share a similar degree of short-term pain relief, though evidence from larger studies suggest the latter may feature a comparatively shorter median latency between treatment and pain relief. Larger, systematic comparison of short-term outcomes between both methodologies may lend further insight into the validity of these findings.

Long-term follow-up of patients following CK therapy suggests sustained pain-relief at most median follow-up times, with the caveat that most long-term follow-up for CK is within 2 years of receiving treatment. In the long-term follow-up for patients from their study, Lim et al. (2005) reported that 78% of patients maintained pain relief after a mean follow-up time of 11 months, compared to the initial 92.7%. Similarly, at a mean follow-up time of 14.7 months, Adler et al. (2009) reported that 72% of patients rated their pain relief as excellent (Boulder-Stanford 1) and 24% as good (Boulder-Stanford 2). With a longer median follow-up time of 28 months, Karam et al. (2014) reported a 72% actuarial rate of freedom from severe pain, defined as BNI scores of 3 or greater, Moreover, at last follow-up, 8% of patients had BNI of 1, 16% had BNI of 2, while 48% had some pain that was managed by medications (BNI 3); 28% had no response to treatment and continued having severe pain (BNI 4 or 5). In Villavicencio et al. (2008), the mean follow-up time was approximately two years. In their study, 47 of the 64 patients who showed preliminary excellent pain relief went on to maintain this response at long-term follow-up; this corresponds to 50% of the total 95-patient sample. Taken together, these early studies suggest that Cyberknife pain-relief remains comparatively robust, though with a progressive decrease over time from the initial rate of response. However, longer-term follow-up beyond the 2-year mark is required to further delineate the extent to which this method of radiosurgery can provide sustained pain relief from trigeminal neuralgia.

While the optimal dosage for Cyberknife treatment is undergoing refinement as longer-term follow-up data is acquired, literature values consistently suggest beneficial outcomes associated with a dose range of 70-90 Gy. As is the case with GKS, higher dose in Cyberknife is frequently associated with the incidence of post-treatment side effects. In Villavicencio et al. (2008), a median maximum dose of 78 Gy was used, with a treatment range from 70 to 85.4 Gy. Additionally, the median length of nerve treated was 6 mm, with a range from 5-12 mm. With these parameters as part of their isocentric technique, the authors found strong initial and favorable long-term pain relief. However, 45 patients in the study reported new post-treatment numbness, with two patients reporting additional dysesthesia. The occurrence of numbness was significantly associated with a history of previous surgical treatments, as well as higher maximum dosage and longer nerve segment irradiation. Other complications in this study included decreased corneal reflex, anesthesia dolorosa, trismus, masticator weakness, diplopia, decreased hearing, dry eye syndrome, and right foot paresis. In contrast, Adler et al. (2009) used a similar median maximum dose of 73.5 Gy, with a range from 71.4 to 86.2 Gy, to irradiate a 6-mm segment of the trigeminal nerve using a non-isocentric approach. In addition to a favorable 72% pain-free response, the authors reported a 17% rate of new-onset facial numbness without any other complications. Cyberknife treatment dosages mirror GKS in the presence of a dose-dependent relationship for both therapeutic efficacy and complication profile. The non-isocentric method of homogenous radiation delivery presents a possible source of clinical utility in achieving comparably high levels of pain relief while reducing the likelihood of complication onset. Additional research is required to determine whether the timing of Cyberknife radiosurgery following symptom onset influences treatment outcomes.

Select case series have demonstrated that recurrence rates for trigeminal neuralgia can extend from 15-30%, suggesting rates of recurrence similar to GKS. In Lim et al. (2005), long-term follow-up revealed that six of the 38 patients who showed initial pain-free response had a recurrence of pain within a median of 6 months following treatment, yielding a recurrence rate of 15.8%. In Villavicencio et al. (2008), 27 of the 87 patients that had initial pain relief had a recurrence of pain symptoms. Factor analysis in this study found that patients who had pre-existing numbness prior to treatment were more likely to experience pain recurrence, and a higher recurrence rate correlated to lower post-treatment numbness. Conversely, however, higher dosage and longer nerve segment irradiation were predictive of a lower recurrence rate. While further evidence regarding the outcomes of repeat CK therapy is needed, Adler et al. (2009) report results for treatment performed in 5 patients. In this case series, 2 patients reported excellent pain relief (Boulder-Stanford 1), 2 reported good pain relief (Boulder-Stanford 2), while 1 reported no pain relief. Notably, in this study, only 1 patient had recurrence of trigeminal neuralgia, and that patient underwent repeat Cyberknife to result in a pain-free response. Although these results suggest repeat Cyberknife may be applied in the clinic for non-responsive or recurrent cases, further analysis is needed to better characterize the complications, outcomes, and optimal dose parameters of secondary Cyberknife therapy.

CONCLUSION

Stereotactic radiosurgery modalities such as Gamma Knife and Cyberknife offer the possibility of pain relief from trigeminal neuralgia through targeted ablation of the trigeminal nerve. Long-term quality of life and patient satisfaction scores following radiosurgical treatment have reported averages of 7.8 and 7.7 out of 10, respectively. Moreover, 87.7% of patients in the same study would recommend radiosurgery (in their case, GKS) to other patients. (Young et al., 2013) Taken alone, these metrics reinforce the inclusion of radiosurgery in possible treatment algorithms for trigeminal neuralgia. When comparing radiosurgery to MVD, radiosurgery is significantly more likely to see older patients and have a shorter follow-up period. However, MVD shows significantly greater likelihood of pain resolution, as well as a lower likelihood of poor pain control, treatment complications, and recurrence of trigeminal neuralgia. (Berger et al., 2017) Moreover, analysis of the cost-effectiveness of surgical modalities used in trigeminal neuralgia reveals the preferred clinical utility of MVD over radiosurgery. Sivakanthan et al. (2014) examined 1582 claims of trigeminal neuralgia from the Medicare claims database and compared MVD, stereotactic radiosurgery, and percutaneous stereotactic rhizotomy. In addition to being the most popular treatment option, MVD produced the highest number of quality-adjusted life-years (QALYs); stereotactic radiosurgery, conversely, produced the least number of QALYs and was the least cost-effective, as defined by cost per QALY. Consequently, although radiosurgery produces significant pain relief outcomes, its high rate of recurrence, low cost-effectiveness, and reduced likelihood of pain relief render it less preferable compared to the gold standard of MVD.

Though it may not replicate the clinical efficacy of MVD, radiosurgery remains an important treatment for chronic pain management in trigeminal neuralgia. Foremost, radiosurgery addresses pain by directly targeting underlying neural structures rather than treating symptoms; thus, unlike medication therapy, pain relief extends beyond the treatment period. Furthermore, the treatment process in radiosurgery is significantly less invasive than open and minimally invasive procedures, and features a treatment protocol that includes same-day discharge with shorter follow-up and little to no post-operative monitoring. Finally, the relatively fewer contraindications associated with radiosurgery make it an ideal treatment modality for patients that are not suitable for open procedures or have medical contraindications.

Moving forward, research into radiosurgery for trigeminal neuralgia must focus on three key issues. First, mechanisms of radiobiological action must be drawn out for clinicians and researchers to better understand how radiosurgery has its pain-relieving effects. Understanding these mechanisms also allows for exploration of the factors that may confer greater or lesser radiosensitivity in specific regions of the trigeminal nerve, as well as the individual factors that influence factors such as treatment latency. Second, target and dose definition must be further refined to better characterize the ideal structures and dose distributions at which the therapeutic effect is maximized, while side effects and complications are most minimized. Finally, longer follow-up of larger patient samples must be performed to determine the duration of a pain-free response, identify risk factors for recurrence, and highlight the ideal time for radiosurgical intervention. By doing so, radiosurgery may be further refined and positioned as a powerful treatment modality in the management of trigeminal neuralgia.

REFERENCES

Adler, J. R. Jr, Bower, R., Gupta, G., Lim, M., Efron, A., Gibbs, I. C., ... Soltys, S. G. (2009). Nonisocentric radiosurgical rhizotomy for trigeminal neuralgia. *Neurosurgery, 64*(2Suppl), A84–A90. doi:10.1227/01.NEU.0000341631.49154.62 PMID:19165079

Adler, J. R. Jr, Chang, S. D., Murphy, M. J., Doty, J., Geis, P., & Hancock, S. L. (1997). The Cyberknife: A frameless robotic system for radiosurgery. *Stereotactic and Functional Neurosurgery, 69*(1–4 Pt 2), 124–128. doi:10.1159/000099863 PMID:9711744

Artico, M., De Caro, G. M., Fraioli, B., & Giuffrè, R. (1997). 1897--celebrating the centennial--Hermann Moritz Gocht and radiation therapy in the treatment of trigeminal neuralgia. *Acta Neurochirurgica, 139*(8), 761–763. doi:10.1007/BF01420050 PMID:9309292

Aubuchon, A. C., Chan, M. D., Lovato, J. F., Balamucki, C. J., Ellis, T. L., Tatter, S. B., … Shaw, E. G. (2011). Repeat Gamma Knife Radiosurgery for Trigeminal Neuralgia. *International Journal of Radiation Oncology, Biology, Physics, 81*(4), 1059–1065. doi:10.1016/j.ijrobp.2010.07.010

Barker, F. G., Jannetta, P. J., Bissonette, D. J., Larkins, M. V., & Jho, H. D. (1996). The Long-Term Outcome of Microvascular Decompression for Trigeminal Neuralgia. *The New England Journal of Medicine, 334*(17), 1077–1084. doi:10.1056/NEJM199604253341701 PMID:8598865

Berger, I., Nayak, N., Schuster, J., Lee, J., Stein, S., & Malhotra, N. R. (2017). Microvascular Decompression Versus Stereotactic Radiosurgery for Trigeminal Neuralgia: A Decision Analysis. *Cureus, 9*(1), e1000. doi:10.7759/cureus.1000 PMID:28280653

Borchers, J. D. III, Yang, H.-J., Sakamoto, G. T., Howes, G. A., Gupta, G., Chang, S. D., & Adler, J. R. Jr. (2009). Cyberknife stereotactic radiosurgical rhizotomy for trigeminal neuralgia: Anatomic and morphological considerations. *Neurosurgery, 64*(2Suppl), A91–A95. doi:10.1227/01.NEU.0000340795.87734.70 PMID:19165080

Casselman, J. W., Kuhweide, R., Deimling, M., Ampe, W., Dehaene, I., & Meeus, L. (1993). Constructive interference in steady state-3DFT MR imaging of the inner ear and cerebellopontine angle. *AJNR. American Journal of Neuroradiology, 14*(1), 47–57. PMID:8427111

Chávez, G.-R. C., & Salles, D. (2005). Three-dimensional Fast Imaging Employing Steady-state Acquisition Magnetic Resonance Imaging for Stereotactic Radiosurgery of Trigeminal Neuralgia. *Neurosurgery*, *56*(3), E628–E628. doi:10.1227/01.NEU.0000154709.44776.50 PMID:15730595

Chen, H. I., & Lee, J. Y. K. (2010). The measurement of pain in patients with trigeminal neuralgia. *Clinical Neurosurgery*, *57*, 129–133. PMID:21280505

Cheuk, A. V., Chin, L. S., Petit, J. H., Herman, J. M., Fang, H.-B., & Regine, W. F. (2004). Gamma knife surgery for trigeminal neuralgia: Outcome, imaging, and brainstem correlates. *International Journal of Radiation Oncology, Biology, Physics*, *60*(2), 537–541. doi:10.1016/j.ijrobp.2004.04.020 PMID:15380590

Cruccu, G., Finnerup, N. B., Jensen, T. S., Scholz, J., Sindou, M., Svensson, P., ... Nurmikko, T. (2016). Trigeminal neuralgia New classification and diagnostic grading for practice and research. *Neurology*, *87*(2), 220–228. doi:10.1212/WNL.0000000000002840 PMID:27306631

Dandy, W. E. (1934). Concerning the cause of trigeminal neuralgia. *American Journal of Surgery*, *24*(2), 447–455. doi:10.1016/S0002-9610(34)90403-7

Deng, J., Ma, C. M., Hai, J., & Nath, R. (2003). Commissioning 6 MV photon beams of a stereotactic radiosurgery system for Monte Carlo treatment planning. *Medical Physics*, *30*(12), 3124–3134. doi:10.1118/1.1624753 PMID:14713079

Descovich, M., Sneed, P. K., Barbaro, N. M., McDermott, M. W., Chuang, C. F., & Barani, I. J., … Lijun, M. (2010). A dosimetric comparison between Gamma Knife and CyberKnife treatment plans for trigeminal neuralgia. *Journal of Neurosurgery*, *113*(Suppl), 199–206. PMID:21222296

Fariselli, L., Marras, C., De Santis, M., Marchetti, M., Milanesi, I., & Broggi, G. (2009). Cyberknife radiosurgery as a first treatment for idiopathic trigeminal neuralgia. *Neurosurgery, 64*(suppl_2), A96–A101. 10.1227/01.NEU.0000341714.55023.8F

Fleetwood, I. G., Innes, A. M., Hansen, S. R., & Steinberg, G. K. (2001). Familial trigeminal neuralgia. Case report and review of the literature. *Journal of Neurosurgery*, *95*(3), 513–517. doi:10.3171/jns.2001.95.3.0513 PMID:11565877

Flickinger, J. C., Pollock, B. E., Kondziolka, D., Phuong, L. K., Foote, R. L., Stafford, S. L., & Lunsford, L. D. (2001). Does increased nerve length within the treatment volume improve trigeminal neuralgia radiosurgery? A prospective double-blind, randomized study. *International Journal of Radiation Oncology, Biology, Physics*, *51*(2), 449–454. doi:10.1016/S0360-3016(01)01606-6 PMID:11567820

Fountas, K. N., Smith, J. R., Lee, G. P., Jenkins, P. D., Cantrell, R. R., & Sheils, W. C. (2007). Gamma Knife stereotactic radiosurgical treatment of idiopathic trigeminal neuralgia: Long-term outcome and complications. *Neurosurgical Focus*, *23*(6), E7. doi:10.3171/FOC-07/12/E8 PMID:18081485

Gorgulho, A. (2012). Radiation mechanisms of pain control in classical trigeminal neuralgia. *Surgical Neurology International*, *3*(2Suppl 1), S17–S25. doi:10.4103/2152-7806.91606 PMID:22826806

Gronseth, G., Cruccu, G., Alksne, J., Argoff, C., Brainin, M., Burchiel, K., ... Zakrzewska, J. M. (2008). Practice Parameter: The diagnostic evaluation and treatment of trigeminal neuralgia (an evidence-based review) Report of the Quality Standards Subcommittee of the American Academy of Neurology and the European Federation of Neurological Societies. *Neurology*, *71*(15), 1183–1190. doi:10.1212/01.wnl.0000326598.83183.04 PMID:18716236

Guo, S., Chao, S. T., Reuther, A. M., Barnett, G. H., & Suh, J. H. (2008). Review of the treatment of trigeminal neuralgia with gamma knife radiosurgery. *Stereotactic and Functional Neurosurgery*, *86*(3), 135–146. doi:10.1159/000120425 PMID:18334855

Hamlyn, P. J., & King, T. T. (1992). Neurovascular compression in trigeminal neuralgia: A clinical and anatomical study. *Journal of Neurosurgery*, *76*(6), 948–954. doi:10.3171/jns.1992.76.6.0948 PMID:1588428

Headache Classification Committee of the International Headache Society (IHS). (2013). The International Classification of Headache Disorders, 3rd edition (beta version). Cephalalgia, 33(9), 629–808. doi:10.1177/0333102413485658

Helis, C. A., Lucas, J. T. Jr, Bourland, J. D., Chan, M. D., Tatter, S. B., & Laxton, A. W. (2015). Repeat Radiosurgery for Trigeminal Neuralgia. *Neurosurgery*, *77*(5), 755–761, discussion 761. doi:10.1227/NEU.0000000000000915 PMID:26214319

Hilton, D. A., Love, S., Gradidge, T., & Coakham, H. B. (1994). Pathological findings associated with trigeminal neuralgia caused by vascular compression. *Neurosurgery*, *35*(2), 299–303. doi:10.1227/00006123-199408000-00017 PMID:7969838

Ho, A., Lo, A. T., Dieterich, S., Soltys, S. G., Gibbs, I. C., Chang, S. G., & Adler, J. R. (2012). Trigeminal neuralgia treatment dosimetry of the Cyberknife. *Medical Dosimetry: Official Journal of the American Association of Medical Dosimetrists*, *37*(1), 42–46. doi:10.1016/j.meddos.2010.12.012 PMID:21723113

Karam, S. D., Tai, A., Snider, J. W., Bhatia, S., Bedrick, E. J., Rashid, A., ... Jean, W. (2014). Refractory trigeminal neuralgia treatment outcomes following CyberKnife radiosurgery. *Radiation Oncology (London, England)*, *9*(1), 257. doi:10.118613014-014-0257-8 PMID:25497053

Katusic, S., Beard, C. M., Bergstralh, E., & Kurland, L. T. (1990). Incidence and clinical features of trigeminal neuralgia, Rochester, Minnesota, 1945-1984. *Annals of Neurology*, *27*(1), 89–95. doi:10.1002/ana.410270114 PMID:2301931

Kondziolka, D., Lacomis, D., Niranjan, A., Mori, Y., Maesawa, S., Fellows, W., & Lunsford, L. D. (2000). Histological effects of trigeminal nerve radiosurgery in a primate model: implications for trigeminal neuralgia radiosurgery. *Neurosurgery, 46*(4), 971-976-977.

Kondziolka, D., Lunsford, L. D., Flickinger, J. C., Young, R. F., Vermeulen, S., Duma, C. M., ... Lindquist, C. (1996). Stereotactic radiosurgery for trigeminal neuralgia: A multiinstitutional study using the gamma unit. *Journal of Neurosurgery*, *84*(6), 940–945. doi:10.3171/jns.1996.84.6.0940 PMID:8847587

Koopman, J. S. H. A., Dieleman, J. P., Huygen, F. J., de Mos, M., Martin, C. G. M., & Sturkenboom, M. C. J. M. (2009). Incidence of facial pain in the general population. *Pain*, *147*(1–3), 122–127. doi:10.1016/j.pain.2009.08.023 PMID:19783099

Kotecha, R., Kotecha, R., Modugula, S., Murphy, E. S., Jones, M., Kotecha, R., ... Chao, S. T. (2016). Trigeminal Neuralgia Treated With Stereotactic Radiosurgery: The Effect of Dose Escalation on Pain Control and Treatment Outcomes. *International Journal of Radiation Oncology, Biology, Physics, 96*(1), 142–148. 10.1016/j.ijrobp.2016.04.013

Lazzara, B. M., Ortiz, O., Bordia, R., Witten, M. R., Haas, J. A., Katz, A. J., & Brown, J. A. (2013). Cyberknife radiosurgery in treating trigeminal neuralgia. *Journal of Neurointerventional Surgery*, *5*(1), 81–85. doi:10.1136/neurintsurg-2011-010125 PMID:22278932

Leksell, L. (1951). The stereotaxic method and radiosurgery of the brain. *Acta Chirurgica Scandinavica*, *102*(4), 316–319. PMID:14914373

Leksell, L. (1971). Sterotaxic radiosurgery in trigeminal neuralgia. *Acta Chirurgica Scandinavica*, *137*(4), 311–314. PMID:4948331

Lettmaier, S. (2014). Radiosurgery in trigeminal neuralgia. *Physica Medica: PM: An International Journal Devoted to the Applications of Physics to Medicine and Biology: Official Journal of the Italian Association of Biomedical Physics*, *30*(5), 592–595. doi:10.1016/j.ejmp.2014.05.006 PMID:24889155

Li, K., & Ma, L. (2004). Selective source blocking for Gamma Knife radiosurgery of trigeminal neuralgia based on analytical dose modelling. *Physics in Medicine and Biology*, *49*(15), 3455–3463. doi:10.1088/0031-9155/49/15/010 PMID:15379025

Lim, M., Villavicencio, A. T., Burneikiene, S., Chang, S. D., Romanelli, P., McNeely, L., ... Adler, J. R. (2005). CyberKnife radiosurgery for idiopathic trigeminal neuralgia. *Neurosurgical Focus*, *18*(5), 1–7. doi:10.3171/foc.2005.18.5.10 PMID:15913285

Lindquist, C., Kihlström, L., & Hellstrand, E. (1991). Functional neurosurgery--a future for the gamma knife? *Stereotactic and Functional Neurosurgery*, *57*(1–2), 72–81. doi:10.1159/000099557 PMID:1725560

Lucas, J. T., Nida, A. M., Isom, S., Marshall, K., Bourland, J. D., Laxton, A. W., ... Chan, M. D. (2014). Predictive Nomogram for the Durability of Pain Relief From Gamma Knife Radiation Surgery in the Treatment of Trigeminal Neuralgia. *International Journal of Radiation Oncology, Biology, Physics*, *89*(1), 120–126. 10.1016/j.ijrobp.2014.01.023

Maarbjerg, S., Gozalov, A., Olesen, J., & Bendtsen, L. (2014). Trigeminal neuralgia – a prospective systematic study of clinical characteristics in 158 patients. *Headache*, *54*(10), 1574–1582. doi:10.1111/head.12441 PMID:25231219

MacDonald, B. K., Cockerell, O. C., Sander, J. W. S., & Shorvon, S. D. (2000). The incidence and lifetime prevalence of neurological disorders in a prospective community-based study in the UK. *Brain*, *123*(4), 665–676. doi:10.1093/brain/123.4.665 PMID:10733998

Maesawa, S., Salame, C., Flickinger, J. C., Pirris, S., Kondziolka, D., & Lunsford, L. D. (2001). Clinical outcomes after stereotactic radiosurgery for idiopathic trigeminal neuralgia. *Journal of Neurosurgery*, *94*(1), 14–20. doi:10.3171/jns.2001.94.1.0014 PMID:11147887

Massager, N., Nissim, O., Murata, N., Devriendt, D., Desmedt, F., Vanderlinden, B., ... Levivier, M. (2006). Effect of beam channel plugging on the outcome of gamma knife radiosurgery for trigeminal neuralgia. *International Journal of Radiation Oncology, Biology, Physics*, *65*(4), 1200–1205. doi:10.1016/j.ijrobp.2006.01.043 PMID:16682146

Mousavi, S. H., Niranjan, A., Huang, M. J., Laghari, F. J., Shin, S. S., Mindlin, J. L., ... Lunsford, L. D. (2015). Early radiosurgery provides superior pain relief for trigeminal neuralgia patients. *Neurology*, *85*(24), 2159–2165. doi:10.1212/WNL.0000000000002216 PMID:26561286

Obermann, M., Yoon, M.-S., Ese, D., Maschke, M., Kaube, H., Diener, H.-C., & Katsarava, Z. (2007). Impaired trigeminal nociceptive processing in patients with trigeminal neuralgia. *Neurology*, *69*(9), 835–841. doi:10.1212/01.wnl.0000269670.30045.6b PMID:17724285

Pan, H.-C., Sheehan, J., Huang, C.-F., Sheu, M.-L., Yang, D.-Y., & Chiu, W.-T. (2010). Quality-of-life outcomes after Gamma Knife surgery for trigeminal neuralgia. *Journal of Neurosurgery*, *113*(Suppl), 191–198. doi:10.3171/2010.8.GKS10879 PMID:21121802

Peker, S., Kurtkaya, O., Uzün, I., & Pamir, M. N. (2006). Microanatomy of the central myelin-peripheral myelin transition zone of the trigeminal nerve. *Neurosurgery*, *59*(2), 354-359. 10.1227/01.NEU.0000223501.27220.69

Régis, J., Tuleasca, C., Resseguier, N., Carron, R., Donnet, A., Gaudart, J., & Levivier, M. (2016). Long-term safety and efficacy of Gamma Knife surgery in classical trigeminal neuralgia: A 497-patient historical cohort study. *Journal of Neurosurgery*, *124*(4), 1079–1087. doi:10.3171/2015.2.JNS142144 PMID:26339857

Rojas-Villabona, A., Kitchen, N., & Paddick, I. (2016). Investigation of dosimetric differences between the TMR 10 and convolution algorithm for Gamma Knife stereotactic radiosurgery. *Journal of Applied Clinical Medical Physics*, *17*(6), 217–229. doi:10.1120/jacmp.v17i6.6347 PMID:27929495

Schwarz, W., & Fox, J. M. (1979). Effects of monochromatic X-radiation on the membrane of nodes of Ranvier under voltage and current clamp conditions. *Experientia*, *35*(9), 1200–1201. doi:10.1007/BF01963288 PMID:314907

Sharim, J., Lo, W.-L., Kim, W., Chivukula, S., Tenn, S., Kaprealian, T., & Pouratian, N. (2017). Radiosurgical target distance from the root entry zone in the treatment of trigeminal neuralgia. *Practical Radiation Oncology*, *7*(4), 221–227. doi:10.1016/j.prro.2016.12.006 PMID:28336479

Sharma, S. C., Ott, J. T., Williams, J. B., & Dickow, D. (2010). Clinical implications of adopting Monte Carlo treatment planning for CyberKnife. *Journal of Applied Clinical Medical Physics*, *11*(1), 3142. doi:10.1120/jacmp.v11i1.3142 PMID:20160699

Siddon, R. L. (1985). Prism representation: A 3D ray-tracing algorithm for radiotherapy applications. *Physics in Medicine and Biology*, *30*(8), 817–824. doi:10.1088/0031-9155/30/8/005 PMID:4048266

Sivakanthan, S., Van Gompel, J. J., Alikhani, P., van Loveren, H., Chen, R., & Agazzi, S. (2014). Surgical management of trigeminal neuralgia: use and cost-effectiveness from an analysis of the Medicare Claims Database. *Neurosurgery, 75*(3), 220-226. 10.1227/NEU.0000000000000430

Smith, K. J., & McDonald, W. I. (1980). Spontaneous and mechanically evoked activity due to central demyelinating lesion. *Nature, 286*(5769), 154–155. doi:10.1038/286154a0 PMID:7402307

Smith, K. J., & Mcdonald, W. I. (1999). The pathophysiology of multiple sclerosis: the mechanisms underlying the production of symptoms and the natural history of the disease. *Philosophical Transactions of the Royal Society of London. Series B, Biological Sciences, 354*(1390), 1649–1673. doi:10.1098/rstb.1999.0510 PMID:10603618

Smith, Z. A., Gorgulho, A. A., Bezrukiy, N., McArthur, D., Agazaryan, N., Selch, M. T., & De Salles, A. A. F. (2011). Dedicated linear accelerator radiosurgery for trigeminal neuralgia: A single-center experience in 179 patients with varied dose prescriptions and treatment plans. *International Journal of Radiation Oncology, Biology, Physics, 81*(1), 225–231. doi:10.1016/j.ijrobp.2010.05.058 PMID:21236592

Smyth, P., Greenough, G., & Stommel, E. (2003). Familial trigeminal neuralgia: Case reports and review of the literature. *Headache, 43*(8), 910–915. doi:10.1046/j.1526-4610.2003.03172.x PMID:12940815

Spina, A., Mortini, P., Alemanno, F., Houdayer, E., & Iannaccone, S. (2017). Trigeminal Neuralgia: Toward a Multimodal Approach. *World Neurosurgery, 103*, 220–230. doi:10.1016/j.wneu.2017.03.126 PMID:28377244

Taich, Z. J., Goetsch, S. J., Monaco, E., Carter, B. S., Ott, K., Alksne, J. F., & Chen, C. C. (2016). Stereotactic Radiosurgery Treatment of Trigeminal Neuralgia: Clinical Outcomes and Prognostic Factors. *World Neurosurgery, 90*(Supplement C), 604–612.e11. doi:10.1016/j.wneu.2016.02.067 PMID:26915701

Tuleasca, C., Carron, R., Resseguier, N., Donnet, A., Roussel, P., & Gaudart, J., … Régis, J. (2014). Repeat Gamma Knife surgery for recurrent trigeminal neuralgia: Long-term outcomes and systematic review. *Journal of Neurosurgery, 121*(Suppl), 210–221. doi:10.3171/2014.8.GKS141487 PMID:25434955

Villavicencio, A. T., Lim, M., Burneikiene, S., Romanelli, P., Adler, J. R., McNeely, L., … Thramann, J. J. (2008). Cyberknife radiosurgery for trigeminal neuralgia treatment: a preliminary multicenter experience. *Neurosurgery, 62*(3), 647-655. 10.1227/01.neu.0000317313.46826.dc

Wolf, A., & Kondziolka, D. (2016). Gamma Knife Surgery in Trigeminal Neuralgia. *Neurosurgery Clinics of North America*, *27*(3), 297–304. doi:10.1016/j.nec.2016.02.006 PMID:27324996

Xu, A. Y., Bhatnagar, J., Bednarz, G., Niranjan, A., Kondziolka, D., Flickinger, J., ... Huq, M. S. (2015). Gamma Knife radiosurgery with CT image-based dose calculation. *Journal of Applied Clinical Medical Physics*, *16*(6), 119–129. doi:10.1120/jacmp.v16i6.5530 PMID:26699563

Yoshino, N., Akimoto, H., Yamada, I., Nagaoka, T., Tetsumura, A., Kurabayashi, T., ... Sasaki, T. (2003). Trigeminal Neuralgia: Evaluation of Neuralgic Manifestation and Site of Neurovascular Compression with 3D CISS MR Imaging and MR Angiography. *Radiology*, *228*(2), 539–545. doi:10.1148/radiol.2282020439 PMID:12802002

Young, B., Shivazad, A., Kryscio, R. J., St Clair, W., & Bush, H. M. (2013). Long-term outcome of high-dose γ knife surgery in treatment of trigeminal neuralgia. *Journal of Neurosurgery*, *119*(5), 1166–1175. doi:10.3171/2013.1.JNS12875 PMID:23600932

Zhao, Z.-F., Yang, L.-Z., Jiang, C.-L., Zheng, Y.-R., & Zhang, J.-W. (2010). Gamma Knife irradiation–induced histopathological changes in the trigeminal nerves of rhesus monkeys. *Journal of Neurosurgery*, *113*(1), 39–44. doi:10.3171/2010.1.JNS091116 PMID:20170304

KEY TERMS AND DEFINITIONS

Barrow Neurological Institute (BNI) Pain Scale: A composite pain scale commonly used in the quantification of trigeminal neuralgia pain; incorporates information about pain severity and use of medication for pain control. Scoring is as follows: I: No pain, no medications, II: Occasional pain, no medications required, III: Some pain, adequately controlled with medications, IV: Some pain, not adequately controlled with medications, V: Severe pain or no pain relief.

Collimator: A device utilized in linear particle accelerator (linac) radiation therapy to shape radiation beams and limit the maximum size of a beam for optimal dose contouring and protection of critical structures.

Cyberknife: A frameless stereotactic radiosurgery modality that uses an arm-mounted external linear particle accelerator to deliver x-ray radiation in an isocentric or non-isocentric manner to targets, with intra-operative adjustments being made using fluoroscopic image guidance.

Gamma Knife: A stereotactic radiosurgery modality that delivers isocentric cobalt-derived gamma ray radiation through a hemispherical collimator unit to patients who are situated in a fixed stereotactic head frame.

Isocenter: The spatial point in a target region through which converging radiation beams, or the central radiation beam, pass (radiation isocenter); the point in space about which the radiation apparatus rotates (mechanical isocenter).

Microvascular Decompression: A surgical procedure done to relive vascular compression of the trigeminal nerve, in which microsurgical instruments are used to isolate the trigeminal nerve, mobilize a compressing vascular loop, and separate the two by placement of a sponge.

Trigeminal Neuralgia: A chronic neuropathic pain condition characterized by paroxysms of lancinating, electric shock-like pain along the distribution of the trigeminal nerve (V1-V3) that may be spontaneous or brought on by innocuous stimuli.

Chapter 11
V2 Rhizotomy

Lucas W. Campos
Summit Pain Alliance, USA

Nicholas Telischak
Stanford University, USA

Huy M. Do
Stanford University, USA

Xiang Qian
Stanford University, USA

ABSTRACT

Trigeminal neuralgia is a facial pain syndrome characterized by excruciating, paroxysmal, electric shock-like pain attacks in the sensory distribution of the trigeminal nerve. Medical management remains the first line of treatment. When this fails, surgical management needs to be considered. Percutaneous interventional procedures such as glycerol rhizotomy, radiofrequency (RF) thermocoagulation, and balloon compression of the trigeminal ganglion and its branches are some of the most commonly used procedures as they avoid exposure to general anesthesia, provide successful short-term results, and are available to people with significant co-morbidities. Of these, RF is the most often used. The V2 and V3 branches of the trigeminal nerve are most commonly affected, and are thus the most frequent targets for RF interventions. These procedures may be performed using conventional fluoroscopic, ultrasound, or CT-guided imaging, including combined flat-panel CT and fluoroscopy. This chapter summarizes these common ablation techniques targeting the V2 branch of the trigeminal nerve.

DOI: 10.4018/978-1-5225-5349-6.ch011

INTRODUCTION

Trigeminal neuralgia (TN) is a severe, neuropathic pain condition affecting the distribution of the trigeminal nerve. The pain is often characterized as electric and sharp as if the face is being stabbed. Pain is often accompanied by a unilateral grimace, which led to the synonym "tic douloureux."(Burchiel & Slavin, 2000). Attacks are most common in the second and third trigeminal divisions, on the right side of the face (Harness & Chase, 1990) . The attacks usually recur with the same intensity and distribution. A brief refractory period of relief typically follows that lasts seconds to hours. This pain can be triggered by stimulating a specific facial area (e.g by light touch or tooth brushing) or can occur spontaneously (Rasmussen, 1991) . The etiology of TN is not fully understood. Dysfunction of the myelin sheath has been the focus of much investigation (Dubner, Sharav, Gracely, & Price, 1987).

Clinical examination, imaging studies, and laboratory tests are usually unremarkable in classic TN (Rasmussen, 1990a). When the signs and symptoms of TN are secondary to another disease process it is called ''symptomatic TN''. The basic pathophysiology of TN remains largely unknown.(Bowsher, 1997; Canavero, Bonicalzi, & Pagni, 1995; Rasmussen, 1990b). Many TN patients suffer pain attacks for months or years before the condition is appropriately diagnosed. Over time, these severe pain attacks have a devastating impact on patients' lives (Rasmussen, 1991). Timely and accurate diagnosis of TN speeds treatment with medication and surgical interventions which can help to limit this negative impact (Tartaro, Stroffolini, & Lepore, 1979).

Aretaeus of Cappadocia is credited with the first clinical description of TN. At the end of the first century, he discovered *heterocrania,* which he described as spasm causing "distortion of the countenance" (Cappadocia.), 1856; Mosberg, 1960). In 1677, the noted American physician and philosopher, John Locke, identified the major clinical features of TN in his work Countess of Northumberland (Mosberg, 1960). It was the first time a physician found that this pain was not caused by dental pathology. In 1773, John Fothergill, an English physician, clearly established the disorder as a discrete syndrome (Eboli, Stone, Aydin, & Slavin, 2009; Pearce, 2003). In 1912, Sir William Osler, one of the four founding professors of Johns Hopkins Hospital, gave the most complete medical description of trigeminal neuralgia for his colleagues, giving new understanding of the disease's pathophysiology (Casey & Jannetta, 2010). Dr. Osler found that specific trigger zones anywhere within the trigeminal distribution, could initiate these severe attacks and tics in the face (Dubner et al., 1987). He found this to be the reason patients avoided touching, washing, and shaving their faces. He also identified intraoral trigger zones, which were stimulated by chewing. This was important because most other facial pains were treated with massage or by applying heat and cold (Türp & Gobetti, 1996).

The overall incidence rate is estimated at approximately three to five cases per year per 100,000 persons. Patients are more likely to be female and older than 50-60 when the first attacks begin (Massager et al., 2007). The age and sex distribution are interesting as most other common chronic headache and facial pain disorders occur at an earlier age (Fraioli, Lisciani, & Fraioli, 2014; Maarbjerg, Di Stefano, Bendtsen, & Cruccu, 2017). The paroxysmal pain usually worsens over time. While there are familial examples, TN does not appear to be increased in any particular ethnic group, geographic region, or climate (Duff, Spinner, Lindor, Dodick, & Atkinson, 1999; Smyth, Greenough, & Stommel, 2003; Maarbjerg et al., 2017).

PATHOPHYSIOLOGY

Compression of the trigeminal nerve root by benign tumors and vascular anomalies can produce symptoms, which are indistinguishable from classic TN. This implies that injury to the nerve root is an important factor in the evolution of the disease (Devor, Amir, & Rappaport, 2002). Early research showed that surgical decompression of the nerve root from vascular anomalies often effectively alleviated the symptoms (Barker, Jannetta, Bissonette, Larkins, & Jho, 1996; Haines, Jannetta, & Zorub, 1980). Damage to the sensory neurons of the trigeminal nerve ganglion causes cascade of changes in the brainstem and likely contributes to the signs and symptoms of TN (Rasminsky, 1978). Following trauma, regenerating peripheral nerve fibers become more depolarized and physiologically excitable. Spontaneous action potentials can originate from multiple sites. In this state, a single action potential may evoke sustained neural depolarizations (Anderson, Vakoula, & Veinote, 2003).

Surgical biopsy specimens from TN patients with vascular compression present on imaging demonstrated evidence of inflammation, demyelination, and close apposition of axons (Deseure & Hans, 2015). Based on these morphologic and physiologic changes, an ''ignition hypothesis'' was formed to explain the principal signs and symptoms in TN. In this model, trigeminal injury induces hyper-excitability of the primary sensory neurons such that any individual neuron depolarization would activate the entire trigeminal system on that laterality. This sudden synchronous discharge according to this hypothesis would be the cause of the sudden lightening jolt of pain during a TN pain attack.

CLINICAL DIAGNOSIS

The diagnosis of trigeminal neuralgia is made from the clinical history alone. No medical imaging or blood marker is available to confirm the diagnosis. Although the hallmark clinical findings of TN have been known for centuries, White and Sweet made a significant contribution by articulating precise and succinct diagnostic criteria for TN (White & Sweet, 1969). Their criteria rapidly gained popular acceptance with clinicians and scientists, and the ''Sweet criteria'' are still commonly used worldwide. The criteria emphasize 5 major clinical findings:

1. The pain is paroxysmal.
2. The pain may be provoked by light touch to the face (trigger zones).
3. The pain is confined to the trigeminal distribution.
4. The pain is unilateral.
5. The clinical sensory examination is normal.

The International Classification of Headache Disorders II establishes classical trigeminal neuralgia as a discrete clinical diagnosis under the general classification of ''cranial neuralgias and central causes of facial pain'' (Flor et al., 2016; Olesen & Steiner, 2004). Criteria for classical TN by this classification are:

1. Paroxysmal attacks of pain lasting from a fraction of a second to 2 minutes, affecting one or more divisions of the trigeminal nerve and fulfilling criteria B and C:
2. Pain has at least one of the following characteristics:
    a. Intense, sharp, superficial or stabbing.
    b. Precipitated from trigger areas or by trigger factors.
3. Attacks are stereotyped in the individual patient.
4. There is no clinically evident neurological deficit.
5. Not attributed to another disorder.

A TN ''trigger zone'' is an area of facial skin or oral mucosa where low-intensity mechanical stimulation (light touch, air puff, hair-bending) can elicit an attack (Rasmussen, 1991) . TN trigger zones are typically only a few millimeters in size and are found in the perioral region (Crue, Shelden, Pudenz, & Freshwater, 1956). Though trigger zones are not always present in TN, the presence of a trigger zone is pathognomonic.

The clinical examination of any patient with TN symptoms should include a comprehensive head and neck examination. The large majority of TN patients will have a normal sensory examination. More detailed quantitative sensory testing may demonstrate mild tactile sensory deficits in some patients (Maarbjerg et al., 2017). A map of any trigger zones should be drawn in the patient's chart as these areas may change over time.

Multiple sclerosis (MS) is another common cause of symptomatic TN, possibly due to demyelination plaques in the trigeminal root (Nurmikko, 2009). MS should be considered in any person with TN symptoms, particularly in younger patients or patients with bilateral TN. TN symptoms can be the first opportunity for the patient to be diagnosed with MS. The neurologic history supporting an MS diagnosis include unexplained episodes of monocular blindness, diplopia, vertigo, ataxia, paraparesis, or lateralized weakness.

DIFFERENTIAL DIAGNOSIS

Glossopharyngeal Neuralgia

Glossopharyngeal neuralgia (GN) is an uncommon craniofacial pain syndrome characterized by severe, transient, stabbing, or burning pain in the ear, base of the tongue, or tonsillar fossa (Revuelta-Gutiérrez, Morales-Martínez, Mejías-Soto, Martínez-Anda, & Ortega-Porcayo, 2016). The pain can spread to other areas of the face, including the external auditory canal or superficial cervical tissue (Blumenfeld & Nikolskaya, 2013). The pain occurs in the distribution of the glossopharyngeal nerve, as well as the auricular and pharyngeal branches of the vagus nerve. This disease can be mistaken for trigeminal neuralgia if a mandibular nerve distribution exists.

GN pain is frequently triggered by chewing, swallowing, talking, yawning, or coughing. The attacks are typically paroxysmal, lightning pains, but some patients have more constant aching, burning, or pressure sensations. GN may be associated with severe bradycardia, hypotension, or transient asystole (Burfield, Ahmad, & Adams, 2016). The diagnosis can be confirmed with pain relief from topical anesthesia or glossopharyngeal block at the jugular foramen (Burfield et al., 2016) or at the styloid process (Telischak et al., 2017). As with trigeminal neuralgia, MRI and evoked potential testing are strongly recommended to rule out secondary causes.

Herpetic and Post-herpetic Neuralgia of the Trigeminal Nerve

Herpetic involvement of the trigeminal nerve is more common in older patients and in immunosuppressed patients. These populations are at higher risk to develop post-herpetic neuralgia (PHN) (O'Neill, Nurmikko, & Sommer, 2017). PHN pain is steady and sustained. The pain often spontaneously regresses within 2 or 3 weeks, but may persist for several months (Maarbjerg et al., 2017). When the pain occurs in persons more than 70 years of age, it may last a year or more. PHN pain is unilateral and is described as both burning and gnawing. It may be accompanied by a paroxysmal sharp, radiating pain caused by light mechanical stimuli (Lovell,

2015). It may occur in any part of the distribution of the trigeminal nerve, but the forehead is most common. PHN hyperalgesia and paresthesia usually begins after the erythema and typical herpetiform lesions erupt (Nair, Gharote, Singh, & Jain-Choudhary, 2014). Patients may have weakness of the masseter and pterygoid muscles on the ipsilateral side (Nair et al., 2014).

Atypical Facial Pain

Atypical facial pain (AFP) or facial pain of unknown cause is characterized by continuous, poorly localized deep burning or aching pain. AFP pain may be unilateral or bilateral and may not follow the distribution of specific peripheral nerves. The pain is often in the nasolabial fold or side of the chin and may spread to the upper or lower jaw or a wider area of the face of neck (Zakrzewska, 2016). Sensory changes, such as allodynia, dysesthesia, and paresthesia are usually present (Türp & Gobetti, 1996) . AFP usually affects middle-aged women. Some patients have a history of trauma or a dental or surgical procedure before the onset of pain (Weiss, Ehrhardt, & Tolba, 2017). Unlike TN, AFP is usually continuous with no periods of remission. Additionally, there are no autonomic symptoms associated with AFP.

MEDICAL MANAGEMENT

Burchiel separated the diagnosis of TN into type 1 and type 2. Type 1 (classic TN) is characterized by unilateral, lancinating, attacks (Eller, Raslan, & Burchiel, 2005). The neurologic examination is normal, and there is a temporary or prolonged response to Carbamazepine. Type 2 (atypical TN) is similar to type 1, but has more constant, aching facial pain between the bouts of paroxysmal pain (Burchiel & Slavin, 2000). Type 2 trigeminal neuralgia may have some facial sensory loss and poor response to medications. It is possible that type 2 trigeminal neuralgia represents an advanced stage of type 1. Both type 1 and type 2 cases are believed to be caused by arterial or venous compression of the trigeminal nerve in the area of transition from central to peripheral myelin (Obersteiner-Redlich zone) near the root entry zone of the nerve to the brainstem (Samadian, Bakhtevari, Nosari, Babadi, & Razaei, 2015).

Initial management of TN is medical. Surgical therapy is considered if medical treatment fails or secondary causes are found during the initial workup of the patient (Larsen, Piepgras, Chyatte, & Rizzolo, 2011). A neurosurgical consultation early in the medical management allow the patient to become educated about treatment options and give them time to contemplate potential interventional treatments should medical therapy prove inadequate or ineffective (Salama et al., 2009). Medical treatment is based on the capacity of the medications to decrease nerve hyperexcitability, either peripherally or centrally. The clinical trials in TN treatment did not provide a full understanding of each medication's impact on this disease (Zakrzewska & Patsalos, 2002).

Generally, medical treatment begins with an antiepileptic medication with known antineuralgic properties. Initial doses are low and titrated up gradually until the patient's pain is satisfactorily reduced or the maximum tolerated dose is reached. Carbamazepine, 100 to 200 mg two or three times daily, is the gold standard treatment and usually provides relief in more than 60-70% of patients. There are multiple medication options available, but a response to carbamazepine is almost diagnostic (Sidebottom & Maxwell, 1995).

If the Carbamazepine is not tolerated, other medications such as Baclofen, Sodium Valproate, Gabapentin, Lamotrigine, Oxcarbazepine, Topiramate, Felbamate, Zonisamide, Vigabatrin, Pregabalin, or Clonazepam may be effective (William P. Cheshire Jr, 2007; W. P. Cheshire, 1995; Fromm, Terrence, & Chattha, 1984; Solaro, Messmer Uccelli, Uccelli, Leandri, & Mancardi, 2000; Solaro, Uccelli, Brichetto, Gaspperini, & Mancardi, 2001; Zakrzewska, 2010). Formal studies of these alternative agents have not been performed (Cheshire Jr, 2007; Zakrzewska, 2010). Trigeminal nerve blocks with local anesthetic and steroid can be extremely effective in the management of the acute pain of trigeminal neuralgia while the patient waits for pharmacologic interventions to become effective (Ro & Chang, 2005). If the patient has been without an attack for several months, slow medication tapering should begin (Larsen et al., 2011). Patients with trigeminal neuralgia often taper the medication themselves, only to have the pain start again (Larsen et al., 2011). Often a combination of antiepileptic medications is needed to relieve pain completely. Surgical options may be considered after multiple medication failures, intolerable of side effects, or pain escalation.

PATIENT SELECTION AND EVALUATION

Surgical treatment of trigeminal neuralgia usually starts percutaneously and is best indicated for Burchiel type 1 TN (Eller et al., 2005). TN is a progressive disease, and classic TN can transform to Burchiel type 2 TN, characterized by more constant pain and sensory impairment. Although some reports have suggested that trials of at least 2 anticonvulsants should be performed before surgical intervention, this no evidence or guideline regarding a minimum duration of medical therapy before moving to an interventional strategy (Gronseth et al., 2008). Many patients experience initial relief with medication, but later develop breakthrough pain. Some studies show that more than 50% of patients with TN eventually undergo invention or surgery

(Dalessio, 1982). Several factors should be taken into consideration when making the choice of which surgical procedure to undertake.

Operations such as microvascular decompression (MVD) directly address the underlying disorder. This procedure requires general anesthesia and a retrosigmoid craniotomy, which can have a prolonged recovery period and so has historically been reserved for the younger, healthy patients. The percutaneous interventions are directed at other areas along the course of the trigeminal pathway, such as the trigeminal tracts in the brainstem, the nerve root, the Gasserian Ganglion, or the peripheral trigeminal nerve distributions (V1 to V3) (Pollock, 2012). Percutaneous procedures directed at the Gasserian Ganglion or trigeminal nerve root include Gamma Knife Radiosurgery (GKRS) of the cisternal portion of the trigeminal nerve. Other percutaneous techniques include glycerol Gasserian rhizotomy, radiofrequency (RF) rhizotomy, and balloon compression of the Gasserian Ganglion (Wang, Bender, & Bettegowda, 2016). The percutaneous procedures produce chemical, thermal, radiation or physical disruption of trigeminal nerve transmission.

Percutaneous procedures are indicated in elderly patients or those with multiple medical comorbidities such that MVD presents a greater risk. Age alone is not an absolute contraindication for craniotomy, MVD has been shown to be well tolerated in patients older than 75 years (Cheng, Lim, Chang, & Barbaro, 2014). RF is not appropriate for patients who cannot tolerate an awake procedure or are unable to cooperate with the necessary localization stimulation (Wang et al., 2016). There is a greater risk of the trigeminal depressor response and hypotension and bradycardia when percutaneous balloon compression (PBC) is used. Thus, PBC is contraindicated in patients with cardiovascular disease (Skirving & Dan, 2001). RF provides more precise lesioning than glycerol rhizotomy (GR) or PBC. Interestingly, many surgeons advocate the use of PBC for isolated first-division pain due to its supposed superior fiber-selective nature (Giovanni Broggi, 2013) .

Atypical facial pain (AFP) has been associated with poorer outcomes in terms of symptom recurrence across several percutaneous and medication treatment modalities (J. M. Zakrzewska, Jassim, & Bulman, 1999). Patients with MS also represent a unique subgroup, because they can suffer from a combination of inflammatory and mechanical demyelination (Cheng, Sanchez-Mejia, Limbo, Ward, & Barbaro, 2005; Pollock, 2012).

HISTORY OF PERCUTANEOUS TREATMENTS

The first attempted percutaneous treatment of TN occurred in 1910, when Harris injected the trigeminal ganglion with alcohol (Harris, 1912). Two years after Harris described his approach, Rethi treated patients with electrocoagulation of the trigeminal nerve and ganglion. The procedure was associated with a high complication rates as a result of unintended injury to the trigeminal nerve and surrounding structures due to limitations in electrode design and temperature control (Wang et al., 2016). In 1914, Hartel described a method for accessing the foramen ovale which is the basis for percutaneous procedures still in use today (Skirving & Dan, 2001) (Wang et al., 2016) . In 1974, Sweet and Wepsic, described RF of the trigeminal rootlets (Sweet & Wepsic, 1974). Their method used short-acting anesthetics to allow for more precise lesion creation using more precise electrical stimulation and temperature monitoring. Over the next few decades, Nugent further refined the RF technique by using a fine cordotomy-type electrode. Tew and Taha introduced curved thermistor-tipped electrodes, which achieved high rates of pain relief with fewer complications (Nugent, 1997; Nugent & Berry, 1974) .

Glycerol rhizotomy (GR) use dates back to the late 19th century, when physicians injected various agents such as chloroform and osmic acid, next to nerve trunks (Cole, Liu, & Apfelbaum, 2005). Although reports indicated that this method was effective in producing pain relief, the effect was transient and often accompanied by significant weakness, sensory loss, and dysesthesias (Cole et al., 2005). GR therapy was refined in 1981 by Hakanson when his team was exploring the use of stereotactic radiotherapy for TN treatment (Lunsford & Bennett, 1984). Glycerol is a trivalent alcohol naturally present in human tissue. Hakanson used the Glycerol as a vehicle to suspend tantalum dust. This solution was then injected into the trigeminal cistern (Dulhunty & Gage, 1973). Hakanson later found that injection of Glycerol alone caused pain relief (Håkanson, 1981). The exact mechanism of action of glycerol is incompletely understood. Studies have suggested its hypertonicity causes a rapid rate of change in intracellular osmolarity, resulting in axonal demyelination and fragmentation (Pal, Dinda, Roy, & Banerji, 1989). GR is widely used for patients with Burchiel type 1, type 2, or multiple sclerosis related trigeminal neuralgia (Kim J. Burchiel, 2003; Håkanson, 1981). Clinical investigations demonstrate that approximately 90% of patients have complete or immediate pain relief following glycerol injection, and 77% have good or excellent pain control after a 10-year follow-up (Jho & Lunsford, 1997). Facial sensory loss may occur following glycerol rhizotomy: 32% to 48% are mild, 13% are moderate, and 6% are dense (Blomstedt & Bergenheim, 2002).

Percutaneous balloon compression (PBC) was discovered in the 1950s when investigator found that scar tissue compressing the trigeminal nerve root was another cause of TN (Taarnhøj, 1952). In 1952, Taarnhøj described his surgical methodology for decompressing the dorsal trigeminal root. Later, Shelden and Pudenz reported their surgical method for decompression of the second and third nerve divisions (Shelden, Pudenz, Freshwater, & Crue, 1955). In working to decompress the trigeminal ganglion, they found that the effectiveness of their technique derived from the resultant injury to the posterior trigeminal root posterior to the ganglion (Shelden et al., 1955). It was not until 1983, when Mullan and Lichtor described compression of the trigeminal ganglion with a percutaneously inserted Fogarty balloon catheter, that PBC became a viable treatment option (Lichtor & Mullan, 1990). Studies in rabbits revealed that compression seems to preferentially affect the medium and large myelinated pain fibers, sparing small fibers, allowing for recovery of motor and sensory function, and preservation of the corneal reflex (Lobato, Rivas, Sarabia, & Lamas, 1990).

Currently, PBC is mainly indicated for patients with Burchiel type 1 or 2 and multiple sclerosis related TN. Pain relief following PBC is usually immediate, but can be delayed by a week after the procedure (Peters & Nurmikko, 2002). Numbness in the V2 and V3 distribution occurs in approximately 80% of patients, but is typically mild and often improves with time (Lichtor & Mullan, 1990). Most patients have some degree of pterygoid weakness, which is also mild and resolves after weeks to months. In rare cases, the unilateral symptomatic jaw weakness is permanent (Skirving & Dan, 2001). The possibility of permanent jaw weakness makes this procedure contraindicated for patients with preexisting contralateral jaw weakness (Lichtor & Mullan, 1990). Theoretically, this complication can also be a problem when this procedure is performed bilaterally, as with MS patients. Pain relief is immediate in 92% to 100% of patients, and recurrence rates are reported as 19% to 32% over 5 to 20 years (Blomstedt & Bergenheim, 2002).

Radiofrequency ablation treatment (RFA) is thought to selectively injure the unmyelinated or poorly myelinated nociceptive nerves, but spare the heavily myelinated fibers associated with touch, proprioception, and motor function. The procedure consists of low-current stimulation to determine the proper position of the electrode over the pathologic trigeminal nerve fibers. This is followed by the creation of a permanent lesion by rapidly vibrating the tissue, which generates enough heat to slowly destroy the selected nerve fibers (Nugent, 1997). Mild paresthesia in the distribution of the facial pain is the goal of RF treatment of trigeminal neuralgia. Significant dysesthesia or sensory loss has been reported in 6% to 28% of treated patients, with loss of the corneal reflex in 3% to 8%, depending on the technique employed (Taha & Tew, 1996). Trigeminal nerve motor weakness has been reported in up to 14% of patients, but is most often mild and transient (Kanpolat, Savas, Bekar, & Berk, 2001). Investigators have reported that 88% to 99% of patients obtain immediate pain relief following RF, with 20% to 27% recurrence rates over a 9- to 14-year follow-up (Taha & Tew, 1996). Patients with a more dense sensory loss from the RF lesion tend to have a lower rate of recurrence, but may develop worsening pain due to anesthesia dolorosa. One clinical report found that 81% of patients obtained excellent pain relief with a second RF treatment (Cheng et al., 2014).

CONVENTIONAL V2 RF RHIZOTOMY

The assumed highly effective nature of RFA treatment is thought to be related to the differential in thermocoagulation of the trigeminal rootlets. Lower temperatures seem to selectively inhibit nociceptive action potentials and spare the nerves that transmit tactile sensation (Son, Kim, Kim, Yang, & Lee, 2011). However, histologic animal studies have indicated that the induced thermal injury affects all sizes of nerve fibers, regardless of their myelination status (Smith, McWhorter, & Challa, 1981). Thus, reducing the overall sensory input to the trigeminal root may be the ultimate mechanism.

The classic approach to RF therapy of the maxillary or mandibular branches of the TN involves placement of the needle through foramen ovale. RF through the foramen ovale can be a difficult and time-consuming procedure for both the physician and the patient due to the need for very precise placement of the needle (Wu, Meng, Xu, Liu, & Wang, 2004). Failure to position the needle properly can lead to treatment failure or serious complications such as nonspecific lesion, intracranial hemorrhage, and infection (Kanpolat et al., 2001). An alternative approach focuses passing through foramen rotundum where V2 nerve branch exits the cranium, and subsequently crosses the pterygopalatine fossa, and enters the orbit through the inferior orbital fissure (Xu, Zhang, Chen, Wu, & Zhou, 2006). Approaching through the foramen rotundum, rather than the foramen ovale, has the potential to simplify targeted treatment of the maxillary branch of the trigeminal nerve in TN patients.

Recent improvements in RF techniques have increased the accuracy of the procedure through the use of intraoperative computed tomography (CT) neuronavigation and frameless stereotactic cannulation of the foramen ovale, with good success (Gusmão, Oliveira, Tazinaffo, & Honey, 2003; Lin et al., 2011). Some investigators reported no difference in surgical outcome or pain relief between CT-guidance with 3D reconstruction and fluoroscopy-guided groups (Yang, Lin, Lee, Weng, & Liao, 2010). However, CT-guidance significantly decreased the median time for needle placement (14 vs 40 min) and intraoperative patient discomfort. Another group proposed a CT-guided technique through the foramen rotundum and found that, compared to an approach through foramen ovale, thermocoagulation through foramen rotundum showed similar results for pain relief immediately and at a 1-year follow-up (Huang et al., 2014). This approach resulted in shorter procedural time and lower incidence of adverse effects such as masseter weakness and loss of corneal reflex.

The RF procedure requires patient cooperation to localize facial stimuli. Avoidance of electrode placement beyond 10 mm of the profile of the clivus, where the trochlear and abducens nerve lie is imperative (Gusmão et al., 2003). Once the needle is in place, the patient can be awakened, and sensory and motor responses tested. Detailed mapping to then occurs to guide lesion placement and minimize sensory and motor side effects (Huang et al., 2014). Lesions are typically made at a maximum 55-60^{c} to 80-90^{C} for 30 - 120 seconds (Xu et al., 2006). The patient can be discharged home on the same day if stable, or observed overnight.

Traditional radiofrequency lesioning of the Gasserian ganglion is thought to destroy the pain fibers at temperatures > 65°C. Pulsed radiofrequency is a nondestructive treatment that delivers short bursts of radiofrequency current from the tip of the electrode at 42°C with long pauses between to allow heat to dissipate in the target tissue. Pulsed RF is thought to cause microscopic damage to axonal microfilaments and microtubules with greater changes occurring in C fibers than in Alpha fibers, minimizing the occurrence of sensory or motor deficit in the surrounding tissues . An electron microscopic analysis comparing the effects of pulsed radiofrequency versus continuous radiofrequency on rabbit dorsal root ganglion found that pulsed radiofrequency was substantially less destructive . However, a recent randomized controlled trial comparing conventional radiofrequency with pulsed radiofrequency found that pulsed radiofrequency was not effective in reducing pain in patients with trigeminal neuralgia .

FLUOROSCOPICALLY GUIDED V2 TREATMENT

During the procedure, the patient is placed in the supine position with the cervical spine in the neutral position. The coronoid notch is identified by palpating the area just anterior and slightly inferior to the acoustic auditory meatus (Lin et al., 2011). The patient holds their mouth in a neutral position. After the skin is prepared with antiseptic solution and local anesthetic, a 22-gauge, 2-inch styletted needle is inserted just below the zygomatic arch directly in the middle of the coronoid notch (Bennett & Giovannitti, 1998). The needle is advanced under the fluoroscopic guidance until the lateral pterygoid plate is encountered. Selective blockade of the maxillary nerve is achieved by redirection anteriorly and slightly superiorly until the needle slips past the anterior margin of the lateral pterygoid plate (Singh, Srivastava, & Dang, 2001). A paresthesia in the distribution of the maxillary nerve is usually elicited about 1 cm deeper than the point at which the lateral pterygoid plate was encountered. After negative aspiration, 3 to 5 mL of local anesthetic and steroid solution is injected in incremental doses. The patient is observed carefully for signs of local anesthetic toxicity. Ablation can then be completed with radiofrequency needles or cryoprobes (Burton M. Onofrio, 1975).

ULTRASOUND GUIDED APPROACH FOR V2 ABLATION

Although x-ray based guidance is still considered the "gold standard" in diagnostics and interventional procedures for head and neck blocks, the use of ultrasonography allows the visualization of soft tissues and surrounding vasculature within the pterygopalatine fossa with real-time needle placement. Ultrasound guidance via the coronoid notch allows identification of the maxilla, lateral pterygoid plate, lateral pterygoid muscle, and the maxillary artery. The ultrasound-guided technique starts with coronoid notch identification. Once identified, a high-frequency, linear ultrasound probe is placed transversely over the coronoid notch (Nader, Kendall, et al., 2013; Nader, Bendok, Prine, & Kendall, 2015; Sola et al., 2012). The coronoid notch provides an acoustic window into the pterygopalatine fossa and allows easy identification of the maxillary nerve. The temporomandibular joint can be identified by locating the ball-shaped mandibular condyle and the mandibular neck (Nader, Schittek, & Kendall, 2013). Under real-time ultrasound guidance, a 22-gauge, 2-inch needle is inserted just below the zygomatic arch directly through the coronoid notch using an out-of-plane approach. The needle is advanced until contact with the lateral pterygoid plate. The needle is redirected toward the pupil of the eye until it slips past the anterosuperior margin of the lateral pterygoid plate and into the pterygopalatine fissure. After negative aspiration, 4 to 5 mL of local anesthetic, with or without 40 to 80 mg of depo-steroid are injected incrementally (Nader et al., 2015). The patient will then be observed carefully for signs of local anesthetic toxicity. Proximity to the sphenopalatine ganglion may cause partial blockade of this structure. This is followed by either a continuous or pulsed RF protocol.

CT GUIDED V2 RF ABLATION

The patient is positioned supine and the head is taped gently to prevent accidental head movement. A positioning grid is placed over the cheek of the painful side. Oblique coronal scanning is conducted with the scanning frame parallel to the plane connecting external acoustic pore to ipsilateral maxillary third molar bone. The resulting CT image frame simultaneously captures the foramen rotundum (FR) and its external and internal openings. The intrinsic ruler of the CT scanner is used to measure the distance from the needle entry point to the external opening of FR or foramen ovale (FO) as well as to determine the needle entry angle. The skin and subcutaneous tissues are anesthetized and a 10 cm 22 gauge radiofrequency needle is inserted and advanced along the predetermined path based on the angle and depth previously measured. Intermittent CT guidance is used until reaching the external opening of the FR or FO. After confirming the absence of blood, cerebral spinal fluid, or paresthesia, a sensory test is performed by stimulating the probe at 100 Hz with pulse width at 500 μS and amplitude at 0.2–0.5 mA until paresthesia concordant to the patient's usual pain is achieved. A motor test is also performed to make certain that the probe was not near any other adjacent nerves. 0.5 mL of 1% lidocaine is injected 2 minutes prior to ablation and either a continuous or pulsed RF protocol is activated. With this approach, when compared with the classic approach through the FO, it appears to be able to not only provide similar pain relief up to at 1 year follow-up visit, but also with fewer adverse effects, except for facial hematoma and facial numbness, which are no worse than the classic approach. CT guidance also lowers procedure duration time and is better tolerated by the patients.

SIDE EFFECTS AND COMPLICATIONS

Because of the highly vascular nature of the pterygopalatine fossa, significant facial hematoma may occur after trigeminal nerve block via the coronoid approach (Singh et al., 2001). This vascularity means use of small, incremental doses of local anesthetic is needed to avoid local anesthetic toxicity. Post-procedure dysesthesia, including anesthesia dolorosa, may occur in a small number of patients who undergo any neurodestructive procedure (Blomstedt & Bergenheim, 2002). These post-procedure symptoms are thought to be due to incomplete destruction of the neural structures. Sloughing of skin in the area of anesthesia also may occur. In addition to disturbances of sensation, blockade or destruction of the branches of the trigeminal nerve may result in abnormal motor function, including weakness of the muscles of mastication and secondary facial asymmetry due to muscle weakness or loss of proprioception. (Kanpolat et al., 2001; Skirving & Dan, 2001) . The patient should be warned that all of these complications may occur. Trigeminal depressor response can also be inadvertently evoked intraoperatively causing bradycardia and possible asystole. Pre- or intra-operative atropine (0.4mg) can be given to prevent such a complication (Wu et al., 2004).

PATIENT OUTCOMES

Pain relief with RF is generally high with most studies reporting greater than 95% or complete pain resolution (G. Broggi, Franzini, Lasio, Giorgi, & Servello, 1990; Tronnier, Rasche, Hamer, Kienle, & Kunze, 2001). Rates of pain control and the duration of pain relief consistently correlate with the degree of sensory loss. A prospective study of 154 patients, found that a high degree of sensory loss predicted a low rates of pain recurrence but the highest rate of dysesthesia (Taha & Tew, 1996). In contrast, patients with mild sensory loss had the highest pain recurrence rates and the lowest rates of dysesthesia (Kanpolat et al., 2001). Most cases of masseter weakness and diplopia resolve by 6 to 12 months (Giovanni Broggi, 2013). In a series of 1600 patients, rates of anesthesia dolorosa ranged from 0% to 12% (Kanpolat et al., 2001). Another study demonstrated rates of corneal anesthesia from 1% to 20.3% (Giovanni Broggi, 2013) Rates of masseter weakness with RF ranged from 3% to 29%.

Few studies have examined predictors of outcomes after RF treatment. Recently, Kosugi found that outcomes were significantly better for patients with isolated V3 vs V2 or multidivisional pain (Kosugi et al., 2015). Taha used a curved, rather than straight, electrode and created more selective lesions which decreased rates of sensory complications (Tew & Taha, 1995).

FUTURE DIRECTIONS

The majority of studies of percutaneous rhizotomy are retrospective, and highly variable in their patient populations, treatment technique, and reported outcomes. Studies include varying numbers of patients with atypical pain, MS, and bilateral TN. Most series also include varying percentages of patients who have had multiple ablative treatments. Although the general technique for each procedure is similar, each type of percutaneous rhizotomy has operator-dependent technical variations that limit comparisons:

1. **GR:** The method for cisternography varies as does the volume of glycerin injected
2. **PBC:** The level of pressure and duration compression
3. **RF:** Type of electrode, delivery of energy, and location of lesioning.

A lack of standardization in pain relief outcomes and definition of complications also limits comparisons of techniques. An additional complicating factor is whether patients require medications postoperatively to achieve complete pain control. Efforts at standardization have been made, including the Barrow Neurological Institute Pain Scale, which grades outcomes on a scale from I to V.

Finally, there is high variability in the duration of follow-up. Although Kaplan-Meier analyses are able to in part control of such variability, the variability in outcomes reporting for TN makes defining the exact time of pain recurrence difficult. All of these factors hamper the use of single-modality studies in comparisons of outcomes across treatment modalities. In addition to incorporating new technical advances, future studies must overcome this patient heterogeneity, procedural variation, and nonstandard outcomes, which limit interpretation and thus advancement of these approaches.

CONCLUSION

Diagnosing TN may require in multiple consultations, and may be preceded by misguided treatments and unnecessary procedures. Once TN has been diagnosed, many therapeutic options become available. The initial treatment is medical management. With many newer pharmacological agents become available, possibilities exist for either monotherapy or polypharmacy. Surgical interventions are available for patients who are intolerant of medication therapy or whose pain is extreme and unremitting. Secondary causes must be explored in all patients because, if such causes are discovered, surgical interventions may supersede medical options.

Each of the medications and each of the surgical procedures is associated with side effects and potential risks. These pitfalls must be weighed based on each individual's medical conditions, lifestyle, age, personal preference, and past therapies. Further reviews of the literature are helping guide the clinical treatment with evidence-based recommendations. The patient must be well-informed about both medical and surgical options as soon as the diagnosis is made. As part of the initial evaluation, the patient should be required to consult with both surgical and medical practitioners. This approach allows for a planned therapeutic attack, with all parties seeking timely and effective pain relief for the patient.

Many elements of percutaneous rhizotomy have remained true to the techniques described by their pioneers. All 3 percutaneous procedures (GN, RF, and PBC) rely on Hartel's landmarks to gain access to the foramen ovale. Much effort has been devoted to improving visualization and navigation to the foramen ovale (Peris-Celda, Graziano, Russo, Mericle, & Ulm, 2013). Although fluoroscopy has been the imaging modality of choice, newer studies have demonstrated the potential usefulness of computed tomography (CT), flat panel CT, ultrasonography and neuronavigation systems, especially for patients with anatomic variants (Aydoseli et al., 2015; Huo et al., 2014). With refinement of electrodes to allow for small lesions, complication rates for RF are still relatively high compared with PBC and GR. The size of the lesion not only depends on the size of the electrode tip and the electrode diameter, as well as the duration of thermocoagulation and the temperature achieved in the tissue (Karol & Karol, 2009). Pulsed RF has been used successfully to treat spinal pain and use in patients with TN has been promising. Erdine and colleagues used pulsed radiofrequency current to treat 5 patients. 60% experienced durable pain relief and no neurologic complications were observed (Erdine et al., 2007).

Percutaneous rhizotomy, in all its forms, offers pain relief for TN that is immediate with varying durability and a generally favorable side effect profile. However, treatment selection remains an inexact science in the absence of high quality outcomes data.

REFERENCES

Anderson, L. C., Vakoula, A., & Veinote, R. (2003). Inflammatory hypersensitivity in a rat model of trigeminal neuropathic pain. *Archives of Oral Biology*, *48*(2), 161–169. doi:10.1016/S0003-9969(02)00203-0 PMID:12642236

Aydoseli, A., Akcakaya, M. O., Aras, Y., Sabanci, P. A., Unal, T. C., Sencer, A., ... Izgi, N. (2015). Neuronavigation-assisted percutaneous balloon compression for the treatment of trigeminal neuralgia: The technique and short-term clinical results. *British Journal of Neurosurgery*, *29*(4), 552–558. doi:10.3109/02688697.2015.1019418 PMID:25807330

Barker, F. G. II, Jannetta, P. J., Bissonette, D. J., Larkins, M. V., & Jho, H. D. (1996). The long-term outcome of microvascular decompression for trigeminal neuralgia. *The New England Journal of Medicine*, *334*(17), 1077–1083. doi:10.1056/NEJM199604253341701 PMID:8598865

Bennett, C. R., & Giovannitti, J. A. Jr. (1998). *Neural blockade of oral and circumoral structures. In Neural Blockade in Clinical Anesthesia and Management of Pain* (3rd ed.; p. 528). Philadelphia: Lippincott Williams & Wilkins.

Blomstedt, P. C., & Bergenheim, A. T. (2002). Technical difficulties and perioperative complications of retrogasserian glycerol rhizotomy for trigeminal neuralgia. *Stereotactic and Functional Neurosurgery*, *79*(3-4), 168–181. doi:10.1159/000070830 PMID:12890975

Blumenfeld, A., & Nikolskaya, G. (2013). Glossopharyngeal neuralgia. *Current Pain and Headache Reports*, *17*(7), 343. doi:10.100711916-013-0343-x PMID:23709235

Bogduk, N. (2006). Pulsed radiofrequency. *Pain Medicine*, *7*(5), 396–407. doi:10.1111/j.1526-4637.2006.00210.x PMID:17014598

Bowsher, D. (1997). Trigeminal neuralgia: An anatomically oriented review. *Clinical Anatomy (New York, N.Y.)*, *10*(6), 409–415. doi: PMID:9358972

Broggi, G. (2013). Percutaneous retrogasserian balloon compression for trigeminal neuralgia. *World Neurosurgery*, *79*(2), 269–270. doi:10.1016/j.wneu.2012.05.015 PMID:22634455

Broggi, G., Franzini, A., Lasio, G., Giorgi, C., & Servello, D. (1990). Long-term results of percutaneous retrogasserian thermorhizotomy for "essential" trigeminal neuralgia: Considerations in 1000 consecutive patients. *Neurosurgery*, *26*(5), 783–786, discussion 786–787. doi:10.1227/00006123-199005000-00008 PMID:2352596

Burchiel, K. J. (2003). A new classification for facial pain. *Neurosurgery*, *53*(5), 1164–1166, discussion 1166–1167. doi:10.1227/01.NEU.0000088806.11659.D8 PMID:14580284

Burchiel, K. J., & Slavin, K. V. (2000). On the natural history of trigeminal neuralgia. *Neurosurgery*, *46*(1), 152–154, discussion 154–155. doi:10.1093/neurosurgery/46.1.152 PMID:10626945

Burfield, L., Ahmad, F., & Adams, J. (2016). Glossopharyngeal neuralgia associated with cardiac syncope. *BMJ Case Reports*, *2016*. doi:10.1136/bcr-2015-214104 PMID:27102416

Canavero, S., Bonicalzi, V., & Pagni, C. A. (1995). The riddle of trigeminal neuralgia. *Pain*, *60*(2), 229–231. doi:10.1016/0304-3959(94)00196-L PMID:7784109

Cappadocia, A. (1856). *The extant works of Aretaeus: the Cappadocian*. Sydenham Society.

Casey, K. F., & Jannetta, P. J. (2010). *History of Trigeminal Neuralgia. Trigeminal Neuralgia, 3*. Oxford University Press.

Cheng, J. S., Lim, D. A., Chang, E. F., & Barbaro, N. M. (2014). A review of percutaneous treatments for trigeminal neuralgia. *Neurosurgery*, *10*(Suppl 1), 25–33, discussion 33. PMID:24509496

Cheng, J. S., Sanchez-Mejia, R. O., Limbo, M., Ward, M. M., & Barbaro, N. M. (2005). Management of medically refractory trigeminal neuralgia in patients with multiple sclerosis. *Neurosurgical Focus*, *18*(5), e13. doi:10.3171/foc.2005.18.5.14 PMID:16419978

Cheshire, W. P. (1995). Felbamate relieved trigeminal neuralgia. *The Clinical Journal of Pain*, *11*(2), 139–142. doi:10.1097/00002508-199506000-00009 PMID:7549170

Cheshire, W. P. Jr. (2007). Trigeminal neuralgia. *Current Pain and Headache Reports*, *11*(1), 69–74. doi:10.100711916-007-0025-7 PMID:17214925

Cole, C. D., Liu, J. K., & Apfelbaum, R. I. (2005). Historical perspectives on the diagnosis and treatment of trigeminal neuralgia. *Neurosurgical Focus*, *18*(5), E4. doi:10.3171/foc.2005.18.5.5 PMID:15913280

Crue, B. L., Shelden, C. H., Pudenz, R. H., & Freshwater, D. B. (1956). Observations on the pain and trigger mechanism in trigeminal neuralgia. *Neurology*, *6*(3), 196–207. doi:10.1212/WNL.6.3.196 PMID:13297120

Dalessio, D. J. (1982). Trigeminal neuralgia. A practical approach to treatment. *Drugs*, *24*(3), 248–255. doi:10.2165/00003495-198224030-00005 PMID:7128480

Deseure, K., & Hans, G. H. (2015). Chronic Constriction Injury of the Rat's Infraorbital Nerve (IoN-CCI) to Study Trigeminal Neuropathic Pain. *Journal of Visualized Experiments*, (103). doi:10.3791/53167 PMID:26437303

Devor, M., Amir, R., & Rappaport, Z. H. (2002). Pathophysiology of trigeminal neuralgia: The ignition hypothesis. *The Clinical Journal of Pain*, *18*(1), 4–13. doi:10.1097/00002508-200201000-00002 PMID:11803297

Dubner, R., Sharav, Y., Gracely, R. H., & Price, D. D. (1987). Idiopathic trigeminal neuralgia: Sensory features and pain mechanisms. *Pain*, *31*(1), 23–33. doi:10.1016/0304-3959(87)90003-0 PMID:3696741

Duff, J. M., Spinner, R. J., Lindor, N. M., Dodick, D. W., & Atkinson, J. L. (1999). Familial trigeminal neuralgia and contralateral hemifacial spasm. *Neurology*, *53*(1), 216–218. doi:10.1212/WNL.53.1.216 PMID:10408564

Dulhunty, A. F., Gage, P. W., & Barry, P. H. (1973). Differential effects of glycerol treatment on membrane capacity and excitation-contraction coupling in toad sartorius fibres. *The Journal of Physiology*, *234*(2), 373–408. doi:10.1113/jphysiol.1973.sp010350 PMID:4203309

Eboli, P., Stone, J. L., Aydin, S., & Slavin, K. V. (2009). Historical characterization of trigeminal neuralgia. *Neurosurgery*, *64*(6), 1183–1186. doi:10.1227/01.NEU.0000339412.44397.76 PMID:19487899

Eller, J. L., Raslan, A. M., & Burchiel, K. J. (2005). Trigeminal neuralgia: Definition and classification. *Neurosurgical Focus*, *18*(5), E3. doi:10.3171/foc.2005.18.5.4 PMID:15913279

Erdine, S., Bilir, A., Cosman, E. R., & Cosman, E. R., Jr. (2009). Ultrastructural changes in axons following exposure to pulsed radiofrequency fields. *Pain Practice: The Official Journal of World Institute of Pain, 9*(6), 407–417.

Erdine, S., Ozyalcin, N. S., Cimen, A., Celik, M., Talu, G. K., & Disci, R. (2007). Comparison of pulsed radiofrequency with conventional radiofrequency in the treatment of idiopathic trigeminal neuralgia. *European Journal of Pain (London, England)*, *11*(3), 309–313. doi:10.1016/j.ejpain.2006.04.001 PMID:16762570

Erdine, S., Yucel, A., Cimen, A., Aydin, S., Sav, A., & Bilir, A. (2005). Effects of pulsed versus conventional radiofrequency current on rabbit dorsal root ganglion morphology. *European Journal of Pain (London, England)*, *9*(3), 251–256. doi:10.1016/j.ejpain.2004.07.002 PMID:15862474

Flor, H., Rasche, D., Islamian, A. P., Rolko, C., Yilmaz, P., Ruppolt, M., & .... (2016). Subtle Sensory Abnormalities Detected by Quantitative Sensory Testing in Patients with Trigeminal Neuralgia. *Pain Physician*, *19*(7), 507–518. PMID:27676667

Fraioli, M. F., Lisciani, D., & Fraioli, C. (2014). Trigeminal neuralgia. *Journal of Neurosurgery*, *120*(1), 288–289. doi:10.3171/2012.12.JNS101876 PMID:24180575

Fromm, G. H., Terrence, C. F., & Chattha, A. S. (1984). Baclofen in the treatment of trigeminal neuralgia: Double-blind study and long-term follow-up. *Annals of Neurology*, *15*(3), 240–244. doi:10.1002/ana.410150306 PMID:6372646

Gronseth, G., Cruccu, G., Alksne, J., Argoff, C., Brainin, M., Burchiel, K., ... Zakrzewska, J. M. (2008). Practice parameter: the diagnostic evaluation and treatment of trigeminal neuralgia (an evidence-based review): report of the Quality Standards Subcommittee of the American Academy of Neurology and the European Federation of Neurological Societies. *Neurology*, *71*(15), 1183–1190. doi:10.1212/01.wnl.0000326598.83183.04 PMID:18716236

Gusmão, S., Oliveira, M., Tazinaffo, U., & Honey, C. R. (2003). Percutaneous trigeminal nerve radiofrequency rhizotomy guided by computerized tomography fluoroscopy. Technical note. *Journal of Neurosurgery*, *99*(4), 785–786. doi:10.3171/jns.2003.99.4.0785 PMID:14567619

Haines, S. J., Jannetta, P. J., & Zorub, D. S. (1980). Microvascular relations of the trigeminal nerve. An anatomical study with clinical correlation. *Journal of Neurosurgery*, *52*(3), 381–386. doi:10.3171/jns.1980.52.3.0381 PMID:7359193

Håkanson, S. (1981). Trigeminal neuralgia treated by the injection of glycerol into the trigeminal cistern. *Neurosurgery*, *9*(6), 638–646. doi:10.1227/00006123-198112000-00005 PMID:7322329

Harness, D. M., & Chase, P. F. (1990). Lateralization of chronic facial pain: Fact or fiction. *Cranio*, *8*(4), 339–341. doi:10.1080/08869634.1990.11678335 PMID:2098197

Harris, W. (1912). Alcohol injection of the Gasserian ganglion for trigeminal neuralgia. *Lancet, 179*(4613), 218–221. doi:10.1016/S0140-6736(01)65362-5 PMID:19975621

Huang, B., Yao, M., Feng, Z., Guo, J., Zereshki, A., Leong, M., & Qian, X. (2014). CT-guided percutaneous infrazygomatic radiofrequency neurolysis through foramen rotundum to treat V2 trigeminal neuralgia. *Pain Medicine, 15*(8), 1418–1428. doi:10.1111/pme.12440 PMID:24716880

Huo, X., Sun, X., Zhang, Z., Guo, W., Guan, N., & Luo, J. (2014). Dyna-CT-assisted percutaneous microballoon compression for trigeminal neuralgia. *Journal of Neurointerventional Surgery, 6*(7), 521–526. doi:10.1136/neurintsurg-2013-010676 PMID:23904451

Jho, H. D., & Lunsford, L. D. (1997). Percutaneous retrogasserian glycerol rhizotomy. Current technique and results. *Neurosurgery Clinics of North America, 8*(1), 63–74. PMID:9018706

Kanpolat, Y., Savas, A., Bekar, A., & Berk, C. (2001). Percutaneous controlled radiofrequency trigeminal rhizotomy for the treatment of idiopathic trigeminal neuralgia: 25-year experience with 1,600 patients. *Neurosurgery, 48*(3), 524–532, discussion 532–534. doi:10.1097/00006123-200103000-00013 PMID:11270542

Karol, E. A., & Karol, M. N. (2009). A multiarray electrode mapping method for percutaneous thermocoagulation as treatment of trigeminal neuralgia. Technical note on a series of 178 consecutive procedures. *Surgical Neurology, 71*(1), 11–17, discussion 17–18. doi:10.1016/j.surneu.2007.09.021 PMID:18328544

Kosugi, S., Shiotani, M., Otsuka, Y., Suzuki, T., Katori, N., Hashiguchi, S., & Morisaki, H. (2015). Long-term outcomes of percutaneous radiofrequency thermocoagulation of gasserian ganglion for 2nd- and multiple-division trigeminal neuralgia. *Pain Practice: The Official Journal of World Institute of Pain, 15*(3), 223–228.

Larsen, A., Piepgras, D., Chyatte, D., & Rizzolo, D. (2011). Trigeminal neuralgia: Diagnosis and medical and surgical management. *JAAPA: Official Journal of the American Academy of Physician Assistants, 24*(7), 20–25. doi:10.1097/01720610-201107000-00005 PMID:21748954

Lichtor, T., & Mullan, J. F. (1990). A 10-year follow-up review of percutaneous microcompression of the trigeminal ganglion. *Journal of Neurosurgery, 72*(1), 49–54. doi:10.3171/jns.1990.72.1.0049 PMID:2294184

Lin, M. H.-C., Lee, M.-H., Wang, T.-C., Cheng, Y.-K., Su, C.-H., Chang, C.-M., & Yang, J.-T. (2011). Foramen ovale cannulation guided by intra-operative computed tomography with integrated neuronavigation for the treatment of trigeminal neuralgia. *Acta Neurochirurgica*, *153*(8), 1593–1599. doi:10.100700701-011-1009-2 PMID:21503836

Lobato, R. D., Rivas, J. J., Sarabia, R., & Lamas, E. (1990). Percutaneous microcompression of the gasserian ganglion for trigeminal neuralgia. *Journal of Neurosurgery*, *72*(4), 546–553. doi:10.3171/jns.1990.72.4.0546 PMID:2319312

Lovell, B. (2015). Trigeminal herpes zoster: Early recognition and treatment are crucial. *BMJ Case Reports*, *2015*(mar20 1), bcr2014208673. doi:10.1136/bcr-2014-208673 PMID:25795749

Lunsford, L. D., & Bennett, M. H. (1984). Percutaneous retrogasserian glycerol rhizotomy for tic douloureux: Part 1. Technique and results in 112 patients. *Neurosurgery*, *14*(4), 424–430. doi:10.1227/00006123-198404000-00006 PMID:6728144

Maarbjerg, S., Di Stefano, G., Bendtsen, L., & Cruccu, G. (2017). Trigeminal neuralgia - diagnosis and treatment. *Cephalalgia: An International Journal of Headache*.

Massager, N., Murata, N., Tamura, M., Devriendt, D., Levivier, M., & Régis, J. (2007). Influence of nerve radiation dose in the incidence of trigeminal dysfunction after trigeminal neuralgia radiosurgery. *Neurosurgery*, *60*(4), 681–687, discussion 687–688. doi:10.1227/01.NEU.0000255393.77538.75 PMID:17415205

Mosberg, W. H., Jr. (1960). Trigeminal Neuralgia: Its History and Treatment. *The Journal of Nervous and Mental Disease*. Retrieved from http://journals.lww.com/jonmd/Citation/1960/07000/Trigeminal_Neuralgia__Its_History_and_Treatment.14.aspx

Nader, A., Bendok, B. R., Prine, J. J., & Kendall, M. C. (2015). Ultrasound-Guided Pulsed Radiofrequency Application via the Pterygopalatine Fossa: A Practical Approach to Treat Refractory Trigeminal Neuralgia. *Pain Physician*, *18*(3), E411–E415. PMID:26000688

Nader, A., Kendall, M. C., De Oliveria, G. S., Chen, J. Q., Vanderby, B., Rosenow, J. M., & Bendok, B. R. (2013). Ultrasound-guided trigeminal nerve block via the pterygopalatine fossa: An effective treatment for trigeminal neuralgia and atypical facial pain. *Pain Physician*, *16*(5), E537–E545. PMID:24077204

Nader, A., Schittek, H., & Kendall, M. C. (2013). Lateral pterygoid muscle and maxillary artery are key anatomical landmarks for ultrasound-guided trigeminal nerve block. *Anesthesiology, 118*(4), 957. doi:10.1097/ALN.0b013e31826d3dfc PMID:23059449

Nair, P., Gharote, H., Singh, P., & Jain-Choudhary, P. (2014). Herpes zoster on the face in the elderly. *BMJ Case Reports, 2014*(1). doi:10.1136/bcr-2013-200101 PMID:25331144

Nugent, G. R. (1997). Radiofrequency treatment of trigeminal neuralgia using a cordotomy-type electrode. A method. *Neurosurgery Clinics of North America, 8*(1), 41–52. PMID:9018704

Nugent, G. R., & Berry, B. (1974). Trigeminal neuralgia treated by differential percutaneous radiofrequency coagulation of the Gasserian ganglion. *Journal of Neurosurgery, 40*(4), 517–523. doi:10.3171/jns.1974.40.4.0517 PMID:4592266

Nurmikko, T. J. (2009). Pathophysiology of MS-related trigeminal neuralgia. *Pain, 143*(3), 165–166. doi:10.1016/j.pain.2009.03.019 PMID:19375226

O'Neill, F., Nurmikko, T., & Sommer, C. (2017). Other facial neuralgias. *Cephalalgia: An International Journal of Headache*.

Olesen, J., & Steiner, T. J. (2004). The International classification of headache disorders, 2nd edn (ICDH-II). *Journal of Neurology, Neurosurgery, and Psychiatry, 75*(6), 808–811. Retrieved from jnnp.bmj.com

Onofrio, B. M. (1975). Radiofrequency percutaneous Gasserian ganglion lesions. *Journal of Neurosurgery, 42*(2), 132–139. doi:10.3171/jns.1975.42.2.0132 PMID:1113146

Pal, H. K., Dinda, A. K., Roy, S., & Banerji, A. K. (1989). Acute effect of anhydrous glycerol on peripheral nerve: An experimental study. *British Journal of Neurosurgery, 3*(4), 463–469. doi:10.3109/02688698909002832 PMID:2803594

Pearce, J. M. S. (2003). Trigeminal neuralgia (Fothergill's disease) in the 17th and 18th centuries. *Journal of Neurology, Neurosurgery, and Psychiatry, 74*(12), 1688. doi:10.1136/jnnp.74.12.1688 PMID:14638891

Peris-Celda, M., Graziano, F., Russo, V., Mericle, R. A., & Ulm, A. J. (2013). Foramen ovale puncture, lesioning accuracy, and avoiding complications: Microsurgical anatomy study with clinical implications. *Journal of Neurosurgery, 119*(5), 1176–1193. doi:10.3171/2013.1.JNS12743 PMID:23600929

Peters, G., & Nurmikko, T. J. (2002). Peripheral and gasserian ganglion-level procedures for the treatment of trigeminal neuralgia. *The Clinical Journal of Pain*, *18*(1), 28–34. doi:10.1097/00002508-200201000-00005 PMID:11803300

Pollock, B. E. (2012). Surgical management of medically refractory trigeminal neuralgia. *Current Neurology and Neuroscience Reports*, *12*(2), 125–131. doi:10.100711910-011-0242-7 PMID:22183181

Rasminsky, M. (1978). Ectopic generation of impulses and cross-talk in spinal nerve roots of "dystrophic" mice. *Annals of Neurology*, *3*(4), 351–357. doi:10.1002/ana.410030413 PMID:208454

Rasmussen, P. (1990a). Facial pain. II. A prospective survey of 1052 patients with a view of: Character of the attacks, onset, course, and character of pain. *Acta Neurochirurgica*, *107*(3-4), 121–128. doi:10.1007/BF01405790 PMID:2077848

Rasmussen, P. (1990b). Facial pain. I. A prospective survey of 1052 patients with a view of: Definition, delimitation, classification, general data, genetic factors, and previous diseases. *Acta Neurochirurgica*, *107*(3-4), 112–120. doi:10.1007/BF01405789 PMID:2077847

Rasmussen, P. (1991). Facial pain. IV. A prospective study of 1052 patients with a view of: Precipitating factors, associated symptoms, objective psychiatric and neurological symptoms. *Acta Neurochirurgica*, *108*(3-4), 100–109. doi:10.1007/BF01418516 PMID:2031469

Revuelta-Gutiérrez, R., Morales-Martínez, A. H., Mejías-Soto, C., Martínez-Anda, J. J., & Ortega-Porcayo, L. A. (2016). Microvascular decompression for glossopharyngeal neuralgia through a microasterional approach: A case series. *Surgical Neurology International*, *7*(1), 51. doi:10.4103/2152-7806.181824 PMID:27213105

Ro, L.-S., & Chang, K.-H. (2005). Neuropathic pain: Mechanisms and treatments. *Chang Gung Medical Journal*, *28*(9), 597–605. PMID:16323550

Salama, H., Ben-Khayal, H., Mohamed, M. A. S., El-Mitwalli, A., Zaher, A. A., Ezzeldin, A., & ... . (2009). Outcome of medical and surgical management in intractable idiopathic trigeminal neuralgia. *Annals of Indian Academy of Neurology*, *12*(3), 173–178. doi:10.4103/0972-2327.56317 PMID:20174498

Samadian, M., Bakhtevari, M. H., Nosari, M. A., Babadi, A. J., & Razaei, O. (2015). Trigeminal Neuralgia Caused by Venous Angioma: A Case Report and Review of the Literature. *World Neurosurgery*, *84*(3), 860–864. doi:10.1016/j.wneu.2015.04.063 PMID:25968963

Shelden, C. H., Pudenz, R. H., Freshwater, D. B., & Crue, B. L. (1955). Compression rather than decompression for trigeminal neuralgia. *Journal of Neurosurgery*, *12*(2), 123–126. doi:10.3171/jns.1955.12.2.0123 PMID:14368343

Sidebottom, A., & Maxwell, S. (1995). The medical and surgical management of trigeminal neuralgia. *Journal of Clinical Pharmacy and Therapeutics*, *20*(1), 31–35. doi:10.1111/j.1365-2710.1995.tb00622.x PMID:7775611

Singh, B., Srivastava, S. K., & Dang, R. (2001). Anatomic considerations in relation to the maxillary nerve block. *Regional Anesthesia and Pain Medicine*, *26*(6), 507–511. doi:10.1097/00115550-200111000-00004 PMID:11707787

Skirving, D. J., & Dan, N. G. (2001). A 20-year review of percutaneous balloon compression of the trigeminal ganglion. *Journal of Neurosurgery*, *94*(6), 913–917. doi:10.3171/jns.2001.94.6.0913 PMID:11409519

Smith, H. P., McWhorter, J. M., & Challa, V. R. (1981). Radiofrequency neurolysis in a clinical model. Neuropathological correlation. *Journal of Neurosurgery*, *55*(2), 246–253. doi:10.3171/jns.1981.55.2.0246 PMID:7252548

Smyth, P., Greenough, G., & Stommel, E. (2003). Familial trigeminal neuralgia: Case reports and review of the literature. *Headache*, *43*(8), 910–915. doi:10.1046/j.1526-4610.2003.03172.x PMID:12940815

Sola, C., Raux, O., Savath, L., Macq, C., Capdevila, X., & Dadure, C. (2012). Ultrasound guidance characteristics and efficiency of suprazygomatic maxillary nerve blocks in infants: A descriptive prospective study. *Paediatric Anaesthesia*, *22*(9), 841–846. doi:10.1111/j.1460-9592.2012.03861.x PMID:22587691

Solaro, C., Messmer Uccelli, M., Uccelli, A., Leandri, M., & Mancardi, G. L. (2000). Low-dose gabapentin combined with either lamotrigine or carbamazepine can be useful therapies for trigeminal neuralgia in multiple sclerosis. *European Neurology*, *44*(1), 45–48. doi:10.1159/000008192 PMID:10894995

Solaro, C., Uccelli, M. M., Brichetto, G., Gaspperini, C., & Mancardi, G. (2001). Topiramate relieves idiopathic and symptomatic trigeminal neuralgia. *Journal of Pain and Symptom Management*, *21*(5), 367–368. doi:10.1016/S0885-3924(01)00275-5 PMID:11398791

Son, B.-C., Kim, H.-S., Kim, I.-S., Yang, S.-H., & Lee, S.-W. (2011). Percutaneous radiofrequency thermocoagulation under fluoroscopic image-guidance for idiopathic trigeminal neuralgia. *Journal of Korean Neurosurgical Society*, *50*(5), 446–452. doi:10.3340/jkns.2011.50.5.446 PMID:22259692

Sweet, W. H., & Wepsic, J. G. (1974). Controlled thermocoagulation of trigeminal ganglion and rootlets for differential destruction of pain fibers: Part 1: Trigeminal neuralgia. *Journal of Neurosurgery*, *40*(2), 143–156. doi:10.3171/jns.1974.40.2.0143 PMID:4587949

Taarnhøj, P. (1952). Decompression of the trigeminal root and the posterior part of the ganglion as treatment in trigeminal neuralgia; preliminary communication. *Journal of Neurosurgery*, *9*(3), 288–290. doi:10.3171/jns.1952.9.3.0288 PMID:14939059

Taha, J. M., & Tew, J. M. Jr. (1996). Comparison of surgical treatments for trigeminal neuralgia: Reevaluation of radiofrequency rhizotomy. *Neurosurgery*, *38*(5), 865–871. doi:10.1097/00006123-199605000-00001 PMID:8727810

Tartaro, S., Stroffolini, F., & Lepore, M. (1979). The importance of etiology for the successful treatment of secondary trigeminal neuralgia. Reviews of some clinical cases. *Journal of Medicine*, *10*(1-2), 121–128. PMID:290724

Tew, J. M., Jr., & Taha, J. M. (1995). Percutaneous rhizotomy in the treatment of intractable facial pain (trigeminal, glossopharyngeal, and vagal nerves). In Operative Neurosurgical Techniques (3rd ed.). Philadelphia: WB Saunders.

Tronnier, V. M., Rasche, D., Hamer, J., Kienle, A. L., & Kunze, S. (2001). Treatment of idiopathic trigeminal neuralgia: Comparison of long-term outcome after radiofrequency rhizotomy and microvascular decompression. *Neurosurgery*, *48*(6), 1261–1267, discussion 1267–1268. PMID:11383728

Türp, J. C., & Gobetti, J. P. (1996). Trigeminal neuralgia versus atypical facial pain. A review of the literature and case report. *Oral Surgery, Oral Medicine, Oral Pathology, Oral Radiology, and Endodontics*, *81*(4), 424–432. doi:10.1016/S1079-2104(96)80018-7 PMID:8705588

Wang, J. Y., Bender, M. T., & Bettegowda, C. (2016). Percutaneous Procedures for the Treatment of Trigeminal Neuralgia. *Neurosurgery Clinics of North America*, *27*(3), 277–295. doi:10.1016/j.nec.2016.02.005 PMID:27324995

Weiss, A. L., Ehrhardt, K. P., & Tolba, R. (2017). Atypical Facial Pain: A Comprehensive, Evidence-Based Review. *Current Pain and Headache Reports*, *21*(2), 8. doi:10.100711916-017-0609-9 PMID:28251523

White, J. C., & Sweet, W. H. (1969). *Pain and the neurosurgeon: A forty-year experience*. Charles C. Thomas.

Wu, C.-Y., Meng, F.-G., Xu, S.-J., Liu, Y.-G., & Wang, H.-W. (2004). Selective percutaneous radiofrequency thermocoagulation in the treatment of trigeminal neuralgia: Report on 1860 cases. *Chinese Medical Journal, 117*(3), 467–470. doi:10.1142/S0192415X04002120 PMID:15043796

Xu, S.-J., Zhang, W.-H., Chen, T., Wu, C.-Y., & Zhou, M. (2006). Neuronavigator-guided percutaneous radiofrequency thermocoagulation in the treatment of intractable trigeminal neuralgia. *Chinese Medical Journal, 119*(18), 1528–1535. PMID:16996006

Yang, J.-T., Lin, M., Lee, M.-H., Weng, H.-H., & Liao, H.-H. (2010). Percutaneous trigeminal nerve radiofrequency rhizotomy guided by computerized tomography with three-dimensional image reconstruction. *Chang Gung Medical Journal, 33*(6), 679–683. PMID:21199613

Zakrzewska, J. M. (2010). Medical management of trigeminal neuropathic pains. *Expert Opinion on Pharmacotherapy, 11*(8), 1239–1254. doi:10.1517/14656561003767449 PMID:20426709

Zakrzewska, J. M. (2016). Chronic/Persistent Idiopathic Facial Pain. *Neurosurgery Clinics of North America, 27*(3), 345–351. doi:10.1016/j.nec.2016.02.012 PMID:27325001

Zakrzewska, J. M., Jassim, S., & Bulman, J. S. (1999). A prospective, longitudinal study on patients with trigeminal neuralgia who underwent radiofrequency thermocoagulation of the Gasserian ganglion. *Pain, 79*(1), 51–58. doi:10.1016/S0304-3959(98)00145-6 PMID:9928776

Zakrzewska, J. M., & Patsalos, P. N. (2002). Long-term cohort study comparing medical (oxcarbazepine) and surgical management of intractable trigeminal neuralgia. *Pain, 95*(3), 259–266. doi:10.1016/S0304-3959(01)00406-7 PMID:11839425

Chapter 12
Pain Psychiatry of Trigeminal Neuralgia

Lily H. Kim
Stanford University School of Medicine, USA

Michael Bret Schneider
Stanford University School of Medicine, USA

ABSTRACT

In addition to the repeated episodes of paroxysmal, electrical facial pain classically associated with the disease, many patients with trigeminal neuralgia (TN) suffer from severe emotional distress. At present, there is no universally agreed pathophysiological explanation for the high incidence of depression and anxiety within this patient population. Despite the unclear understanding, the psychiatric comorbidities should be addressed as a part of comprehensive, multi-modal approach. Anticonvulsants or serotonin and norepineprhine reuptake inhibitors are viable pharmacological options that can supplement the currently used carbamazepine therapy. For medically refractory cases, surgical interventions are being suggested as effective alternatives in managing both the pain and the psychiatric complaints of TN. Examples include microvascular decompression, stereotactic radiosurgery, and repetitive transcranial magnetic stimulation. Continued research to understand TN should take into account the psychiatric burden in this population in order to promote a holistic treatment approach.

INTRODUCTION

Once called the "suicide disease" (Adams et al., 2011), trigeminal neuralgia (TN) is historically known to accompany significant emotional and mental distress. Many studies have suggested association between TN and psychiatric illnesses, namely, depression and anxiety disorders (Lee, Yeung, Wong, & McMillan, 2008) (Yap,

DOI: 10.4018/978-1-5225-5349-6.ch012

Tan, Chua, & Tan, 2002) (Mongini, Ciccone, Ceccarelli, Baldi, & Ferrero, 2007). This chapter will explore the comorbitiy links between TN and psychiatric illness, as well as candidates for a shared neural substrate, and promising new treatments. In particular, the authors argue for a multi-modal approach to treat both the pain and psychiatric aspects of this complex illness.

BACKGROUND

TN is one of the many pain conditions associated with the fifth cranial nerve. It is differentiated from trigeminal autonomic cephalgias, migraines, temporomandibular joint disorders, and post-herpetic neuralgia (Goadsby et al, Moskowitz et al, Karatas et al, Cook et al, Watson et al) (Watson, Evans, Watt, & Birkett, 1988) by clinical diagnostic criteria, which at least in part, seem to represent the specific pathogenesis of the pain. In TN, any one or more of the three branches of trigeminal nerve—V1 (ophthalmic nerve), V2 (maximally nerve), V3 (mandibular nerve)—may be involved. Historically, TN was also known as "tic douloureux," which means painful tic in French (Cole, Liu, & Apfelbaum, 2005). This term captures the nature of pain associated with TN; the brief yet excruciating pain causes patients to grimace or make flinching facial expression that can be mistaken for tic disorders or Tourette syndrome. The initially poorly understood disease has been under the scrutiny of many researchers, and although we still have imperfect explanation for the underlying cause of the disease, we now have several treatment options, both medical and surgical, to relieve the pain.

The characteristic of facial pain experienced by TN patients can be described as sudden, intermittent, and stabbing kind of pain that is maximal at onset and often unilateral. Innocuous activities such as brushing teeth and chewing become triggers of extreme pain for patients with TN. Each episode is usually fairly brief, as short as few seconds and usually not longer than several minutes. But there may be hundreds of these episodes per day with variable pattern of remission, which can lead to severe limitation in daily function and significant impairment in quality of life (Zakrzewska & Linskey, 2016; Nurmikko & Eldridge, 2001).

Although not a part of diagnostic criteria, nonpainful symptoms can also be experienced in many TN patients. Approximately one-third of TN patients have symptoms like excessive tearing and rhinorrhea from dysregulation of autonomic system, such as those experienced by patients with trigeminal autonomic cephalgia. Abnormal sensory exam findings such as hypesthesia are equally common (Maarbjerg, Gozalov, Olesen, & Bendtsen, 2014).

Emotional disturbance is another clinical feature among TN patient population, which will be the focus of the rest of this chapter. Mood disorders like depression and anxiety disorders are some of the most common mental illness categories in the general population. The prevalence of these conditions is even higher in patients with patients with chronic pain (Tsang et al., 2008; McWilliams, Cox, & Enns, 2003).

Unipolar depression (to distinguish from bipolar disorder that has components of both depression and mania) is a clinical diagnosis made by the prolongation of depressed mood that leads to diminished interest, sense of guilt, hopelessness, sleep disturbances, psychomotor retardation, and even suicidal ideation (American Psychiatric Association, 2013). Also called major depressive disorder (MDD), depression may be secondary to preexisting illnesses, some of the classic causes being neurodegenerative conditions such as Huntington disease and Alzheimer disease (Reus et al., 2016).

Anxiety disorders is an equally broad group of diagnoses with abnormally heightened sense of nervousness and fear. In fact, depression and anxiety may co-exist in significant percentage of people (Talkovsky, Green, Osegueda, & Norton, 2017). Up to 85% of depression patients also have anxiety and 90% of patients with anxiety disorders have depression. For patients diagnosed with both depression and anxiety disorder, the clinical picture is more severe, which correlates with increased morbidity and mortality (Tiller, 2013).

PSYCHIATRIC COMORBIDITIES

Many studies to date have either directly or indirectly supported a tight association of TN and psychiatric disturbances. Although chronic pain in general has been linked to disorders such as depression, the pain psychiatry of TN in particular has been the focus of interest to many researchers due to the high coincidence of psychiatric diagnoses within TN patient population. In a study of 30 patients in a Brazilian hospital, patients with facial pain, namely those diagnosed with TN or temporomandibular disorder (TMD), were more likely to complain of depressive or anxiety symptoms as measured by Hospital Anxiety Depression scale, compared to other patients in the clinic. On average, patients with TN or TMD had "moderate" level of anxiety and "mild" level of depression. Most of these patients rated their level of limitation due to pain as "severe" (Castro, Siqueira, Perissinotti, & Siqueira, 2008). Not surprisingly, higher pain severity has been shown to positively correlate with lower daily functioning and subjective assessment of personal well-being, as measured by modified Short Form Brief Pain Inventory and EuroQol Survey (Tolle, Dukes, & Sadosky, 2006).

However, even among TN patients, there seem to be a difference in the levels of comorbid psychological illnesses depending on the nature of the pain. In some cases, TN may be accompanied by low-intensity facial pain in the background, known as "trigeminal neuralgia with concomitant pain," according to the International Classification for Headache Disorders (Zakrzewska & Linskey, 2016). Patients in this specific subgroup of TN are more likely to suffer from depression and anxiety, compared to TN patients without chronic orofacial pain. In a study published in 2011, patients who experience dull yet persistent pain in addition to paroxysmal pain episodes tended to experience more limitation in their daily functioning, as measured by the Sheehan Disability Scale (SDS), more severe anxiety as demonstrated by Covi's Anxiety Scale (CAS), and more significant depression accordng to the Beck Depression Inventory (BDI), than their counterparts. Some of the psychologically disturbing symptoms that the TN patients with chronic pain complained of included the following: awakening (83.3%), worry (76.7%), sleep disturbance (73.3%), fear (66.7%), tiredness (56.7%), and anorexia (56.7%). In fact, among the chronic pain group, only 1 patient out of 30 was free from any depressive symptoms while most others had either moderate or severe depression. In a logistic regression analysis, the authors identified severe depressive symptoms as risk factors for intensity of pain perception (Macianskyte, Januzis, Kubilius, Adomaitiene, & Sciupokas, 2011).

In a large retrospective study using Taiwanese national database, patients with TN were shown to have a higher incidence of depression, anxiety disorders, and sleep disorders diagnosed by psychiatrists, compared to the general population without TN. The risk of developing these psychiatric disorders persisted beyond the first year of TN diagnosis. Hence, it is not only the newly diagnosed patients "coping" with the sudden change in their lives who struggle emotionally – patients in different stages of disease course are all at risk of developing psychological disturbances (Wu et al., 2015).

Interestingly, in the aforementioned study, there was no difference in the risk of schizophrenia or bipolar disorders between TN patients and the controls. It seems that TN increases the risks of developing a few specific, and not all, psychiatric illnesses (Wu et al., 2015). It should be noted, however, that carbamazepine, the first-line treatment for TN, is also used as an alternative treatment of bipolar disorders in chronic pain patients, especially for those who cannot tolerate lithium (Rahman, Campbell, O'Connell, & Nallapula, 2014; Muzina & Calabrese, 2005; Fountoulakis, Balaris, Nikolaou, & Nuimatoudis, 2016). The fact that many TN patients are on carbamazepine treatment may lead to underestimation of prevalence of comorbid bipolar disorders in this population.

PATHOPHYSIOLOGY

The most widely known pathophysiology of TN is vascular compression of the trigeminal nerve root. This belief serves as the basis for performing microvascular decompression (MVD) for TN patients who fail medical management. Although it is thought be highly successful in controlling pain, this surgical intervention does not produce optimal results for a considerable number of patients. This implies that neurovascular conflict alone falls short in explaining all types of TN, and the pathophysiology of TN remains unclear at best (Jia & Li, 2010; Cheng, Long, Hui, Lei, & Zhang, 2017; Gubian & Rosahl, 2017).

Chronic pain has been long known to be one of the physical manifestations of psychological disorders (Dworkin, Hetzel, & Banks, 1999), but it remains unclear whether the debilitating pain associated with TN causes depression or whether depression predisposes patients to experience more pain with TN (Macianskyte et al., 2011). Wu et al provides several different theories that may explain the high comorbidities of depression and anxiety disorders in TN patients (Wu et al., 2015). Among those hypotheses is the role of neurotransmitters and cytokines. Examination of CSF in TN patients showed decreased levels of norepinephrine and serotonin, which are key monoaminergic neurotransmitters implicated in depression and anxiety (Strittmatter et al., 1997). Chronic inflammation and upregulation of cytokines is also known to underlie TN pathology (Sabalys, Juodzbalys, & Wang, 2013) as well as depression and anxiety (Kronfol & Remick, 2000). The problem with this latter theory is that presence of inflammatory dysregulation has also been shown in patients in schizophrenia (Leza et al., 2015) and bipolar disorder (Patel & Frey, 2015), which are psychiatric illnesses with no currently established link to TN.

Among the candidates for shared biological substrate of chronic pain, depression, and anxiety is the ventral tegmental area, a region within the midbrain that contains dopamine-synthesizing neurons that has been known to be activated in chronic pain. Previously, this had been widely presumed to be a compensatory response to the pain, an analgesic reward. However, Zhang et al recently demonstrated that the firing of the ventral tegmental area is a signal of chronic pain, propagated via projections to the nucleus accumbens, and that brain-derived neurotrophic factor may help the nucleus accumbens to acquire hypersensitivity to pain signals (H. Zhang et al., 2017).

In the case of TN specifically, the trigeminal nerve itself and its midbrain efferents are of interest. In a pilot study by Cook et al, patients with medically refractory MDD were treated with repeated trigeminal nerve stimulations, which involved daily stimulation of V1 branch for 8 weeks. After this trial period, a statistically significant improvement in depressive symptoms was observed, with 4 out of 11 patients achieving remission (Cook et al., 2013). This promising result seems to suggest that that there may be a pathophysiological link between depression and TN involving the trigeminal nerve (Wang et al., 2016). The trigeminal nerve is a prominent site of efferent projections to different parts of the brain, in addition to the sensory cortex. Signals are also relayed from the trigeminal nerve to the nucleus tractus solitarius in the brainstem and beyond via projections to the locus coeruleus, the raphe nuclei, the thalamus, the amygdala, hypothalamus, insular cortex, and medial and orbital prefrontal cortices (Contreras, Beckstead, & Norgren, 1982; Ray & Price, 1992; Tokita, Inoue, & Boughter, 2009; Karatas et al., 2013; Wang et al., 2017).

Animal studies have attempted to explore the association between TN and depression in a molecular level. In both the mouse models that underwent constriction of the infraorbital nerve to simulate neuropathic pain in TN and the models with learned helplessness, the Huntington's disease signaling pathway was up-regulated. Seven proteins were up-regulated in both mouse models while one protein was down-regulated in both models. The shared changes in molecular signaling provide a possible mechanism underlying the high rate of co-occurrence of TN and depression (Guo et al., 2017).

It is interesting to note that several studies have shown that women are more likely to have TN than men with a gender ratio approximating 1:1.7 (Maarbjerg, Di Stefano, Bendtsen, & Cruccu, 2017; Katusic, Beard, Bergstralh, & Kurland, 1990). Likewise, depression and anxiety have long known to have a higher prevalence in women whereas schizophrenia and bipolar disorder with more maniac episodes, the risks of which are not increased by having TN, are more common in men. In fact, female gender and severe pain intensity are known to be risk factors for developing depression and anxiety among TN patients. In one study, female patients with TN were 2.4 times more likely to experience depression and 3.5 times more likely to suffer anxiety than male TN patients (Cheng et al., 2017). To see whether depression and anxiety in the general population share other risk factors with those in TN patients, additional population-based epidemiological studies are needed.

Chronic pain patients, including those suffering from TN, are unable to distinguish between pain that signals imminent danger and pain that results from a disease of aberrant connectivity and reinforcement in pain and fear pathways. This leads to malaptive thoughts, conditioned anxieties, and avoidant behaviors that are widely shared among patients with chronic pain but also typical of TN-associated suffering (Rachman, 1977; Salkovskis, 1991; Stroud, Thorn, Jensen, & Boothby, 2000; Baller & Ross, 2017).

Although TN pain is typically described as brief, in the scale of seconds and minutes, many patients have 50-100 of these episodes scattered throughout the day. In consequence, patients often have anticipatory stress even before the onset of painful episodes. The anticipation of adverse events has long been associated with heightened pain sensation, which then leads to significant psychological distress, contributing to the vicious cycle of pain (Turk & Rudy, 1986).

The unpredictability of TN pain further contributes to the psychological distress over time. TN pain can be touch-evoked but the remission and reemergence of symptoms are essentially unpredictable (Katusic et al., 1990) (Cheshire, 2007). It has been known for a long time that loss of control and declining sense of mastery over self contributes to development of depression and anxiety (Rehm, 1977; Rudy, Kerns, & Turk, 1988; Mineka & Kelly, 1989; Fuchs & Rehm, 1977). However, these previously well-understood connections in stressful life events (specifically, chronic pain) and associated psychological disorders have not been explicitly studied among TN patients.

NON-INVASIVE TREATMENT

Currently, sodium channel blockers, namely, carbamezepine, is widely used for treating TN based on previous studies that showed clinically significant efficacy (Taylor, Brauer, & Espir, 1981; Sindrup & Jensen, 2002; Attal et al., 2006; Cruccu et al., 2008). While carbamezapine may be the first-line treatment for TN, it is by no means the only option. Oxcarbazepine, another sodium channel blocker with similar mechanism, can be used when patients do not respond to carbamezepine (Gomez-Arguelles et al., 2008; Beydoun, Schmidt, & D'souza, 2002). However, other pharmacotherapy options may need to be tried due to the limited efficacy of these agents, side effect profile, and general lack of utility as an antidepressant and an anxiolytic (Alves, Azevedo, & Carvalho, 2004; Backonja, 2002). Although oxcarbazepine is generally better tolerated than carbamezepine, both drugs share similar side effects including sedation, dizziness, cognitive impairement, hyponatremia, and rash (Zakrzewska & Patsalos, 1989; Nicol, 1969).

In theory, the simplest possible drug regimen that would adequately addresses both the pain and depression and/or anxiety would be ideal. For the currently available medical therapy, serotonin and norepinephrine reuptake inhibitors (SNRIs) may be safe and effective for TN patients not only to alleviate the depressive and anxiety symptoms but also to address the pain itself. Duloxetine has long been used as a medication for depression and neuropathic pain such as diabetic neuropathy. In a small study of 15 TN patients, duloxetine therapy resulted in significant pain relief regardless of coexisting psychiatric illnesses (Anand, Dhikav, Prasad, & Shewtengna, 2011).

Even SNRIs not currently approved as antidepressants may help TN patients. In a case report, a patient who had to discontinue carbamazapine due to hepatoxic side effect was given milnacipran, a SNRI approved for treating fibromyalgia and neuropathic pain but not for depression in the USA. With this treatment substition, the patient was once again able to achieve symptom control without further side effects (Ito, Yoshida, Kimura, Ozaki, & Kurita, 2007). Other medical treatment options include anticonvulsants. In particular, lamotrigine has been positively rated for refractory TN and is also known to be an effective antidepressant (Solmi et al., 2016; Alves et al., 2004).

In case of pharmacotherapy failure, other treatment methods are sought. Repetitive transcranial magnetic stimulation (rTMS) is a non-invasive neuromodulatory modality with a demonstrated strong antidepressant effect (O'Reardon et al., 2007; George, Taylor, & Short, 2013; George et al., 2010). There is also a growing evidence on the efficacy of rTMS in TN patients (Leung et al., 2009; Weber, 2017). The dual effect of targeting both the neuropathic pain and depression makes rTMS a reasonable option for TN patients with mood disorders who respond poorly to medications.

SURGICAL TREATMENT

Depression and anxiety disorders in patients with TN have been shown to have implications in surgical success rate. In a study of young patients under the age of 30 with medically unresponsive TN who received MVD surgery, comorbid psychological conditions were associated with repeated procedures in multiple medical centers. Even with more aggressive surgical interventions, young patients with depression or anxiety were more likely to experience major complications, such as, hearing loss, pulmonary embolism, and cavernous sinus thrombosis, while being less likely to remain pain-free post-surgery. This study suggests that repeated MVDs may be ineffective in TN patients with comorbid psychiatric symptoms, especially in younger populations (Mousavi, Sekula, Gildengers, Gardner, & Lunsford, 2016).

However, a different study of older TN patients (with mean age of 47.5 years) argues otherwise. In a prospective study of 128 patients, MVD provided a significant improvement in depression and anxiety as measured by Beck Depression Inventory (BDI) and Beck Anxiety Inventory (BAI). This may be partly explained by the fact that the majority of the study patients experienced complete pain relief following the surgery (Cheng et al., 2017).

Another surgical intervention with a reported psychological benefit in TN patients is stereotactic radiosurgery (SRS). Following this minimally invasive procedure, patients reported significantly lower scores on Patient Health Questionnaire 9 (PHQ-9), which is a widely used screening tool for depression. In addition to the improvement of mood, the surgery achieved successful pain control in 89% of participants, who remained pain free at 12-month follow-up (Kotecha et al., 2017). Similarly, in a study of 167 patients who underwent percutaneous trigeminal ganglion radiofrequency thermocoagulation, depression and anxiety in patients with TN improved significantly following the procedure (Tang et al., 2016).

THE IMPORTANCE OF NEUROPSYCHOLOGICAL SUPPORT

Given the high incidence of comorbid psychiatric conditions in TN patients, neuropsychological support for the patients should be considered in addition to the current medical and surgical treatment targeting the neuropathic pain, as was proposed in a recent literature review (Spina, Mortini, Alemanno, Houdayer, & Iannaccone, 2017). This is especially important given that despite the high incidence of psychiatric comorbidities in this population, only limited number of patients consult with psychiatrists and receive antidepressants (Macianskyte et al., 2011). European countries were shown to have a higher number of TN patients who are treated for their psychiatric symptoms, with approximately one-third of them on either on antidepressants, anxiotylitics, or medications for sleep disturbances (Tolle et al., 2006).

A recent review article suggested a multimodal approach to treating TN, given the high incidence of comorbid psychological disturbances and psychiatric diagnoses among this patient population. Given that pain is inherently subjective and personal experience unique to each patient, the authors propose that providers pay more attention to understanding patients' perception of pain. Various pain scales, such as the McGill Pain Scale, the Numerical Rating Scale, the Brief Pain Inventory, and the recently introduced Penn Facial Pain Scale are some of the tools that can help clinicians with assessment of pain (Spina et al., 2017).

One study to date has explored the potential cognitive decline in TN patients (Meskal, Rutten, Beute, Salden, & Sitskoorn, 2014). The high incidence of anxiety and depression may partly account for the risk of cognitive impairement in TN patients, further compromising the subjective quality of life in this population already experiencing debilitating pain. In fact, chronic mood disorders and anxiety disorders, especially those that are undertreated, have been associated with cognitive decline (Salagre et al., 2017) (McAllister-Williams et al., 2017). Despite lack of evidence in the current literature, it would benefit patients if providers could identify TN patients who may benefit from additional neuropsychological support through formal testing prior to initiating the commonly used carbamazepine treatment as this medication can impair alertness and cause drowsiness in some patients (Killian & Fromm, 1968; Campbell, Graham, & Zilkha, 1966). In consideration of additional support, younger patients should not be excluded. Although more reports have shown that elderly population with depression and anxiety are especially vulnerable to cognitive impairment (Mantella et al., 2007; Sinoff & Werner, 2003), younger population has also been shown to be subject to memory loss and execute dysfunction associated with long-term mental disorders (Castaneda, Tuulio-Henriksson, Marttunen, Suvisaari, & Lonnqvist, 2008).

In a similar vein, cognitive behavioral therapy (CBT) has emerged as an effective modality to help patients who are suffering from chronic pain, including TN. CBT help patients realize that common reactions to the seriousness and unstoppable nature of chronic pain can lead to emotions of depression, anxiety, hopelessness, and helplessness. Patients often develop avoidant behaviors, such as refusing to get out of bed, dropping out of work, and not participating in activities that could bring pleasure and distraction—behaviors that are not only impairing unto themselves but may also worsen the underlying pain condition. By encouraging exercise, behavioral activation, cognitive reframing, and relaxation, CBT allows patients to break the cycle of negative reinforcement. CBT allows patients to learn that many of their fears—while understandable—are often unwarranted (i.e., their imagined situation may be worse thant the reality) and counterproductive to their long-term recovery (Murphy et al., 2014; Gold, 2015).

Even in patients with disabling chronic pain who have already limited many parts of daily living including cessation of work, CBT has shown to effective in reversing life patterns to incorportate more physical activity while dramatically improving symptoms of depression and anxiety (McCracken, MacKichan, & Eccleston, 2007). Mindfulness-based cognitive therapy, a variation of the classic CBT, is another technique that produces significant improvement of clinical symptoms, even in treatment-resistant depression (Eisendrath et al., 2016). Regardless of the different types, cognitive therapies in general are the least invasive treatment approach with no known side effects and should be recommended for all patients suffering from TN.

FUTURE RESEARCH DIRECTIONS

Current medical treatment of TN patients with depression and/or anxiety disorders commonly combines anticonvulsants and antidepressants. However, current medicine lacks knowledge of whether the depression and anxiety that co-present with TN should be treated in the same way as depression and anxiety that occur independent of TN. Therefore, treatments in the future should seek to capitalize on our growing understanding of the shared neurological substrate of TN, anxiety, and depression. This way, we may be able to identify a pharmacological target for a tailored therapy to address the psychiatric disorders prevalent in TN patient population.

Refined surgical techniques and novel approaches are continously being explored. A recently published study reported the favorable result of adding nerve combing method for patients who initially failed the convenitonal MVD procedure. Compared to patients who underwent repeat MVD only, those who received an adjunct nerve combing tended to have better long-term pain control (X. Zhang et al., 2017). Although most of these studies do not explore the psychiatric benefits post-surgery, future studies should investigate whether these new pain-relieving surgeries also improve depression or anxiety. This will be especially important given that considerable number of TN patients with depression and/or anxiety do not respond well to current surgical approaches (Mousavi et al., 2016).

In the field of alternative medicine, *Hypericum perforatum* (St. John's Wort) has been suggested as a treatment option for TN patients. There has been a case report of a patient with a TN who had reported a remission of pain following this remedy, but evidence is sparse and limited. Given its use in depression, however, *Hypericum perforatum* might be able to serve as an adjunct treatment for both conditions (Assiri, Alyami, Uyanik, & Romero-Reyes, 2017).

Future studies should also investigate the efficacy of trigeminal nerve stimulation in treating MDD in TN patients. Stimulation targeting the fifth cranial nerve is not a new technique. As early as in the 1970s, trigeminal nerve stimulation has been tried to alleviate neuropathic pain with demonstrated success (Hellsing, 1976; Augustinsson et al., 1977; Reuter, Krekeler, Krainick, Thoden, & Doerr, 1976). As was previously introduced in this chapter, recently this stimulation method is being explored as a treatment for medically refractory MDD cases (Cook et al., 2013). However, no attempt has been made to study the efficacy of this treatment in a specific subgroup of TN patients with concomittant depression that is unresponsive to pharmacotherapy.

CONCLUSION

The current practice of medicine often involves treating medical and psychiatric diseases as separate entities. This traditional school of thought, although convenient, falls short in managing complex, multifactorial disease processes such as TN. Emerging evidence shows that there may be either anatomical or functional pathophysiological commonality shared between the physical pain and the psychological disturbances in TN. The presence of concurrent psychiatric complaints in a substantial percentage of patients with TN may render many of the current treatment options aimed solely at pain control insufficient for comprehensive management.

Possibly because of its complex nature, TN was a disease of particular interest to the pioneering neurosurgeon Harvey Cushing. As early as 1890s, Cushing began treating TN patients via Gasserian ganglion extirpation, avulsion of sensory root or the nerve itself, or alcohol injection (Adams et al., 2011). Cushing's tireless research into treatment and subsequent reflection of cases may have stemmed from his deep understanding of the physical and emotional distress felt by the patients plagued by this rare and mysterious disease. This spirit very much holds true at present even when the technicality of his surgical methods may not be applicable.

In fact, psychiatric symptoms of TN has only recently started to gain attention, before which little was known and hence largely dismissed (Cheng et al., 2017). With the collective evidence from current literature supporting the severity of psychological burden in TN patients, providers should employ an empathetic and creative management approach that incorporates psychiatric support in addition to the traditional medical treatment while constantly eliciting patient feedback.

REFERENCES

Adams, H., Pendleton, C., Latimer, K., Cohen-Gadol, A. A., Carson, B. S., & Quinones-Hinojosa, A. (2011). Harvey Cushing's case series of trigeminal neuralgia at the Johns Hopkins Hospital: A surgeon's quest to advance the treatment of the 'suicide disease'. *Acta Neurochirurgica, 153*(5), 1043–1050. doi:10.100700701-011-0975-8 PMID:21409517

Alves, T. C., Azevedo, G. S., & Carvalho, E. S. (2004). Tratamento famacológico da neuralgia do trigêmeo: Revisão sistemática e metanálise. *Revista Brasileira de Anestesiologia, 54*(6), 836–849. doi:10.1590/S0034-70942004000600015 PMID:19471799

American Psychiatric Association. (2013). *Diagnostic and statistical manual of mental disorders (DSM-5®)*. American Psychiatric Pub.

Anand, K. S., Dhikav, V., & Prasad, A., & Shewtengna. (2011). Efficacy, safety and tolerability of duloxetine in idiopathic trigeminal neuralgia. *Journal of the Indian Medical Association, 109*(4), 264–266. PMID:22187799

Assiri, K., Alyami, Y., Uyanik, J. M., & Romero-Reyes, M. (2017). Hypericum perforatum (St. John's Wort) as a possible therapeutic alternative for the management of trigeminal neuralgia (TN) - A case report. *Complementary Therapies in Medicine, 30*, 36–39. doi:10.1016/j.ctim.2016.10.014 PMID:28137525

Attal, N., Cruccu, G., Haanpaa, M., Hansson, P., Jensen, T. S., Nurmikko, T., ... Wiffen, P. (2006). EFNS guidelines on pharmacological treatment of neuropathic pain. *European Journal of Neurology, 13*(11), 1153–1169. doi:10.1111/j.1468-1331.2006.01511.x PMID:17038030

Augustinsson, L. E., Bohlin, P., Bundsen, P., Carlsson, C. A., Forssman, L., Sjoberg, P., & Tyreman, N. O. (1977). Pain relief during delivery by transcutaneous electrical nerve stimulation. *Pain, 4*(1Supp C), 59–65. doi:10.1016/0304-3959(77)90087-2 PMID:927881

Backonja, M.-M. (2002). Use of anticonvulsants for treatment of neuropathic pain. *Neurology*, *59*(5suppl 2), S14–S17. doi:10.1212/WNL.59.5_suppl_2.S14 PMID:12221151

Baller, E. B., & Ross, D. A. (2017). Your System Has Been Hijacked: The Neurobiology of Chronic Pain. *Biological Psychiatry*, *82*(8), e61–e63. doi:10.1016/j.biopsych.2017.08.009 PMID:28935098

Beydoun, A., Schmidt, D., & D'souza, J. (2002). *Oxcarbazepine versus carbamazepine in trigeminal neuralgia: a meta-analysis of three double-blind comparative trials.* Paper presented at the Neurology.

Campbell, F. G., Graham, J. G., & Zilkha, K. J. (1966). Clinical trial of carbazepine (tegretol) in trigeminal neuralgia. *Journal of Neurology, Neurosurgery, and Psychiatry*, *29*(3), 265–267. doi:10.1136/jnnp.29.3.265 PMID:5327969

Castaneda, A. E., Tuulio-Henriksson, A., Marttunen, M., Suvisaari, J., & Lonnqvist, J. (2008). A review on cognitive impairments in depressive and anxiety disorders with a focus on young adults. *Journal of Affective Disorders*, *106*(1-2), 1–27. doi:10.1016/j.jad.2007.06.006 PMID:17707915

Castro, A. R., Siqueira, S. R., Perissinotti, D. M., & Siqueira, J. T. (2008). Psychological evaluation and cope with trigeminal neuralgia and temporomandibular disorder. *Arquivos de Neuro-Psiquiatria*, *66*(3b3B), 716–719. doi:10.1590/S0004-282X2008000500021 PMID:18949269

Cheng, J., Long, J., Hui, X., Lei, D., & Zhang, H. (2017). Effects of microvascular decompression on depression and anxiety in trigeminal neuralgia: A prospective cohort study focused on risk factors and prognosis. *Clinical Neurology and Neurosurgery*, *161*, 59–64. doi:10.1016/j.clineuro.2017.08.011 PMID:28858633

Cheshire, W. P. (2007). Trigeminal neuralgia: For one nerve a multitude of treatments. *Expert Review of Neurotherapeutics*, *7*(11), 1565–1579. doi:10.1586/14737175.7.11.1565 PMID:17997704

Cole, C. D., Liu, J. K., & Apfelbaum, R. I. (2005). Historical perspectives on the diagnosis and treatment of trigeminal neuralgia. *Neurosurgical Focus*, *18*(5), E4. doi:10.3171/foc.2005.18.5.5 PMID:15913280

Contreras, R. J., Beckstead, R. M., & Norgren, R. (1982). The central projections of the trigeminal, facial, glossopharyngeal and vagus nerves: An autoradiographic study in the rat. *Journal of the Autonomic Nervous System*, *6*(3), 303–322. doi:10.1016/0165-1838(82)90003-0 PMID:7169500

Cook, I. A., Schrader, L. M., Degiorgio, C. M., Miller, P. R., Maremont, E. R., & Leuchter, A. F. (2013). Trigeminal nerve stimulation in major depressive disorder: Acute outcomes in an open pilot study. *Epilepsy & Behavior*, *28*(2), 221–226. doi:10.1016/j.yebeh.2013.05.008 PMID:23773978

Cruccu, G., Gronseth, G., Alksne, J., Argoff, C., Brainin, M., Burchiel, K., ... Zakrzewska, J. M.European Federation of Neurological, Society. (2008). AAN-EFNS guidelines on trigeminal neuralgia management. *European Journal of Neurology*, *15*(10), 1013–1028. doi:10.1111/j.1468-1331.2008.02185.x PMID:18721143

Dworkin, R. H., Hetzel, R. D., & Banks, S. M. (1999). Toward a model of the pathogenesis of chronic pain. *Seminars in Clinical Neuropsychiatry*, *4*(3), 176–185. doi:10.153/SCNP00400176 PMID:10498785

Eisendrath, S. J., Gillung, E., Delucchi, K. L., Segal, Z. V., Nelson, J. C., McInnes, L. A., ... Feldman, M. D. (2016). A Randomized Controlled Trial of Mindfulness-Based Cognitive Therapy for Treatment-Resistant Depression. *Psychotherapy and Psychosomatics*, *85*(2), 99–110. doi:10.1159/000442260 PMID:26808973

Fountoulakis, K. N., Balaris, D., Nikolaou, V., & Nuimatoudis, J. (2016). Non-conventional pharmacological agents for the treatment of bipolar disorder: A systematic review of the evidence. *Psychiatriki*, *27*(4), 253–263. doi:10.22365/jpsych.2016.274.253 PMID:28114089

Fuchs, C. Z., & Rehm, L. P. (1977). A self-control behavior therapy program for depression. *Journal of Consulting and Clinical Psychology*, *45*(2), 206–215. doi:10.1037/0022-006X.45.2.206 PMID:850005

George, M. S., Lisanby, S. H., Avery, D., McDonald, W. M., Durkalski, V., Pavlicova, M., ... Sackeim, H. A. (2010). Daily left prefrontal transcranial magnetic stimulation therapy for major depressive disorder: A sham-controlled randomized trial. *Archives of General Psychiatry*, *67*(5), 507–516. doi:10.1001/archgenpsychiatry.2010.46 PMID:20439832

George, M. S., Taylor, J. J., & Short, E. B. (2013). The expanding evidence base for rTMS treatment of depression. *Current Opinion in Psychiatry*, *26*(1), 13–18. doi:10.1097/YCO.0b013e32835ab46d PMID:23154644

Gold, P. W. (2015). The organization of the stress system and its dysregulation in depressive illness. *Molecular Psychiatry*, *20*(1), 32–47. doi:10.1038/mp.2014.163 PMID:25486982

Gomez-Arguelles, J. M., Dorado, R., Sepulveda, J. M., Herrera, A., Arrojo, F. G., Aragon, E., ... Anciones, B. (2008). Oxcarbazepine monotherapy in carbamazepine-unresponsive trigeminal neuralgia. *Journal of Clinical Neuroscience*, *15*(5), 516–519. doi:10.1016/j.jocn.2007.04.010 PMID:18378142

Gubian, A., & Rosahl, S. K. (2017). Meta-Analysis on Safety and Efficacy of Microsurgical and Radiosurgical Treatment of Trigeminal Neuralgia. *World Neurosurgery*, *103*, 757–767. doi:10.1016/j.wneu.2017.04.085 PMID:28435111

Guo, Q. H., Tong, Q. H., Lu, N., Cao, H., Yang, L., & Zhang, Y. Q. (2017). Proteomic Analysis of the Hippocampus in Mouse Models of Trigeminal Neuralgia and Inescapable Shock-Induced Depression. *Neuroscience Bulletin*. doi:10.100712264-017-0131-4 PMID:28424990

Hellsing, G. (1976). [Transcutaneous neural stimulation (TNS) in chronic pain in patients with temporomandibular joint disorders. A clinical report]. *Tandlakartidningen*, *68*(13-14), 789–793. PMID:1077220

Ito, M., Yoshida, K., Kimura, H., Ozaki, N., & Kurita, K. (2007). Successful treatment of trigeminal neuralgia with milnacipran. *Clinical Neuropharmacology*, *30*(3), 183–185. doi:10.1097/wnf.0b013e31803bb3da PMID:17545752

Jia, D. Z., & Li, G. (2010). Bioresonance hypothesis: A new mechanism on the pathogenesis of trigeminal neuralgia. *Medical Hypotheses*, *74*(3), 505–507. doi:10.1016/j.mehy.2009.09.056 PMID:19900765

Karatas, H., Erdener, S. E., Gursoy-Ozdemir, Y., Lule, S., Eren-Kocak, E., Sen, Z. D., & Dalkara, T. (2013). Spreading depression triggers headache by activating neuronal Panx1 channels. *Science*, *339*(6123), 1092–1095. doi:10.1126cience.1231897 PMID:23449592

Katusic, S., Beard, C. M., Bergstralh, E., & Kurland, L. T. (1990). Incidence and clinical features of trigeminal neuralgia, Rochester, Minnesota, 1945-1984. *Annals of Neurology*, *27*(1), 89–95. doi:10.1002/ana.410270114 PMID:2301931

Killian, J. M., & Fromm, G. H. (1968). Carbamazepine in the treatment of neuralgia. Use of side effects. *Archives of Neurology*, *19*(2), 129–136. doi:10.1001/archneur.1968.00480020015001 PMID:4877400

Kotecha, R., Miller, J. A., Modugula, S., Barnett, G. H., Murphy, E. S., Reddy, C. A., ... Chao, S. T. (2017). Stereotactic Radiosurgery for Trigeminal Neuralgia Improves Patient-Reported Quality of Life and Reduces Depression. *International Journal of Radiation Oncology, Biology, Physics*, *98*(5), 1078–1086. doi:10.1016/j.ijrobp.2017.04.008 PMID:28721891

Kronfol, Z., & Remick, D. G. (2000). Cytokines and the brain: Implications for clinical psychiatry. *The American Journal of Psychiatry*, *157*(5), 683–694. doi:10.1176/appi.ajp.157.5.683 PMID:10784457

Lee, L. T., Yeung, R. W., Wong, M. C., & McMillan, A. S. (2008). Diagnostic subtypes, psychological distress and psychosocial dysfunction in southern Chinese people with temporomandibular disorders. *Journal of Oral Rehabilitation*, *35*(3), 184–190. doi:10.1111/j.1365-2842.2007.01792.x PMID:18254795

Leung, A., Donohue, M., Xu, R., Lee, R., Lefaucheur, J. P., Khedr, E. M., ... Chen, R. (2009). rTMS for suppressing neuropathic pain: A meta-analysis. *The Journal of Pain*, *10*(12), 1205–1216. doi:10.1016/j.jpain.2009.03.010 PMID:19464959

Leza, J. C., Garcia-Bueno, B., Bioque, M., Arango, C., Parellada, M., Do, K., ... Bernardo, M. (2015). Inflammation in schizophrenia: A question of balance. *Neuroscience and Biobehavioral Reviews*, *55*, 612–626. doi:10.1016/j.neubiorev.2015.05.014 PMID:26092265

Maarbjerg, S., Di Stefano, G., Bendtsen, L., & Cruccu, G. (2017). Trigeminal neuralgia - diagnosis and treatment. *Cephalalgia*, *37*(7), 648–657. doi:10.1177/0333102416687280 PMID:28076964

Maarbjerg, S., Gozalov, A., Olesen, J., & Bendtsen, L. (2014). Trigeminal neuralgia--a prospective systematic study of clinical characteristics in 158 patients. *Headache*, *54*(10), 1574–1582. doi:10.1111/head.12441 PMID:25231219

Macianskyte, D., Januzis, G., Kubilius, R., Adomaitiene, V., & Sciupokas, A. (2011). Associations between chronic pain and depressive symptoms in patients with trigeminal neuralgia. *Medicina (Kaunas, Lithuania)*, *47*(7), 386–392. PMID:22112988

Mantella, R. C., Butters, M. A., Dew, M. A., Mulsant, B. H., Begley, A. E., Tracey, B., ... Lenze, E. J. (2007). Cognitive impairment in late-life generalized anxiety disorder. *The American Journal of Geriatric Psychiatry*, *15*(8), 673–679. doi:10.1097/JGP.0b013e31803111f2 PMID:17426260

McAllister-Williams, R. H., Bones, K., Goodwin, G. M., Harrison, J., Katona, C., Rasmussen, J., ... Young, A. H. (2017). Analysing UK clinicians' understanding of cognitive symptoms in major depression: A survey of primary care physicians and psychiatrists. *Journal of Affective Disorders*, *207*, 346–352. doi:10.1016/j.jad.2016.09.036 PMID:27743537

McCracken, L. M., MacKichan, F., & Eccleston, C. (2007). Contextual cognitive-behavioral therapy for severely disabled chronic pain sufferers: Effectiveness and clinically significant change. *European Journal of Pain (London, England)*, *11*(3), 314–322. doi:10.1016/j.ejpain.2006.05.004 PMID:16762571

McWilliams, L. A., Cox, B. J., & Enns, M. W. (2003). Mood and anxiety disorders associated with chronic pain: An examination in a nationally representative sample. *Pain*, *106*(1-2), 127–133. doi:10.1016/S0304-3959(03)00301-4 PMID:14581119

Meskal, I., Rutten, G. J., Beute, G. N., Salden, M. E., & Sitskoorn, M. M. (2014). Cognitive deficits in patients with trigeminal neuralgia: Opportunities to improve care and quality of life. *Acta Neurochirurgica*, *156*(8), 1565–1566. doi:10.100700701-014-2100-2 PMID:24809528

Mineka, Susan, & Kelly, Kelly A. (1989). The relationship between anxiety, lack of control and loss of control.

Mongini, F., Ciccone, G., Ceccarelli, M., Baldi, I., & Ferrero, L. (2007). Muscle tenderness in different types of facial pain and its relation to anxiety and depression: A cross-sectional study on 649 patients. *Pain*, *131*(1-2), 106–111. doi:10.1016/j.pain.2006.12.017 PMID:17258397

Mousavi, S. H., Sekula, R. F., Gildengers, A., Gardner, P., & Lunsford, L. D. (2016). Concomitant depression and anxiety negatively affect pain outcomes in surgically managed young patients with trigeminal neuralgia: Long-term clinical outcome. *Surgical Neurology International*, *7*(1), 98. doi:10.4103/2152-7806.194145 PMID:28168085

Murphy, J. L., McKellar, J. D., Raffa, S. D., Clark, M. E., Kerns, R. D., & Karlin, B. E. (2014). *Cognitive behavioral therapy for chronic pain among veterans: therapist manual*. Washington, DC: US Department of Veterans Affairs.

Muzina, D. J., & Calabrese, J. R. (2005). Maintenance therapies in bipolar disorder: Focus on randomized controlled trials. *The Australian and New Zealand Journal of Psychiatry*, *39*(8), 652–661. doi:10.1080/j.1440-1614.2005.01649.x PMID:16050919

Nicol, C. F. (1969). A four year double-blind study of tegretol in facial pain. *Headache*, *9*(1), 54–57. doi:10.1111/j.1526-4610.1969.hed0901054.x PMID:4896266

Nurmikko, T. J., & Eldridge, P. R. (2001). Trigeminal neuralgia—pathophysiology, diagnosis and current treatment. *BJA: British Journal of Anaesthesia*, *87*(1), 117–132. doi:10.1093/bja/87.1.117 PMID:11460800

O'Reardon, J. P., Solvason, H. B., Janicak, P. G., Sampson, S., Isenberg, K. E., Nahas, Z., ... Sackeim, H. A. (2007). Efficacy and safety of transcranial magnetic stimulation in the acute treatment of major depression: A multisite randomized controlled trial. *Biological Psychiatry, 62*(11), 1208–1216. doi:10.1016/j.biopsych.2007.01.018 PMID:17573044

Patel, J. P., & Frey, B. N. (2015). Disruption in the Blood-Brain Barrier: The Missing Link between Brain and Body Inflammation in Bipolar Disorder? *Neural Plasticity, 708306*. doi:10.1155/2015/708306 PMID:26075104

Rachman, S. (1977). The conditioning theory of fear-acquisition: A critical examination. *Behaviour Research and Therapy, 15*(5), 375–387. doi:10.1016/0005-7967(77)90041-9 PMID:612338

Rahman, T., Campbell, A., O'Connell, C. R., & Nallapula, K. (2014). Carbamazepine in bipolar disorder with pain: Reviewing treatment guidelines. *The Primary Care Companion for CNS Disorders, 16*(5). doi:10.4088/PCC.14r01672 PMID:25667814

Ray, J. P., & Price, J. L. (1992). The organization of the thalamocortical connections of the mediodorsal thalamic nucleus in the rat, related to the ventral forebrain-prefrontal cortex topography. *The Journal of Comparative Neurology, 323*(2), 167–197. doi:10.1002/cne.903230204 PMID:1401255

Rehm, L. P. (1977). A self-control model of depression. *Behavior Therapy, 8*(5), 787–804. doi:10.1016/S0005-7894(77)80150-0

Reus, G. Z., Titus, S. E., Abelaira, H. M., Freitas, S. M., Tuon, T., Quevedo, J., & Budni, J. (2016). Neurochemical correlation between major depressive disorder and neurodegenerative diseases. *Life Sciences, 158*, 121–129. doi:10.1016/j.lfs.2016.06.027 PMID:27370938

Reuter, E., Krekeler, G., Krainick, J. U., Thoden, U., & Doerr, M. (1976). [Pain suppression in the trigeminal region by means of transcutaneous nerve stimulation]. *Deutsche Zahnarztliche Zeitschrift, 31*(3), 274–276. PMID:1082811

Rudy, T. E., Kerns, R. D., & Turk, D. C. (1988). Chronic pain and depression: Toward a cognitive-behavioral mediation model. *Pain, 35*(2), 129–140. doi:10.1016/0304-3959(88)90220-5 PMID:3237427

Sabalys, G., Juodzbalys, G., & Wang, H. L. (2013). Aetiology and pathogenesis of trigeminal neuralgia: A comprehensive review. *Journal of Oral & Maxillofacial Research, 3*(4), e2. doi:10.5037/jomr.2012.3402 PMID:24422020

Salagre, E., Sole, B., Tomioka, Y., Fernandes, B. S., Hidalgo-Mazzei, D., Garriga, M., ... Grande, I. (2017). Treatment of neurocognitive symptoms in unipolar depression: A systematic review and future perspectives. *Journal of Affective Disorders*, *221*, 205–221. doi:10.1016/j.jad.2017.06.034 PMID:28651185

Salkovskis, P. M. (1991). The importance of behaviour in the maintenance of anxiety and panic: A cognitive account. *Behavioural and Cognitive Psychotherapy*, *19*(1), 6–19. doi:10.1017/S0141347300011472

Sindrup, S. H., & Jensen, T. S. (2002). Pharmacotherapy of trigeminal neuralgia. *The Clinical Journal of Pain*, *18*(1), 22–27. doi:10.1097/00002508-200201000-00004 PMID:11803299

Sinoff, G., & Werner, P. (2003). Anxiety disorder and accompanying subjective memory loss in the elderly as a predictor of future cognitive decline. *International Journal of Geriatric Psychiatry*, *18*(10), 951–959. doi:10.1002/gps.1004 PMID:14533128

Solmi, M., Veronese, N., Zaninotto, L., van der Loos, M. L., Gao, K., Schaffer, A., ... Correll, C. U. (2016). Lamotrigine compared to placebo and other agents with antidepressant activity in patients with unipolar and bipolar depression: A comprehensive meta-analysis of efficacy and safety outcomes in short-term trials. *CNS Spectrums*, *21*(5), 403–418. doi:10.1017/S1092852916000523 PMID:27686028

Spina, A., Mortini, P., Alemanno, F., Houdayer, E., & Iannaccone, S. (2017). Trigeminal Neuralgia: Toward a Multimodal Approach. *World Neurosurgery*, *103*, 220–230. doi:10.1016/j.wneu.2017.03.126 PMID:28377244

Strittmatter, M., Grauer, M., Isenberg, E., Hamann, G., Fischer, C., Hoffmann, K. H., ... Schimrigk, K. (1997). Cerebrospinal fluid neuropeptides and monoaminergic transmitters in patients with trigeminal neuralgia. *Headache*, *37*(4), 211–216. doi:10.1046/j.1526-4610.1997.3704211.x PMID:9150615

Stroud, M. W., Thorn, B. E., Jensen, M. P., & Boothby, J. L. (2000). The relation between pain beliefs, negative thoughts, and psychosocial functioning in chronic pain patients. *Pain*, *84*(2-3), 347–352. doi:10.1016/S0304-3959(99)00226-2 PMID:10666540

Talkovsky, A. M., Green, K. L., Osegueda, A., & Norton, P. J. (2017). Secondary depression in transdiagnostic group cognitive behavioral therapy among individuals diagnosed with anxiety disorders. *Journal of Anxiety Disorders*, *46*, 56–64. doi:10.1016/j.janxdis.2016.09.008 PMID:27707524

Tang, Y., Ma, L., Li, N., Guo, Y., Yang, L., Wu, B., ... Ni, J. X. (2016). Percutaneous trigeminal ganglion radiofrequency thermocoagulation alleviates anxiety and depression disorders in patients with classic trigeminal neuralgia: A cohort study. *Medicine; Analytical Reviews of General Medicine, Neurology, Psychiatry, Dermatology, and Pediatries*, *95*(49), e5379. doi:10.1097/MD.0000000000005379 PMID:27930513

Taylor, J. C., Brauer, S., & Espir, M. L. (1981). Long-term treatment of trigeminal neuralgia with carbamazepine. *Postgraduate Medical Journal*, *57*(663), 16–18. doi:10.1136/pgmj.57.663.16 PMID:7279817

Tiller, J. W. (2013). Depression and anxiety. *The Medical Journal of Australia*, *199*(6Suppl), S28–S31. PMID:25370281

Tokita, K., Inoue, T., & Boughter, J. D. Jr. (2009). Afferent connections of the parabrachial nucleus in C57BL/6J mice. *Neuroscience*, *161*(2), 475–488. doi:10.1016/j.neuroscience.2009.03.046 PMID:19327389

Tolle, T., Dukes, E., & Sadosky, A. (2006). Patient burden of trigeminal neuralgia: Results from a cross-sectional survey of health state impairment and treatment patterns in six European countries. *Pain Practice*, *6*(3), 153–160. doi:10.1111/j.1533-2500.2006.00079.x PMID:17147591

Tsang, A., Von Korff, M., Lee, S., Alonso, J., Karam, E., Angermeyer, M. C., ... Watanabe, M. (2008). Common chronic pain conditions in developed and developing countries: Gender and age differences and comorbidity with depression-anxiety disorders. *The Journal of Pain*, *9*(10), 883–891. doi:10.1016/j.jpain.2008.05.005 PMID:18602869

Turk, D. C., & Rudy, T. E. (1986). Assessment of cognitive factors in chronic pain: A worthwhile enterprise? *Journal of Consulting and Clinical Psychology*, *54*(6), 760–768. doi:10.1037/0022-006X.54.6.760 PMID:3540044

Wang, Y., Cao, D. Y., Remeniuk, B., Krimmel, S., Seminowicz, D. A., & Zhang, M. (2017). Altered brain structure and function associated with sensory and affective components of classic trigeminal neuralgia. *Pain*, *158*(8), 1561–1570. doi:10.1097/j.pain.0000000000000951 PMID:28520647

Wang, Y., Li, D., Bao, F., Guo, C., Ma, S., & Zhang, M. (2016). Microstructural abnormalities of the trigeminal nerve correlate with pain severity and concomitant emotional dysfunctions in idiopathic trigeminal neuralgia: A randomized, prospective, double-blind study. *Magnetic Resonance Imaging*, *34*(5), 609–616. doi:10.1016/j.mri.2015.11.013 PMID:26747406

Watson, C. P., Evans, R. J., Watt, V. R., & Birkett, N. (1988). Post-herpetic neuralgia: 208 cases. *Pain*, *35*(3), 289–297. doi:10.1016/0304-3959(88)90139-X PMID:2852344

Weber, K. (2017). Neuromodulation and Devices in Trigeminal Neuralgia. *Headache*, *57*(10), 1648–1653. doi:10.1111/head.13166 PMID:28905370

Wu, T. H., Hu, L. Y., Lu, T., Chen, P. M., Chen, H. J., Shen, C. C., & Wen, C. H. (2015). Risk of psychiatric disorders following trigeminal neuralgia: A nationwide population-based retrospective cohort study. *The Journal of Headache and Pain*, *16*(1), 64. doi:10.118610194-015-0548-y PMID:26174508

Yap, A. U., Tan, K. B., Chua, E. K., & Tan, H. H. (2002). Depression and somatization in patients with temporomandibular disorders. *The Journal of Prosthetic Dentistry*, *88*(5), 479–484. doi:10.1067/mpr.2002.129375 PMID:12473996

Zakrzewska, J. M., & Linskey, M. E. (2016). Trigeminal Neuralgia. (1532-0650 (Electronic)).

Zakrzewska, J. M., & Patsalos, P. N. (1989). Oxcarbazepine: A new drug in the management of intractable trigeminal neuralgia. *Journal of Neurology, Neurosurgery, and Psychiatry*, *52*(4), 472–476. doi:10.1136/jnnp.52.4.472 PMID:2738589

Zhang, H., Qian, Y. L., Li, C., Liu, D., Wang, L., Wang, X. Y., ... Cao, J. L. (2017). Brain-Derived Neurotrophic Factor in the Mesolimbic Reward Circuitry Mediates Nociception in Chronic Neuropathic Pain. *Biological Psychiatry*, *82*(8), 608–618. doi:10.1016/j.biopsych.2017.02.1180 PMID:28390647

Zhang, X., Xu, L., Zhao, H., Tang, Y. D., Zhu, J., Yuan, Y., ... Li, S. T. (2017). Long-term efficacy of nerve combing for the patients with trigeminal neuralgia who failed prior microvascular decompression. *World Neurosurgery*, *108*, 711–715. doi:10.1016/j.wneu.2017.09.081

KEY TERMS AND DEFINITIONS

Anxiety Disorders: A category of mental illnesses within Diagnostic and Statistical Manual of Mental Disorders (DSM) classification system that is characterized by excessive degree of anxiety and worry, which can be generalized or situation-specific.

Mood (Affective) Disorders: A category of mental illnesses within Diagnostic and Statistical Manual of Mental Disorders (DSM) classification system that is characterized by inappropriate emotional responses to a situation, which can be overly elevated, depressed, or a combination of the two.

Multi-Modal Treatment: An approach of managing a disease that incorporates various aspects of the condition, such as the physical, emotional, and social impairments, often by actively inviting patient's perspective and when needed, by including a team of different specialists.

Neuropsychological Support: A systematic approach to help patients who experience neurological and psychological challenges with early identification and pharmacological or behavioral therapies as indicated, often by involving necessary specialists and inviting patient perspectives.

Orofacial Pain: A broad category of pain that involves the sensitive areas of face and mouth, of which TN is one well-known type. Because of the rich innervations in these areas, the pain is often severe, and for reasons not clearly understood, may be associated with psychological distress.

Pain Psychiatry: The medical sub-specialty of a applying the principles of psychiatry the specifics of pain. Biological, psychological and social factors are considered. As an example of psychological factors, thought process and emotional understanding of pain as a subjective experience, which, when maladaptive, may lead to the development of chronic psychological distress and exacerbate physical pain.

Psychiatric Comorbidity: The psychiatric conditions, both diagnosed and undiagnosed, that tend to accompany another medical condition.

Compilation of References

Abdennebi, B., & Guenane, L. (2014). Technical considerations and outcome assessment in retrogasserian balloon compression for treatment of trigeminal neuralgia. Series of 901 patients. *Surgical Neurology International*, *5*(1), 118. doi:10.4103/2152-7806.137838 PMID:25101213

Adams, H., Pendleton, C., Latimer, K., Cohen-Gadol, A. A., Carson, B. S., & Quinones-Hinojosa, A. (2011). Harvey Cushing's case series of trigeminal neuralgia at the Johns Hopkins Hospital: a surgeon's quest to advance the treatment of the 'suicide disease'. In *Acta neurochirurgica* (Vol. 153, pp. 1043–1050). Academic Press. doi:10.1007/s00701-011-0975-8

Adams, C. B., Kaye, A. H., & Teddy, P. J. (1982). The treatment of trigeminal neuralgia by posterior fossa microsurgery. *Journal of Neurology, Neurosurgery, and Psychiatry*, *45*(11), 1020–1026. doi:10.1136/jnnp.45.11.1020 PMID:7175525

Adler, J. R. Jr, Bower, R., Gupta, G., Lim, M., Efron, A., Gibbs, I. C., ... Soltys, S. G. (2009). Nonisocentric radiosurgical rhizotomy for trigeminal neuralgia. *Neurosurgery*, *64*(2Suppl), A84–A90. doi:10.1227/01.NEU.0000341631.49154.62 PMID:19165079

Adler, J. R. Jr, Chang, S. D., Murphy, M. J., Doty, J., Geis, P., & Hancock, S. L. (1997). The Cyberknife: A frameless robotic system for radiosurgery. *Stereotactic and Functional Neurosurgery*, *69*(1–4 Pt 2), 124–128. doi:10.1159/000099863 PMID:9711744

Alafaci, C., Granata, F., Cutugno, M., Marino, D., Conti, A., & Tomasello, F. (2015). Glossopharyngeal neuralgia caused by a complex neurovascular conflict: Case report and review of the literature. *Surgical Neurology International*, *6*(1), 19. doi:10.4103/2152-7806.150810 PMID:25709856

Alberico, R. A., Fenstermaker, R. A., & Lobel, J. (2001). Focal enhancement of cranial nerve V after radiosurgery with the Leksell gamma knife: Experience in 15 patients with medically refractory trigeminal neuralgia. *AJNR. American Journal of Neuroradiology*, *22*(10), 1944–1948. PMID:11733329

Alves, T. C., Azevedo, G. S., & Carvalho, E. S. (2004). Tratamento famacológico da neuralgia do trigêmeo: Revisão sistemática e metanálise. *Revista Brasileira de Anestesiologia*, *54*(6), 836–849. doi:10.1590/S0034-70942004000600015 PMID:19471799

Amagasaki, K., Abe, S., Watanabe, S., Naemura, K., & Nakaguchi, H. (2014). Trigeminal neuralgia caused by a trigeminocerebellar artery. *Journal of Neurosurgery*, *121*(4), 940–943. doi:10.3171/2014.6.JNS132292 PMID:25014438

Ameli, N. O. (1965). Avicenna and trigeminal neuralgia. *Journal of the Neurological Sciences*, *2*(2), 105–107. doi:10.1016/0022-510X(65)90074-2 PMID:4862205

American Psychiatric Association. (2013). *Diagnostic and statistical manual of mental disorders (DSM-5®)*. American Psychiatric Pub.

Ammori, M. B., King, A. T., Siripurapu, R., Herwadkar, A. V., & Rutherford, S. A. (2013). Factors Influencing Decision-making and Outcome in the Surgical Management of Trigeminal Neuralgia. *Journal of Neurological Surgery. Part B, Skull Base*, *74*(2), 75–81. doi:10.1055-0033-1333617 PMID:24436892

Anand, K. S., Dhikav, V., & Prasad, A., & Shewtengna. (2011). Efficacy, safety and tolerability of duloxetine in idiopathic trigeminal neuralgia. *Journal of the Indian Medical Association*, *109*(4), 264–266. PMID:22187799

Anand, K., Khikav, V., & Prasad, A., & Shewtengna. (2011). Efficacy, safety, and tolerability of duloxetine in idiopathic trigeminal neuralgia. *Journal of the Indian Medical Association*, *109*(4), 264–266. PMID:22187799

Anderson, L. C., Vakoula, A., & Veinote, R. (2003). Inflammatory hypersensitivity in a rat model of trigeminal neuropathic pain. *Archives of Oral Biology*, *48*(2), 161–169. doi:10.1016/S0003-9969(02)00203-0 PMID:12642236

André, N. (1756). *Observations pratiques sur les maladies de l' urèthre et sur plusiers faits convulsifs, & la guérison de plusiers maladies chirurgicales, avec la décomposition d'un remède propre à réprimer la dissolution gangréneuse & cancéreuse, & à la réparer; avec des*. Paris: Delaguette.

Antoni, A. A., & Johnson, J. H. (1958). Treatment of tic douloureux with stilbamidine isethionate. *Journal of Oral Surgery*, *16*(3), 226–230. Retrieved from http://www.ncbi.nlm.nih.gov/pubmed/13526059 PMID:13526059

Antonini, G., Di Pasquale, A., Cruccu, G., Truini, A., Morino, S., Saltelli, G., ... Bozzao, A. (2014). Magnetic resonance imaging contribution for diagnosing symptomatic neurovascular contact in classical trigeminal neuralgia: A blinded case-control study and meta-analysis. *Pain*, *155*(8), 1464–1471. doi:10.1016/j.pain.2014.04.020 PMID:24785270

Aoki, K. (2005). Review of a proposed mechanism for the antinocicpetive action of botulinum toxin type A. *Neurtoxicology*, *26*(5), 785–793. doi:10.1016/j.neuro.2005.01.017 PMID:16002144

Apfelbaum, R. I. (1977). A comparision of percutaneous radiofrequency trigeminal neurolysis and microvascular decompression of the trigeminal nerve for the treatment of tic douloureux. *Neurosurgery*, *1*(1), 16–21. doi:10.1227/00006123-197707000-00004 PMID:615946

Aretaeus. (1856). *The extant works of Aretaeus, the Cappadocian* (F. Adams, Ed.). London: Sydenham Society.

Arias, M. J. (1986). Percutaneous retrogasserian glycerol rhizotomy for trigeminal neuralgia. A prospective study of 100 cases. *Journal of Neurosurgery*, *65*(1), 32–36. doi:10.3171/jns.1986.65.1.0032 PMID:3712027

Artico, M., De Caro, G. M., Fraioli, B., & Giuffrè, R. (1997). 1897--celebrating the centennial--Hermann Moritz Gocht and radiation therapy in the treatment of trigeminal neuralgia. *Acta Neurochirurgica*, *139*(8), 761–763. doi:10.1007/BF01420050 PMID:9309292

Artz, G. J., Hux, F. J., Larouere, M. J., Bojrab, D. I., Babu, S., & Pieper, D. R. (2008). Endoscopic vascular decompression. *Otology & Neurotology*, *29*(7), 995–1000. doi:10.1097/MAO.0b013e318184601a PMID:18698270

Aspevall, O., Hillebrant, E., Linderoth, B., & Rylander, M. (1991). Meningitis due to Gemella haemolysans after neurosurgical treatment of trigeminal neuralgia. *Scandinavian Journal of Infectious Diseases*, *23*(4), 503–505. doi:10.3109/00365549109075101 PMID:1957134

Asplund, P., Blomstedt, P., & Bergenheim, A. T. (2016). Percutaneous Balloon Compression vs Percutaneous Retrogasserian Glycerol Rhizotomy for the Primary Treatment of Trigeminal Neuralgia. *Neurosurgery*, *78*(3), 421–428, discussion 428. doi:10.1227/NEU.0000000000001059 PMID:26465639

Asplund, P., Linderoth, B., & Bergenheim, A. T. (2010). The predictive power of balloon shape and change of sensory functions on outcome of percutaneous balloon compression for trigeminal neuralgia. *Journal of Neurosurgery*, *113*(3), 498–507. doi:10.3171/2010.2.JNS091466 PMID:20345223

Assiri, K., Alyami, Y., Uyanik, J. M., & Romero-Reyes, M. (2017). Hypericum perforatum (St. John's Wort) as a possible therapeutic alternative for the management of trigeminal neuralgia (TN) - A case report. *Complementary Therapies in Medicine*, *30*, 36–39. doi:10.1016/j.ctim.2016.10.014 PMID:28137525

Attal, N., Cruccu, G., Haanpaa, M., Hansson, P., Jensen, T. S., Nurmikko, T., ... Wiffen, P. (2006). EFNS guidelines on pharmacological treatment of neuropathic pain. *European Journal of Neurology*, *13*(11), 1153–1169. doi:10.1111/j.1468-1331.2006.01511.x PMID:17038030

Aubuchon, A. C., Chan, M. D., Lovato, J. F., Balamucki, C. J., Ellis, T. L., Tatter, S. B., … Shaw, E. G. (2011). Repeat Gamma Knife Radiosurgery for Trigeminal Neuralgia. *International Journal of Radiation Oncology, Biology, Physics*, *81*(4), 1059–1065. doi:10.1016/j.ijrobp.2010.07.010

Auger, R. G., & Whisnant, J. P. (1990). Hemifacial spasm in Rochester and Olmsted County, Minnesota, 1960 to 1984. *Archives of Neurology*, *47*(11), 1233–1234. doi:10.1001/archneur.1990.00530110095023 PMID:2241620

Augustinsson, L. E., Bohlin, P., Bundsen, P., Carlsson, C. A., Forssman, L., Sjoberg, P., & Tyreman, N. O. (1977). Pain relief during delivery by transcutaneous electrical nerve stimulation. *Pain*, *4*(1Supp C), 59–65. doi:10.1016/0304-3959(77)90087-2 PMID:927881

Averbuch, M., & Katzper, M. (2004). Assessment of visual analog versus categorical scale for measurement of osteoarthritis pain. *Journal of Clinical Pharmacology*, *44*(4), 368–372. doi:10.1177/0091270004263995 PMID:15051743

Aydoseli, A., Akcakaya, M. O., Aras, Y., Sabanci, P. A., Unal, T. C., Sencer, A., ... Izgi, N. (2015). Neuronavigation-assisted percutaneous balloon compression for the treatment of trigeminal neuralgia: The technique and short-term clinical results. *British Journal of Neurosurgery*, *29*(4), 552–558. doi:10.3109/02688697.2015.1019418 PMID:25807330

Backonja, M.-M. (2002). Use of anticonvulsants for treatment of neuropathic pain. *Neurology*, *59*(5suppl 2), S14–S17. doi:10.1212/WNL.59.5_suppl_2.S14 PMID:12221151

Baller, E. B., & Ross, D. A. (2017). Your System Has Been Hijacked: The Neurobiology of Chronic Pain. *Biological Psychiatry*, *82*(8), e61–e63. doi:10.1016/j.biopsych.2017.08.009 PMID:28935098

Banczerowski, P., Czigléczki, G., & Nyáry, I. (2014). Long-term effectiveness of an ad hoc tailored titanium implant as a spacer for microvascular decompression in the treatment of trigeminal neuralgia caused by megadolichoectatic basilar artery anomaly: 9-year follow-up. *Journal of Neurosurgery*, *121*(6), 1492–1496. doi:10.3171/2014.8.JNS132445 PMID:25259563

Barker, F. G., Jannetta, P. J., Bissonette, D. J., Larkins, M. V., & Jho, H. D. (1996). The Long-Term Outcome of Microvascular Decompression for Trigeminal Neuralgia. *The New England Journal of Medicine*, *334*(17), 1077–1084. doi:10.1056/NEJM199604253341701 PMID:8598865

Bartholow, R. (1873). Therapeutics of the Nervous System and Mind. In The Chicago Journal of Nervous and Mental Disease (pp. 100–104). Chicago.

Bartholow, R. (1876). *A practical treatise on materia medica and therapeutics*. New York: D. Appleton and Company. Retrieved from https://archive.org/details/apracticaltreat03bartgoog

Batisti, J. P. M., Kleinfelder, A. D. F., Galli, N. B., Moro, A., Munhoz, R. P., & Teive, H. A. G. (2017). Treatment of hemifacial spasm with botulinum toxin type a: Effective, long lasting and well tolerated. *Arquivos de Neuro-Psiquiatria*, *75*(2), 87–91. doi:10.1590/0004-282x20160191 PMID:28226076

Baxter, D. W., & Schacherl, U. (1962). Experimental studies on the morphological changes produced by intrathecal phenol. *Canadian Medical Association Journal*, *86*, 1200–1205. PMID:13866009

Beck, D. W., Olson, J. J., & Urig, E. J. (1986). Percutaneous retrogasserian glycerol rhizotomy for treatment of trigeminal neuralgia. *Journal of Neurosurgery*, *65*(1), 28–31. doi:10.3171/jns.1986.65.1.0028 PMID:3712026

Becker, M., Kohler, R., Vargas, M. I., Viallon, M., & Delavelle, J. (2008). Pathology of the trigeminal nerve. *Neuroimaging Clinics of North America*, *18*(2), 283–307. doi:10.1016/j.nic.2007.11.002

Bederson, J. B., & Wilson, C. B. (1989). Evaluation of microvascular decompression and partial sensory rhizotomy in 252 cases of trigeminal neuralgia. *Journal of Neurosurgery*, *71*(3), 359–367. doi:10.3171/jns.1989.71.3.0359 PMID:2769387

Behrman, S. (1960). John Lizars. Centenary of a forgotten pioneer of the surgery of trigeminal neuralgia. *British Medical Journal*, *2*(5213), 1665–1666. Retrieved from http://www.ncbi.nlm.nih.gov/pubmed/13688719 PMID:13688719

Bellotti, C., Medina, M., Oliveri, G., Ettorre, F., Barrale, S., Sturiale, C., & Melcarne, A. (1988). Neuralgia of the intermediate nerve combined with trigeminal neuralgia: Case report. *Acta Neurochirurgica*, *91*(3-4), 142–143. doi:10.1007/BF01424571 PMID:2457298

Bender, M., Pradilla, G., Batra, S., See, A., Bhutiani, N., James, C., . . . Lim, M. (2012). Effectiveness of repeat glycerol rhizotomy in treating recurrent trigeminal neuralgia. *Neurosurgery, 70*(5), 1125-1133.

Bender, M. T., Pradilla, G., Batra, S., See, A. P., James, C., Pardo, C. A., ... Lim, M. (2013). Glycerol rhizotomy and radiofrequency thermocoagulation for trigeminal neuralgia in multiple sclerosis. *Journal of Neurosurgery*, *118*(2), 329–336. doi:10.3171/2012.9.JNS1226 PMID:23121430

Bender, M. T., Pradilla, G., James, C., Raza, S., Lim, M., & Carson, B. S. (2011). Surgical treatment of pediatric trigeminal neuralgia: Case series and review of the literature. *Child's Nervous System*, *27*(12), 2123–2129. doi:10.100700381-011-1593-8 PMID:21965150

Bender, M., Pradilla, G., Batra, S., See, A., Bhutiani, N., James, C., ... Lim, M. (2012). Effectiveness of Repeat Glycerol Rhizotomy in Treating Recurrent Trigeminal Neuralgia. *Neurosurgery*, *70*(5), 1125–1134. doi:10.1227/NEU.0b013e31823f5eb6 PMID:22067421

Bennett, C. R., & Giovannitti, J. A. Jr. (1998). *Neural blockade of oral and circumoral structures. In Neural Blockade in Clinical Anesthesia and Management of Pain* (3rd ed.; p. 528). Philadelphia: Lippincott Williams & Wilkins.

Bennett, M. H., & Jannetta, P. J. (1983). Evoked potentials in trigeminal neuralgia. *Neurosurgery*, *13*(3), 242–247. doi:10.1227/00006123-198309000-00005 PMID:6312364

Bennett, M. H., & Lunsford, L. D. (1984). Percutaneous retrogasserian glycerol rhizotomy for tic douloureux: Part 2. Results nd implications of trigeminal evoked potential studies. *Neurosurgery*, *14*(4), 431–435. doi:10.1227/00006123-198404000-00007 PMID:6728145

Bergenheim, A. T., Asplund, P., & Linderoth, B. (2013). Percutaneous Retrogasserian Balloon Compression for Trigeminal Neuralgia: Review of Critical Technical Details and Outcomes. *World Neurosurgery*, *79*(2), 359–368. doi:10.1016/j.wneu.2012.03.014 PMID:22480980

Bergenheim, A. T., & Hariz, M. I. (1995). Influence of previous treatment on outcome after glycerol rhizotomy for trigeminal neuralgia. *Neurosurgery*, *36*(2), 303–309, discussion 309–310. doi:10.1227/00006123-199502000-00009 PMID:7731510

Bergenheim, A. T., Hariz, M. I., & Laitinen, L. V. (1991). Selectivity of retrogasserian glycerol rhizotomy in the treatment of trigeminal neuralgia. *Stereotactic and Functional Neurosurgery*, *56*(3), 159–165. doi:10.1159/000099402 PMID:1796220

Bergenheim, A. T., Hariz, M. I., & Laitinen, L. V. (1993). Retrogasserian glycerol rhizotomy and its selectivity in the treatment of trigeminal neuralgia. *Acta Neurochirurgica. Supplementum*, *58*, 174–177. PMID:8109286

Berger, I., Nayak, N., Schuster, J., Lee, J., Stein, S., & Malhotra, N. R. (2017). Microvascular Decompression Versus Stereotactic Radiosurgery for Trigeminal Neuralgia: A Decision Analysis. *Cureus*, *9*(1), e1000. doi:10.7759/cureus.1000 PMID:28280653

Beydoun, A., Schmidt, D., & D'Souza, J. (2002). Oxcarbazepine versus carbamazepine in trigeminal neuralgia: a meta-analysis of three double blind comparative trials. *Neurology*, *58*(suppl 3).

Beydoun, A., Schmidt, D., & D'souza, J. (2002). *Oxcarbazepine versus carbamazepine in trigeminal neuralgia: a meta-analysis of three double-blind comparative trials.* Paper presented at the Neurology.

Beydoun, A. (2000). Safety and efficacy of oxcarbazepine: Results of randomized, double-blind trials. *Pharmacotherapy*, *20*(8), 152–158. doi:10.1592/phco.20.12.152S.35254 PMID:10937814

Blom, S. (1962). Trigeminal neuralgia: Its treatment with a new anticonvulsant drug (G-32883). *Lancet (London, England)*, *1*(7234), 839–840. PMID:13870089

Blom, S. (1962). Trigeminal Neuralgia: Its Treatment with a New Anti-Convulsant Drug (G-32883). *Lancet*, *279*(7234), 839–840. doi:10.1016/S0140-6736(62)91847-0 PMID:13870089

Blom, S. (1963). Tic Douloureux Treated With New Anticonvulsant. *Archives of Neurology*, *9*(3), 285–290. doi:10.1001/archneur.1963.00460090091009 PMID:14049402

Blomstedt, P. C., & Bergenheim, A. T. (2002). Technical difficulties and perioperative complications of retrogasserian glycerol rhizotomy for trigeminal neuralgia. *Stereotact Funct Neurosurg, 79*(3-4), 168-181. doi: 7083070830

Blomstedt, P. C., & Bergenheim, A. T. (2002). Technical difficulties and perioperative complications of retrogasserian glycerol rhizotomy for trigeminal neuralgia. *Stereotactic and Functional Neurosurgery*, *79*(3-4), 168–181. doi:10.1159/000070830 PMID:12890975

Blumenfeld, A., & Nikolskaya, G. (2013). Glossopharyngeal neuralgia. *Current Pain and Headache Reports*, *17*(7), 343. doi:10.100711916-013-0343-x PMID:23709235

Bobek, M. P., & Sagher, O. (1999). Aseptic meningitis caused by Teflon implantation for microvascular decompression. Case report. *Journal of Neurosurgery*, *90*(1), 145–147. doi:10.3171/jns.1999.90.1.0145 PMID:10413169

Bogduk, N. (2006). Pulsed radiofrequency. *Pain Medicine*, *7*(5), 396–407. doi:10.1111/j.1526-4637.2006.00210.x PMID:17014598

Bohman, L. E., Pierce, J., Stephen, J. H., Sandhu, S., & Lee, J. Y. (2014). Fully endoscopic microvascular decompression for trigeminal neuralgia: Technique review and early outcomes. *Neurosurgical Focus*, *37*(4), E18. doi:10.3171/2014.7.FOCUS14318 PMID:25270137

Borchers, J. D. III, Yang, H.-J., Sakamoto, G. T., Howes, G. A., Gupta, G., Chang, S. D., & Adler, J. R. Jr. (2009). Cyberknife stereotactic radiosurgical rhizotomy for trigeminal neuralgia: Anatomic and morphological considerations. *Neurosurgery*, *64*(2Suppl), A91–A95. doi:10.1227/01.NEU.0000340795.87734.70 PMID:19165080

Borges, A., & Casselman, J. (2010). Imaging the trigeminal nerve. *European Journal of Radiology*, *74*(2), 323–340. doi:10.1016/j.ejrad.2010.02.006 PMID:20227216

Bowsher, D. (1997). Trigeminal neuralgia: An anatomically oriented review. *Clinical Anatomy (New York, N.Y.)*, *10*(6), 409–415. doi: PMID:9358972

Braham, J., & Saiz, A. (1960). Phenytoin in the treatment of trigeminal and other neuralgias. *Lancet*, *2*(7156), 892–893. doi:10.1016/S0140-6736(60)91959-0

Bretschneider, H. (1847). *Versuch einer Begründung der Pathologie und Therapie der äusseren Neuralgieen*. Jena: Mauke.

Brisman, R. (2007). Microvascular decompression vs. gamma knife radiosurgery for typical trigeminal neuralgia: Preliminary findings. *Stereotactic and Functional Neurosurgery*, *85*(2-3), 94–98. doi:10.1159/000097925 PMID:17167238

Brisman, R., Khandji, A. G., & Mooij, R. B. (2002). Trigeminal nerve-blood vessel relationship as revealed by high-resolution magnetic resonance imaging and its effect on pain relief after gamma knife radiosurgery for trigeminal neuralgia. *Neurosurgery*, *50*(6), 1261–1267. PMID:12015844

Brock, S., Scaioli, V., Ferroli, P., & Broggi, G. (2004). Neurovascular decompression in trigeminal neuralgia: Role of intraoperative neurophysiological monitoring in the learning period. *Stereotactic and Functional Neurosurgery*, *82*(5-6), 199–206. doi:10.1159/000082446 PMID:15583464

Broggi, G. (2013). Percutaneous retrogasserian balloon compression for trigeminal neuralgia. *World Neurosurgery*, *79*(2), 269–270. doi:10.1016/j.wneu.2012.05.015 PMID:22634455

Broggi, G., Franzini, A., Lasio, G., Giorgi, C., & Servello, D. (1990). Long-term results of percutaneous retrogasserian thermorhizotomy for "essential" trigeminal neuralgia: Considerations in 1000 consecutive patients. *Neurosurgery*, *26*(5), 783–786, discussion 786–787. doi:10.1227/00006123-199005000-00008 PMID:2352596

Broggi, M., Acerbi, F., Ferroli, P., Tringali, G., Schiariti, M., & Broggi, G. (2013). Microvascular decompression for neurovascular conflicts in the cerebello-pontine angle: Which role for endoscopy? *Acta Neurochirurgica*, *155*(9), 1709–1716. doi:10.100700701-013-1824-8 PMID:23884611

Brown, J. A., Coursaget, C., Preul, M. C., & Sangvai, D. (1999). Mercury water and cauterizing stones: Nicolas André and tic douloureux. *Journal of Neurosurgery*, *90*(5), 977–981. doi:10.3171/jns.1999.90.5.0977 PMID:10223470

Brown, J. A., McDaniel, M. D., & Weaver, M. T. (1993). Percutaneous trigeminal nerve compression for treatment of trigeminal neuralgia: Results in 50 patients. *Neurosurgery, 32*(4), 570–573. doi:10.1227/00006123-199304000-00012 PMID:7682678

Brown, J. A., & Pilitsis, J. G. (2005). Percutaneous balloon compression for the treatment of trigeminal neuralgia: Results in 56 patients based on balloon compression pressure monitoring. *Neurosurgical Focus, 18*(5), E10. doi:10.3171/foc.2005.18.5.11 PMID:15913277

Brown, J. A., & Pilitsis, J. G. (2005). Percutaneous balloon compression for trigeminal neuralgia: Reduced dysesthesias and masseter weakness using intraluminal compression pressure monitoring in a consecutive series of 56 patients. *Neurosurgery, 57*(2), 414–414. doi:10.1093/neurosurgery/57.2.414a

Bruyn, G. W. (1984). Nervus intermedius neuralgia (Hunt). *Cephalalgia: an International Journal of Headache, 4*(1), 71–78. doi:10.1046/j.1468-2982.1984.0401071.x PMID:6370459

Burchiel, K. J. (1988). Percutaneous retrogasserian glycerol rhizolysis in the management of trigeminal neuralgia. *Journal of Neurosurgery, 69*(3), 361–366. doi:10.3171/jns.1988.69.3.0361 PMID:3404233

Burchiel, K. J. (2003). A new classification for facial pain. *Neurosurgery, 53*(5), 1164–1166, discussion 1166–1167. doi:10.1227/01.NEU.0000088806.11659.D8 PMID:14580284

Burchiel, K. J., & Russell, L. C. (1985). Glycerol neurolysis: Neurophysiological effects of topical glycerol application on rat saphenous nerve. *Journal of Neurosurgery, 63*(5), 784–788. doi:10.3171/jns.1985.63.5.0784 PMID:4056882

Burchiel, K. J., & Slavin, K. V. (2000). On the natural history of trigeminal neuralgia. *Neurosurgery, 46*(1), 152–154, discussion 154–155. doi:10.1093/neurosurgery/46.1.152 PMID:10626945

Burfield, L., Ahmad, F., & Adams, J. (2016). Glossopharyngeal neuralgia associated with cardiac syncope. *BMJ Case Reports, 2016*. doi:10.1136/bcr-2015-214104 PMID:27102416

Butler, R. (1962). Sir Charles Bell. *Resenha Médica, 3*(2), 56–62. doi:10.2218/resmedica.v3i2.389

Bymaster, F. P., Lee, T. C., Knadler, M. P., Detke, M. K., & Lyengar, S. (2005). The dual transporter inhibitor duloxetine: A review of its preclinical pharmacology, pharmacokinetic profile, and clinical results in depression. *Current Pharmocology Design, 11*(12), 1475–1493. doi:10.2174/1381612053764805 PMID:15892657

Campbell, F. G., Graham, J. G., & Zilkha, K. J. (1966). Clinical trial of carbazepine (tegretol) in trigeminal neuralgia. *Journal of Neurology, Neurosurgery, and Psychiatry, 29*(3), 265–267. doi:10.1136/jnnp.29.3.265 PMID:5327969

Campos-Benitez, M., & Kaufmann, A. M. (2008). Neurovascular compression findings in hemifacial spasm. *Journal of Neurosurgery, 109*(3), 416–420. doi:10.3171/JNS/2008/109/9/0416 PMID:18759570

Canavero, S., & Bonicalzi, V. (1997). Lamotrigine control of trigeminal neuralgia: An expanded study. *Journal of Neurology, 244*(8), 527–532. doi:10.1007004150050137 PMID:9309561

Canavero, S., Bonicalzi, V., & Pagni, C. A. (1995). The riddle of trigeminal neuralgia. *Pain, 60*(2), 229–231. doi:10.1016/0304-3959(94)00196-L PMID:7784109

Capelle, H. H., Brandis, A., Tschan, C. A., & Krauss, J. K. (2010). Treatment of recurrent trigeminal neuralgia due to Teflon granuloma. *The Journal of Headache and Pain, 11*(4), 339–344. doi:10.100710194-010-0213-4 PMID:20419329

Cappadocia, A. (1856). *The extant works of Aretaeus: the Cappadocian.* Sydenham Society.

Carnochan, J. M. (1858). Exsection of the Trunk of the Second Branch of the Fifth Pair of Nerves, beyond the Ganglion of Meckel, for Severe Neuralgia of the Face: With Three Cases. *The Southern Medical and Surgical Journal, 14*, 126–136. Retrieved from https://archive.org/stream/southern1858medi/southern1858medi_djvu.txt

Casey, K. F., & Jannetta, P. J. (2010). *History of Trigeminal Neuralgia. Trigeminal Neuralgia, 3*. Oxford University Press.

Casselman, J. W., Kuhweide, R., Deimling, M., Ampe, W., Dehaene, I., & Meeus, L. (1993). Constructive interference in steady state-3DFT MR imaging of the inner ear and cerebellopontine angle. *AJNR. American Journal of Neuroradiology, 14*(1), 47–57. PMID:8427111

Castaneda, A. E., Tuulio-Henriksson, A., Marttunen, M., Suvisaari, J., & Lonnqvist, J. (2008). A review on cognitive impairments in depressive and anxiety disorders with a focus on young adults. *Journal of Affective Disorders, 106*(1-2), 1–27. doi:10.1016/j.jad.2007.06.006 PMID:17707915

Castro, A. R., Siqueira, S. R., Perissinotti, D. M., & Siqueira, J. T. (2008). Psychological evaluation and cope with trigeminal neuralgia and temporomandibular disorder. *Arquivos de Neuro-Psiquiatria, 66*(3b3B), 716–719. doi:10.1590/S0004-282X2008000500021 PMID:18949269

Cavanagh, J. B., & Buxton, P. H. (1989). Trichloroethylene cranial neuropathy: Is it really a toxic neuropathy or does it activate latent herpes virus. *Journal of Neurology, Neurosurgery, and Psychiatry, 52*(3), 297–303. doi:10.1136/jnnp.52.3.297 PMID:2538571

Chandra, B. (1976). The use of clonazepam in the treatment of trigeminal neuralgia. *Proceedings of the Australian Association of Neurologists, 13*, 119-22.

Chang, C.-S., Chuang, C.-C., Wu, M.-F., Liu, W.-S., Tu, H.-T., & Huang, C.-F. (2012). Gamma Knife surgery for hemifacial spasm related to cerebellopontine angle tumors. *Journal of Neurosurgery, 117*(Suppl), 170–174. doi:10.3171/2012.7.GKS12999 PMID:23205806

Chaudhry, N., Srivastava, A., & Joshi, L. (2015). Hemifacial spasm: The past, present and future. *Journal of the Neurological Sciences, 356*(1-2), 27–31. doi:10.1016/j.jns.2015.06.032 PMID:26111430

Chávez, G.-R. C., & Salles, D. (2005). Three-dimensional Fast Imaging Employing Steady-state Acquisition Magnetic Resonance Imaging for Stereotactic Radiosurgery of Trigeminal Neuralgia. *Neurosurgery, 56*(3), E628–E628. doi:10.1227/01.NEU.0000154709.44776.50 PMID:15730595

Cheng, J. S., Lim, D. A., Chang, E. F., & Barbaro, N. M. (2014). A review of percutaneous treatments for trigeminal neuralgia. *Neurosurgery, 10*(1), 25–33. doi:10.1227/NEU.0000000000001687

Chen, G. Q., Wang, X. S., Wang, L., & Zheng, J. P. (2014). Arterial compression of nerve is the primary cause of trigeminal neuralgia. *Neurological Sciences, 35*(1), 61–66. doi:10.100710072-013-1518-2 PMID:23963805

Cheng, J. S., Lim, D. A., Chang, E. F., & Barbaro, N. M. (2014). A review of percutaneous treatments for trigeminal neuralgia. *Neurosurgery, 10*(Suppl 1), 25–33, discussion 33. doi:10.1227/NEU.0000000000000168700006123-201403001-00003 PMID:24509496

Cheng, J. S., Sanchez-Mejia, R. O., Limbo, M., Ward, M. M., & Barbaro, N. M. (2005). Management of medically refractory trigeminal neuralgia in patients with multiple sclerosis. *Neurosurgical Focus, 18*(5), e13. doi:10.3171/foc.2005.18.5.14 PMID:16419978

Cheng, J., Long, J., Hui, X., Lei, D., & Zhang, H. (2017). Effects of microvascular decompression on depression and anxiety in trigeminal neuralgia: A prospective cohort study focused on risk factors and prognosis. *Clinical Neurology and Neurosurgery, 161*, 59–64. doi:10.1016/j.clineuro.2017.08.011 PMID:28858633

Cheng, T. M., Cascino, T. L., & Onofrio, B. M. (1993). Comprehensive study of diagnosis and treatment of trigeminal neuralgia secondary to tumors. *Neurology, 43*(11), 2298–2302. doi:10.1212/WNL.43.11.2298 PMID:8232946

Chen, H. I., & Lee, J. Y. (2010). The measurement of pain in patients with trigeminal neuralgia. *Clinical Neurosurgery, 57*, 129–133. PMID:21280505

Chen, J.-F., Tu, P.-H., & Lee, S.-T. (2012). Repeated Percutaneous Balloon Compression for Recurrent Trigeminal Neuralgia: A Long-Term Study. *World Neurosurgery, 77*(2), 352–356. doi:10.1016/j.wneu.2011.06.013 PMID:22120364

Chen, J., Lee, S., Lui, T., Yeh, Y., Chen, T., & Tzaan, W. (2000). Teflon granuloma after microvascular decompression for trigeminal neuralgia. *Surgical Neurology, 53*(3), 281–287. doi:10.1016/S0090-3019(00)00169-5 PMID:10773262

Chen, L., Xu, M., & Zou, Y. (2010). Treatment of Trigeminal Neuralgia with Percutaneous Glycerol Injection into Meckel's Cavity: Experience in 4012 Patients. *Cell Biochemistry and Biophysics, 58*(2), 85–89. doi:10.100712013-010-9094-z PMID:20717747

Cheshire, W. (2015). Cranial Neuralgias. *Confinia Neurologica, 21*(4), 1072–1085. PMID:26252592

Cheshire, W. P. (1995). Felbamate relieved trigeminal neuralgia. *The Clinical Journal of Pain, 11*(2), 139–142. doi:10.1097/00002508-199506000-00009 PMID:7549170

Cheshire, W. P. (2007). Trigeminal neuralgia: For one nerve a multitude of treatments. *Expert Review of Neurotherapeutics*, *7*(11), 1565–1579. doi:10.1586/14737175.7.11.1565 PMID:17997704

Cheshire, W. P. Jr. (2007). Trigeminal neuralgia. *Current Pain and Headache Reports*, *11*(1), 69–74. doi:10.100711916-007-0025-7 PMID:17214925

Cheshire, W. Jr. (2001). Fosphenytoin: An intravenous option for the management of acute trigeminal neuralgia crisis. *Journal of Pain and Symptom Management*, *21*(6), 506–510. doi:10.1016/S0885-3924(01)00269-X PMID:11397609

Chesire, W. (2002). Defining the role for gabapentin in the treatment of trigeminal neuralgia: A retrospective study. *The Journal of Pain*, *3*(2), 137–142. doi:10.1054/jpai.2002.122944 PMID:14622800

Cheuk, A. V., Chin, L. S., Petit, J. H., Herman, J. M., Fang, H.-B., & Regine, W. F. (2004). Gamma knife surgery for trigeminal neuralgia: Outcome, imaging, and brainstem correlates. *International Journal of Radiation Oncology, Biology, Physics*, *60*(2), 537–541. doi:10.1016/j.ijrobp.2004.04.020 PMID:15380590

Chiu, W. A., Jinot, J., Scott, C. S., Makris, S. L., Cooper, G. S., Dzubow, R. C., ... Caldwell, J. C. (2012). Human Health Effects of Trichloroethylene: Key Findings and Scientific Issues. *Environmental Health Perspectives*, *121*(3), 303–311. doi:10.1289/ehp.1205879 PMID:23249866

Cho, D. Y., Chang, C. G., Wang, Y. C., Wang, F. H., Shen, C. C., & Yang, D. Y. (1994). Repeat operations in failed microvascular decompression for trigeminal neuralgia. *Neurosurgery*, *35*(4), 665–669, discussion 669–670. doi:10.1227/00006123-199410000-00012 PMID:7808609

Chun-Cheng, Q., Qing-Shi, Z., Ji-Qing, Z., & Zhi-Gang, W. (2009). A single-blinded pilot study assessing neurovascular contact by using high-resolution MR imaging in patients with trigeminal neuralgia. *European Journal of Radiology*, *69*(3), 459–463. doi:10.1016/j.ejrad.2007.10.010 PMID:18035511

Cohen-Gadol, A. A. (2011). Microvascular decompression surgery for trigeminal neuralgia and hemifacial spasm: Naunces of the technique based on experiences with 100 patients and review of the literature. *Clinical Neurology and Neurosurgery*, *113*(10), 844–853. doi:10.1016/j.clineuro.2011.06.003 PMID:21752534

Cole, C. D., Liu, J. K., & Apfelbaum, R. I. (2005). Historical perspectives on the diagnosis and treatment of trigeminal neuralgia. *Neurosurgical Focus*, *18*(5), E4. Retrieved from http://www.ncbi.nlm.nih.gov/pubmed/15913280. doi:10.3171/foc.2005.18.5.5 PMID:15913280

Contreras, R. J., Beckstead, R. M., & Norgren, R. (1982). The central projections of the trigeminal, facial, glossopharyngeal and vagus nerves: An autoradiographic study in the rat. *Journal of the Autonomic Nervous System*, *6*(3), 303–322. doi:10.1016/0165-1838(82)90003-0 PMID:7169500

Cook, I. A., Schrader, L. M., Degiorgio, C. M., Miller, P. R., Maremont, E. R., & Leuchter, A. F. (2013). Trigeminal nerve stimulation in major depressive disorder: Acute outcomes in an open pilot study. *Epilepsy & Behavior*, *28*(2), 221–226. doi:10.1016/j.yebeh.2013.05.008 PMID:23773978

Corrêa, C. F., & Teixeira, M. J. (1998). Balloon compression of the Gasserian ganglion for the treatment of trigeminal neuralgia. *Stereotactic and Functional Neurosurgery*, *71*(2), 83–89. doi:10.1159/000029651 PMID:10087472

Cosnett, J. E. (1990). Therapeutics in retrospect: Iron carbonate in chorea and tic douloureux. *Journal of the Royal Society of Medicine*, *83*, 390–391. Retrieved from https://www.ncbi.nlm.nih.gov/pmc/articles/PMC1292693/pdf/jrsocmed00135-0060.pdf PMID:2199675

Costa, J., Espírito-Santo, C., Borges, A., Ferreira, J. J., Coelho, M., Moore, P., & Sampaio, C. (2005). Botulinum toxin type A therapy for hemifacial spasm. *The Cochrane Database of Systematic Reviews, 40*(1). doi:10.1002/14651858.CD004899.pub2

Court, J. E., & Kase, C. S. (1976). Treatment of tic douloureux with a new anticonvulsant (clonazepam). *Journal of Neurology, Neurosurgery, and Psychiatry*, *39*(3), 297–299. doi:10.1136/jnnp.39.3.297 PMID:932745

Cruccu, G., Finnerup, N. B., Jensen, T. S., Scholz, J., Sindou, M., Svensson, P., ... Nurmikko, T. (2016). Trigeminal neuralgia: New classification and diagnostic grading for practice and research. *Neurology*, *87*(2), 220–228. doi:10.1212/WNL.0000000000002840 PMID:27306631

Cruccu, G., Gronseth, G., Alksne, J., Argoff, C., Brainin, M., Burchiel, K., ... Zakrzewska, J. M.European Federation of Neurological, Society. (2008). AAN-EFNS guidelines on trigeminal neuralgia management. *European Journal of Neurology*, *15*(10), 1013–1028. doi:10.1111/j.1468-1331.2008.02185.x PMID:18721143

Cruccu, G., & Truini, A. (2013). Refractory trigeminal neuralgia. Non-surgical treatment options. *CNS Drugs*, *27*(2), 91–96. doi:10.100740263-012-0023-0 PMID:23225488

Crue, B. L., Shelden, C. H., Pudenz, R. H., & Freshwater, D. B. (1956). Observations on the pain and trigger mechanism in trigeminal neuralgia. *Neurology*, *6*(3), 196–207. doi:10.1212/WNL.6.3.196 PMID:13297120

Cui, M., Khanijou, S., Rubino, J., & Aoki, K. R. (2004). Subcutaneous administration of botulinum toxin type A reduces formalin-induced pain. *Pain*, *107*(1-2), 125–133. doi:10.1016/j.pain.2003.10.008 PMID:14715398

Culbertson, J. C. (1887). Artificial production of peripheral neuritis. *The Cincinnati Lancet, 58*. Retrieved from https://books.google.com/books?id=fktAAQAAMAAJ&pg=PA146&lpg=PA146&dq=Pitres+Vaillard+alcohol&source=bl&ots=18Qxur5Jbx&sig=a3wDF56ZUBkz-Lf7A16czA6mjWo&hl=en&sa=X&ved=0ahUKEwjSvLKFr5zRAhXDQSYKHStGCBMQ6AEIIjAD#v=onepage&q=PitresVaillardalcohol&f=false

Cushing, H. (1920). The role of deep alcohol injections in the treatment of trigeminal neuralgia. *Journal of the American Medical Association*, *75*(7), 441. doi:10.1001/jama.1920.02620330001001

Cushing, H., & Keen, W. W. (1983). A Method of Total Extirpation of the Gasserian Ganglion for Trigeminal Neuralgia. *Journal of the American Medical Association*, *250*(4), 519. doi:10.1001/jama.1983.03340040059035 PMID:6345823

Cutbush, K., & Atkinson, R. L. (1994). Treatment of trigeminal neuralgia by posterior fossa microvascular decompression. *The Australian and New Zealand Journal of Surgery*, *64*(3), 173–176. doi:10.1111/j.1445-2197.1994.tb02171.x PMID:8117193

Dalessio, D. J. (1982). Trigeminal neuralgia. A practical approach to treatment. *Drugs*, *24*(3), 248–255. doi:10.2165/00003495-198224030-00005 PMID:7128480

Dandy, W. (1929). An operation for the cure of tic douloureux: Partial section of the sensory root at the pons. *Archives of Surgery*, *18*(2), 687–734. doi:10.1001/archsurg.1929.04420030081005

Dandy, W. E. (1932). The treatment of trigeminal neuralgia by the cerebellar route. *Annals of Surgery*, *96*(4), 787–795. doi:10.1097/00000658-193210000-00026 PMID:17866870

Dandy, W. E. (1934). Concerning the cause of trigeminal neuralgia. *American Journal of Surgery*, *24*(2), 447–455. doi:10.1016/S0002-9610(34)90403-7

Dannenbaum, M., Lega, B. C., Suki, D., Harper, R. L., & Yoshor, D. (2008). Microvascular decompression for hemifacial spasm: Long-term results from 114 operations performed without neurophysiological monitoring. *Journal of Neurosurgery*, *109*(3), 410–415. doi:10.3171/JNS/2008/109/9/0410 PMID:18759569

Davidoff, L. M. (1950). *Trifacial neuralgia. Oral Surgery, Oral Medicine, Oral Pathology* (Vol. 3). Mosby. 10.1016/0030-4220(50)90372-0

de Bondt, B.-J., Stokroos, R., & Casselman, J. (2007). Persistent trigeminal artery associated with trigeminal neuralgia: Hypothesis of neurovascular compression. *Neuroradiology*, *49*(1), 23–26. doi:10.100700234-006-0150-8 PMID:17089114

Defazio, G., Abbruzzese, G., Girlanda, P., Vacca, L., Currà, A., De Salvia, R., ... Berardelli, A. (2002). Botulinum toxin A treatment for primary hemifacial spasm: A 10-year multicenter study. *Archives of Neurology*, *59*(3), 418–420. doi:10.1001/archneur.59.3.418 PMID:11890846

Deng, J., Ma, C. M., Hai, J., & Nath, R. (2003). Commissioning 6 MV photon beams of a stereotactic radiosurgery system for Monte Carlo treatment planning. *Medical Physics*, *30*(12), 3124–3134. doi:10.1118/1.1624753 PMID:14713079

Derry, S., Wiffen, PJ., Aldrington, D., & Moore, R.A. (2015). Nortriptyline for neuropathic pain in adults. *Cochrane Database Systematic Reviews*, *8*(1).

Descovich, M., Sneed, P. K., Barbaro, N. M., McDermott, M. W., Chuang, C. F., & Barani, I. J., … Lijun, M. (2010). A dosimetric comparison between Gamma Knife and CyberKnife treatment plans for trigeminal neuralgia. *Journal of Neurosurgery*, *113*(Suppl), 199–206. PMID:21222296

Deseure, K., & Hans, G. H. (2015). Chronic Constriction Injury of the Rat's Infraorbital Nerve (IoN-CCI) to Study Trigeminal Neuropathic Pain. *Journal of Visualized Experiments*, (103). doi:10.3791/53167 PMID:26437303

Deshmukh, Hott, Tabrizi, Nakaji, Feiz-Erfan, & Spetzler. (2005). Cavernous malformation of the trigeminal nerve manifesting with trigeminal neuralgia: case report. *Neurosurgery*, *56*(3).

Devor, M., Amir, R., & Rappaport, Z. H. (2002). Pathophysiology of trigeminal neuralgia: The ignition hypothesis. *The Clinical Journal of Pain*, *18*(1), 4–13. doi:10.1097/00002508-200201000-00002 PMID:11803297

Dewhurst, K. (1957). A Symposium on Trigemonal Neuralgia With Contributions by Kocke, Sydenham, and other Eminent Seventeenth Century Physicians. *Journal of the History of Medicine and Allied Sciences*, *XII*(1), 21–36. doi:10.1093/jhmas/XII.1.21 PMID:13406256

Dhople, Adams, Maggio, Naqvi, Regine, & Kwok. (2009). *Long-term outcomes of Gamma Knife radiosurgery for classic trigeminal neuralgia: implications of treatment and critical review of the literature.* Academic Press. doi:10.3171/2009.2.JNS08977

Dieckmann, G., Bockermann, V., Heyer, C., Henning, J., & Roesen, M. (1987). Five-and-a-half years' experience with percutaneous retrogasserian glycerol rhizotomy in treatment of trigeminal neuralgia. *Applied Neurophysiology*, *50*(1-6), 401–413. PMID:3502439

Domingues, R., Kuster, G., & Aquino, C. (2007). Treatment of trigeminal neuralgia with low doses of topiramate. *Arquivos de Neuro-Psiquiatria*, *65*(3b), 792–794. doi:10.1590/S0004-282X2007000500011 PMID:17952282

Dubner, R., Sharav, Y., Gracely, R. H., & Price, D. D. (1987). Idiopathic trigeminal neuralgia: Sensory features and pain mechanisms. *Pain*, *31*(1), 23–33. doi:10.1016/0304-3959(87)90003-0 PMID:3696741

Duff, J. M., Spinner, R. J., Lindor, N. M., Dodick, D. W., & Atkinson, J. L. (1999). Familial trigeminal neuralgia and contralateral hemifacial spasm. *Neurology*, *53*(1), 216–218. doi:10.1212/WNL.53.1.216 PMID:10408564

Dulhunty, A. F., Gage, P. W., & Barry, P. H. (1973). Differential effects of glycerol treatment on membrane capacity and excitation-contraction coupling in toad sartorius fibres. *The Journal of Physiology*, *234*(2), 373–408. doi:10.1113/jphysiol.1973.sp010350 PMID:4203309

Dvorak, T., Finn, A., Price, L. L., Mignano, J. E., Fitzek, M. M., Wu, J. K., & Yao, K. C. (2009). Retreatment of trigeminal neuralgia with Gamma Knife radiosurgery: Is there an appropriate cumulative dose? Clinical article. *Journal of Neurosurgery*, *111*(2), 359–364. doi:10.3171/2008.11.JNS08770 PMID:19326978

Dworkin, R. H., Hetzel, R. D., & Banks, S. M. (1999). Toward a model of the pathogenesis of chronic pain. *Seminars in Clinical Neuropsychiatry*, *4*(3), 176–185. doi:10.153/SCNP00400176 PMID:10498785

Eadie, M. J. (2012). *Headaches: Through the Centuries*. Oxford University Press. doi:10.1093/med/9780199860975.001.0001

Eboli, P., Stone, J. L., Aydin, S., & Slavin, K. V. (2009). Historical characterization of trigeminal neuralgia. *Neurosurgery*, *64*(6), 1183–1187. doi:10.1227/01.NEU.0000339412.44397.76 PMID:19487899

Eide, P. K., & Stubhaug, A. (1997). Sensory perception in patients with trigeminal neuralgia: Effects of percutaneous retrogasserian glycerol rhizotomy. *Stereotactic and Functional Neurosurgery*, *68*(1-4 Pt 1), 207–211. doi:10.1159/000099925 PMID:9711718

Eisendrath, S. J., Gillung, E., Delucchi, K. L., Segal, Z. V., Nelson, J. C., McInnes, L. A., ... Feldman, M. D. (2016). A Randomized Controlled Trial of Mindfulness-Based Cognitive Therapy for Treatment-Resistant Depression. *Psychotherapy and Psychosomatics*, *85*(2), 99–110. doi:10.1159/000442260 PMID:26808973

Elahi, F., & Ho, K. W. (2014). Anesthesia dolorosa of trigeminal nerve, a rare complication of acoustic neuroma surgery. *Case Reports in Neurological Medicine*, *496794*. doi:10.1155/2014/496794 PMID:25328729

El-Ghandour, N. M. F. (2010). Microvascular decompression in the treatment of trigeminal neuralgia caused by vertebrobasilar ectasia. *Neurosurgery*, *67*(2), 330–337. doi:10.1227/01.NEU.0000371978.86528.60 PMID:20644418

Eller, J. L., Raslan, A. M., & Burchiel, K. J. (2005). Trigeminal neuralgia: Definition and classification. *Neurosurgical Focus*, *18*(5), E3. doi:10.3171/foc.2005.18.5.4 PMID:15913279

Elster, P. (1951). Symptoms and diagnosis of trigeminal neuralgia and conclusions regarding essential and symptomatic trigeminal neuralgia. *Psychiatrie, Neurologie, und Medizinische Psychologie*, *3*(4), 86–93. PMID:14844533

El-Tallawy, H. N., Farghaly, W. M., Rageh, T. A., Shehata, G. A., Abdel Hakeem, M. N., Badry, R., & Kandil, M. R. (2013). Prevalence of trigeminal neuralgia in Al-Quseir city (Red sea Governorate), Egypt. *Clinical Neurology and Neurosurgery*, *115*(9), 1792–1794. doi:10.1016/j.clineuro.2013.04.014 PMID:23692870

Emril, D. R., & Ho, K.-Y. (2010). Treatment of trigeminal neuralgia: Role of radiofrequency ablation. *Journal of Pain Research*, *3*, 249–254. doi:10.2147/JPR.S14455 PMID:21311718

Engh, J. A., Horowitz, M., Burkhart, L., Chang, Y.-F., & Kassam, A. (2005). Repeat microvascular decompression for hemifacial spasm. *Journal of Neurology, Neurosurgery, and Psychiatry*, *76*(11), 1574–1580. doi:10.1136/jnnp.2004.056861 PMID:16227555

Epstein, J. B., & Marcoe, J. H. (1994). Topical application of capsaicin for treatment of oral neuropathic pain and trigeminal neuralgia. *Oral Surgery, Oral Medicine, and Oral Pathology*, *77*(2), 135–140. doi:10.1016/0030-4220(94)90275-5 PMID:8139830

Erdem, E., & Alkan, A. (2001). Peripheral glycerol injections in the treatment of idiopathic trigeminal neuralgia: Retrospective analysis of 157 cases. *Journal of Oral and Maxillofacial Surgery*, *59*(10), 1176–1179. doi:10.1053/joms.2001.26721 PMID:11573175

Erdine, S., Bilir, A., Cosman, E. R., & Cosman, E. R., Jr. (2009). Ultrastructural changes in axons following exposure to pulsed radiofrequency fields. *Pain Practice: The Official Journal of World Institute of Pain*, *9*(6), 407–417.

Erdine, S., Ozyalcin, N. S., Cimen, A., Celik, M., Talu, G. K., & Disci, R. (2007). Comparison of pulsed radiofrequency with conventional radiofrequency in the treatment of idiopathic trigeminal neuralgia. *European Journal of Pain (London, England)*, *11*(3), 309–313. doi:10.1016/j.ejpain.2006.04.001 PMID:16762570

Erdine, S., Yucel, A., Cimen, A., Aydin, S., Sav, A., & Bilir, A. (2005). Effects of pulsed versus conventional radiofrequency current on rabbit dorsal root ganglion morphology. *European Journal of Pain (London, England)*, *9*(3), 251–256. doi:10.1016/j.ejpain.2004.07.002 PMID:15862474

Eseonu, C. I., Goodwin, C. R., Zhou, X., Theodros, D., Bender, M. T., Mathios, D., ... Lim, M. (2015). Reduced CSF leak in complete calvarial reconstructions of microvascular decompression craniectomies using calcium phosphate cement. *Journal of Neurosurgery*, *123*(6), 1476–1479. doi:10.3171/2015.1.JNS142102 PMID:26230465

Fardy, M. J., & Patton, D. W. (1994). Complications associated with peripheral alcohol injections in the management of trigeminal neuralgia. *British Journal of Oral & Maxillofacial Surgery*, *32*(6), 387–391. doi:10.1016/0266-4356(94)90031-0 PMID:7849000

Fardy, M. J., Zakrzewska, J. M., & Patton, D. W. (1994). Peripheral surgical techniques for the management of trigeminal neuralgia?Alcohol and glycerol injections. *Acta Neurochirurgica*, *129*(3–4), 181–184. doi:10.1007/BF01406500 PMID:7531385

Fariselli, L., Marras, C., De Santis, M., Marchetti, M., Milanesi, I., & Broggi, G. (2009). Cyberknife radiosurgery as a first treatment for idiopathic trigeminal neuralgia. *Neurosurgery, 64*(suppl_2), A96–A101. 10.1227/01.NEU.0000341714.55023.8F

Febles, C., Werner-Wasik, M., Rosenwasser, R. H., Goldman, W. H., Curran, W. J., & Andrews, D. W. (n.d.). A comparison of treatment outcomes with Gamma Knife radiosurgery versus Glycerol Rhizotomy in the management of trigeminal neuralgia. *International Journal of Radiation Oncology, Biology, Physics, 57*(2), S253. doi: 10.1016/s0360-3016(03)01087-3

Feletti, A., Santi, G. Z., Sammartino, F., Bevilacqua, M., Cisotto, P., & Longatti, P. (2013). Peripheral trigeminal nerve field stimulation: Report of 6 cases. *Neurosurgical Focus*, *35*(3), E10. doi:10.3171/2013.7.FOCUS13228 PMID:23991813

Ferguson, G. G., Brett, D. C., Peerless, S. J., Barr, H. W., & Girvin, J. P. (1981). Trigeminal neuralgia: a comparison of the results of percutaneous rhizotomy and microvascular decompression. *The Canadian Journal of Neurological Sciences, 8*(3), 207–14. Retrieved from http://www.ncbi.nlm.nih.gov/pubmed/6169418

Fernandez-Conejero, I., Ulkatan, S., Sen, C., & Deletis, V. (2012). Intra-operative neurophysiology during microvascular decompression for hemifacial spasm. *Clinical Neurophysiology*, *123*(1), 78–83. doi:10.1016/j.clinph.2011.10.007 PMID:22136736

Ferrell, P., & McLeod, H. (2008). Carbamazepine, HLA-B*1502 and risk of Stevens-Johnson syndrome and toxic epidermal necrolysis: US FDA recommendations. *Pharmacogenomics*, *9*(10), 1543–1546. doi:10.2217/14622416.9.10.1543 PMID:18855540

Ferroli, Acerbi, Broggi, & Broggi. (2010). Arteriovenous micromalformation of the trigeminal root: intraoperative diagnosis with indocyanine green videoangiography: case report. *Neurosurgery, 67*(3 Suppl).

Figueiredo, P. C., Brock, M., De Oliveira, A. M. J., & Prill, A. (1989). Arteriovenous malformation in the cerebellopontine angle presenting as trigeminal neuralgia. *Arquivos de Neuro-Psiquiatria, 47*(1), 61–71. doi:10.1590/S0004-282X1989000100008 PMID:2669692

Fleetwood, I. G., Innes, A. M., Hansen, S. R., & Steinberg, G. K. (2001). Familial trigeminal neuralgia. Case report and review of the literature. *Journal of Neurosurgery, 95*(3), 513–517. doi:10.3171/jns.2001.95.3.0513 PMID:11565877

Flickinger, J. C., Pollock, B. E., Kondziolka, D., Phuong, L. K., Foote, R. L., Stafford, S. L., & Lunsford, L. D. (2001). Does increased nerve length within the treatment volume improve trigeminal neuralgia radiosurgery? A prospective double-blind, randomized study. *International Journal of Radiation Oncology, Biology, Physics, 51*(2), 449–454. doi:10.1016/S0360-3016(01)01606-6 PMID:11567820

Flor, H., Rasche, D., Islamian, A. P., Rolko, C., Yilmaz, P., Ruppolt, M., & … . (2016). Subtle Sensory Abnormalities Detected by Quantitative Sensory Testing in Patients with Trigeminal Neuralgia. *Pain Physician, 19*(7), 507–518. PMID:27676667

Fothergill, J. (1773). Of a painful affection of the face. *Medical Observations and Inquiries by a Society of Physicians, 5*, 129–142. Retrieved from https://archive.hshsl.umaryland.edu/bitstream/10713/3435/1/Fothergill1940.pdf

Fothergill, J. (1776). *Of a painful affection of the face*. Academic Press.

Fountas, K. N., Smith, J. R., Lee, G. P., Jenkins, P. D., Cantrell, R. R., & Sheils, W. C. (2007). Gamma Knife stereotactic radiosurgical treatment of idiopathic trigeminal neuralgia: Long-term outcome and complications. *Neurosurgical Focus, 23*(6), E7. doi:10.3171/FOC-07/12/E8 PMID:18081485

Fountoulakis, K. N., Balaris, D., Nikolaou, V., & Nuimatoudis, J. (2016). Non-conventional pharmacological agents for the treatment of bipolar disorder: A systematic review of the evidence. *Psychiatriki, 27*(4), 253–263. doi:10.22365/jpsych.2016.274.253 PMID:28114089

Fowler, G. R. (1886). I. The Operative Treatment of Facial Neuralgia. *Annals of Surgery, 3*(4), 269–320. doi:10.1097/00000658-188603000-00026 PMID:17856059

Fraioli, B., Esposito, V., Guidetti, B., Cruccu, G., & Manfredi, M. (1989). Treatment of Trigeminal Neuralgia by Thermocoagulation, Glycerolization, and Percutaneous Compression of the Gasserian Ganglion and or Retrogasserian Rootlets - Long-Term Results and Therapeutic Protocol. *Neurosurgery, 24*(2), 239–245. doi:10.1227/00006123-198902000-00014 PMID:2783993

Fraioli, M. F., Lisciani, D., & Fraioli, C. (2014). Trigeminal neuralgia. *Journal of Neurosurgery, 120*(1), 288–289. doi:10.3171/2012.12.JNS101876 PMID:24180575

Fraioli, M. F., Moschettoni, L., Fraioli, C., & Strigari, L. (2010). Treatment of idiopathic hemifacial spasm with radiosurgery or hypofractionated stereotactic radiotherapy: Preliminary results. *Minimally Invasive Neurosurgery: MIN*, *53*(1), 34–36. doi:10.1055-0030-1247584 PMID:20376743

Frazier, C. H. (1928). Operation for the radical cure of trigeminal neuralgia: Analysis of five hundred cases. *Annals of Surgery*, *88*(3), 534–547. doi:10.1097/00000658-192809000-00021 PMID:17865965

Freeman, A. R., Reuben, J. P., Brandt, P. W., & Grundfest, H. (1966). Osmometrically determined characteristics of the cell membrane of squid and lobster giant axons. *The Journal of General Physiology*, *50*(2), 423–445. doi:10.1085/jgp.50.2.423 PMID:11526838

Fromm, G. H., Terrence, C. F., & Chattha, A. S. (1984). Baclofen in the treatment of trigeminal neuralgia: Double-blind study and long-term follow-up. *Annals of Neurology*, *15*(3), 240–244. doi:10.1002/ana.410150306 PMID:6372646

Fromm, G., Aumentado, D., & Terrence, C. (1993). A clinical and experimental investigation of the effects of tizanidine in trigeminal neuralgia. *Pain*, *53*(3), 265–271. doi:10.1016/0304-3959(93)90222-B PMID:8351156

Fromm, G., & Terrence, C. (1987). Comparison of L-baclofen and racemic baclofen in trigeminal neuralgia. *Neurology*, *37*(11), 1725–1728. doi:10.1212/WNL.37.11.1725 PMID:3313099

Fuchs, C. Z., & Rehm, L. P. (1977). A self-control behavior therapy program for depression. *Journal of Consulting and Clinical Psychology*, *45*(2), 206–215. doi:10.1037/0022-006X.45.2.206 PMID:850005

Fujimaki, T., Fukushima, T., & Miyazaki, S. (1990). Percutaneous retrogasserian glycerol injection in the management of trigeminal neuralgia: Long-term follow-up results. *Journal of Neurosurgery*, *73*(2), 212–216. doi:10.3171/jns.1990.73.2.0212 PMID:2195139

Fusco, B., & Alessandri, M. (1992). Analgesic Effect of Capsaicin in idiopathic trigeminal neuralgia. *Anesthesia and Analgesia*, *74*(3), 375–377. doi:10.1213/00000539-199203000-00011 PMID:1539818

Gardner, W. J., & Miklos, M. V. (1959). Response of trigeminal neuralgia to decompression of sensory root; discussion of cause of trigeminal neuralgia. *Journal of the American Medical Association*, *170*(15).

Gardner, W. J. (1959). Response of trigeminal neuralgia to decompression of sensory root; discussion of cause of trigeminal neuralgia. *Journal of the American Medical Association*, *170*(15), 1773. doi:10.1001/jama.1959.03010150017004 PMID:13672767

Gardner, W. J. (1962). Concerning the Mechanism of Trigeminal Neuralgia and Hemifacial Spasm. *Journal of Neurosurgery*, *19*(11), 947–958. doi:10.3171/jns.1962.19.11.0947 PMID:13946557

Gardner, W. J., & Sava, G. A. (1962). Hemifacial Spasm—a Reversible Pathophysiologic State. *Journal of Neurosurgery*, *19*(3), 240–247. doi:10.3171/jns.1962.19.3.0240

Gaul, C., Hastreiter, P., Duncker, A., & Naraghi, R. (2011). Diagnosis and neurosurgical treatment of glossopharyngeal neuralgia: Clinical findings and 3-D visualization of neurovascular compression in 19 consecutive patients. *The Journal of Headache and Pain*, *12*(5), 527–534. doi:10.100710194-011-0349-x PMID:21567138

George, M. S., Lisanby, S. H., Avery, D., McDonald, W. M., Durkalski, V., Pavlicova, M., ... Sackeim, H. A. (2010). Daily left prefrontal transcranial magnetic stimulation therapy for major depressive disorder: A sham-controlled randomized trial. *Archives of General Psychiatry*, *67*(5), 507–516. doi:10.1001/archgenpsychiatry.2010.46 PMID:20439832

George, M. S., Taylor, J. J., & Short, E. B. (2013). The expanding evidence base for rTMS treatment of depression. *Current Opinion in Psychiatry*, *26*(1), 13–18. doi:10.1097/YCO.0b013e32835ab46d PMID:23154644

Giovanelli, M., Marini, G., & Marossero, F. (1963). Typical Trigeminal Neuralgia in the Presence of Macroscopic Organic Lesions of the Central Nervous System. *Minerva Neurochirurgica*, *54*, 124–130. PMID:14125306

Goerss, S. J., Atkinson, J. L. D., & Kallmes, D. F. (2009). Variable size percutaneous balloon compression of the gasserian ganglion for trigeminal neuralgia. *Surgical Neurology*, *71*(3), 388–390. doi:10.1016/j.surneu.2007.09.040 PMID:18291447

Gold, P. W. (2015). The organization of the stress system and its dysregulation in depressive illness. *Molecular Psychiatry*, *20*(1), 32–47. doi:10.1038/mp.2014.163 PMID:25486982

Gomez-Arguelles, J. M., Dorado, R., Sepulveda, J. M., Herrera, A., Arrojo, F. G., Aragon, E., ... Anciones, B. (2008). Oxcarbazepine monotherapy in carbamazepine-unresponsive trigeminal neuralgia. *Journal of Clinical Neuroscience*, *15*(5), 516–519. doi:10.1016/j.jocn.2007.04.010 PMID:18378142

Goodwin, C. R., Yang, J. X., Bettegowda, C., Hwang, B., James, C., Biser, A., ... Lim, M. (2013). Glycerol rhizotomy via a retrosigmoid approach as an alternative treatment for trigeminal neuralgia. *Clinical Neurology and Neurosurgery*, *115*(12), 2454–2456. doi:10.1016/j.clineuro.2013.09.009 PMID:24161889

Gorgulho, A. (2012). Radiation mechanisms of pain control in classical trigeminal neuralgia. *Surgical Neurology International*, *3*(2Suppl 1), S17–S25. doi:10.4103/2152-7806.91606 PMID:22826806

Graham, J. G., & Zilkha, K. J. (1966). Treatment of trigeminal neuralgia with carbamazepine: A follow-up study. *British Medical Journal*, *1*(5481), 210–211. doi:10.1136/bmj.1.5481.210 PMID:5901730

Green, M., & Selman, J. (1991). Review Article: The Medical Management of Trigeminal Neuralgia. *Headache*, *31*(9), 588–592. doi:10.1111/j.1526-4610.1991.hed3109588.x PMID:1774173

Gronseth, G., Crucu, G., Alksne, J., Argoff, C., Brainin, M., Burchiel, K., ... Zakrzewska, J. (2008). Practice Parameter: The diagnostic evaluation and treatment of trigeminal neuralgia (an evidence-based review). *Neurology, 71*(15), 1183–1190. doi:10.1212/01.wnl.0000326598.83183.04 PMID:18716236

Guardinani, E., Sadoughi, B., Blitzer, A., & Sirois, D. (2013). A new treatment paradigm for trigeminal neuralgia using botulinum toxin type A. *The Laryngoscope, 124*(2), 413–417. doi:10.1002/lary.24286 PMID:23818108

Gubian, A., & Rosahl, S. K. (2017). Meta-Analysis on Safety and Efficacy of Microsurgical and Radiosurgical Treatment of Trigeminal Neuralgia. *World Neurosurgery, 103*, 757–767. doi:10.1016/j.wneu.2017.04.085 PMID:28435111

Guidetti, B. (1950). Essential trigeminal neuralgia; section of the descending bulbar trigeminal tract according to Sjoqvist's method. *Sistema Nervoso, 2*(4), 247–257. PMID:14809416

Guo, Q. H., Tong, Q. H., Lu, N., Cao, H., Yang, L., & Zhang, Y. Q. (2017). Proteomic Analysis of the Hippocampus in Mouse Models of Trigeminal Neuralgia and Inescapable Shock-Induced Depression. *Neuroscience Bulletin*. doi:10.100712264-017-0131-4 PMID:28424990

Guo, S., Chao, S. T., Reuther, A. M., Barnett, G. H., & Suh, J. H. (2008). Review of the treatment of trigeminal neuralgia with gamma knife radiosurgery. *Stereotactic and Functional Neurosurgery, 86*(3), 135–146. doi:10.1159/000120425 PMID:18334855

Gusmão, S., Oliveira, M., Tazinaffo, U., & Honey, C. R. (2003). Percutaneous trigeminal nerve radiofrequency rhizotomy guided by computerized tomography fluoroscopy. *Journal of Neurosurgery, 99*(4), 785–786. doi:10.3171/jns.2003.99.4.0785 PMID:14567619

Habeych, M. E., Shah, A. C., Nikonow, T. N., Balzer, J. R., Crammond, D. J., Thirumala, P. D., ... Horowitz, M. (2011). Effect of botulinum neurotoxin treatment in the lateral spread monitoring of microvascular decompression for hemifacial spasm. *Muscle & Nerve, 44*(4), 518–524. doi:10.1002/mus.22104 PMID:21826681

Haines, S. J., Jannetta, P. J., & Zorub, D. S. (1980). Microvascular relations of the trigeminal nerve: An anatomical study with clinical correlation. *Journal of Neurosurgery, 52*(3), 381–386. doi:10.3171/jns.1980.52.3.0381 PMID:7359193

Håkanson, S., & Leksell, L. (1979). Stereotactic radiosurgery in trigeminal neuralgia. In G. F. Pauser G., Gross D. (Ed.), Gesichtsschmerz: Schmerzstudien (pp. 231-237). New York: Gustav Fischer Verlag.

Håkanson, S. (1981). Trigeminal neuralgia treated by the injection of glycerol into the trigeminal cistern. *Neurosurgery, 9*(6), 638–646. doi:10.1227/00006123-198112000-00005 PMID:7322329

Håkanson, S. (1983). Retrogasserian glycerol injection as treatment of tic douloureux. *Advances in Pain Research and Therapy, 5*, 927–933.

Håkanson, S. (1991). In G. H. Fromm (Ed.), *Surgical treatment: retrogasserian glycerol injection*. Boston: ButterworthHeinemann.

Haller, S., Etienne, L., Kövari, E., Varoquaux, A. D., Urbach, H., & Becker, M. (2016). Imaging of Neurovascular Compression Syndromes: Trigeminal Neuralgia, Hemifacial Spasm, Vestibular Paroxysmia, and Glossopharyngeal Neuralgia. *AJNR. American Journal of Neuroradiology, 37*(8), 1384–1392. doi:10.3174/ajnr.A4683 PMID:26892985

Halpern, C. H., Lang, S.-S., & Lee, J. Y. (2013). Fully endoscopic microvascular decompression: Our early experience. *Minimally Invasive Surgery*. PMID:24083024

Hamlyn, P. J. (1997). Neurovascular relationships in the posterior cranial fossa, with special reference to trigeminal neuralgia. 2. Neurovascular compression of the trigeminal nerve in cadaveric controls and patients with trigeminal neuralgia: Quantification and influence of method. *Clinical Anatomy (New York, N.Y.), 10*(6), 380–388. doi: PMID:9358968

Hamlyn, P. J., & King, T. T. (1992). Neurovascular compression in trigeminal neuralgia: A clinical and anatomical study. *Journal of Neurosurgery, 76*(6), 948–954. doi:10.3171/jns.1992.76.6.0948 PMID:1588428

Hanakita, J., & Kondo, A. (1988). Serious complications of microvascular decompression operations for trigeminal neuralgia and hemifacial spasm. *Neurosurgery, 22*(2), 348–352. doi:10.1227/00006123-198802000-00012 PMID:3352885

Han, K. R., & Kim, C. (2010). The Long-Term Outcome of Mandibular Nerve Block with Alcohol for the Treatment of Trigeminal Neuralgia. *Anesthesia and Analgesia, 111*(2), 550–553. doi:10.1213/ANE.0b013e3181e4204c PMID:20584871

Han, K. W., Zhang, D. F., Chen, J. G., & Hou, L. J. (2016). Presurgical visualization of the neurovascular relationship in trigeminal neuralgia with 3D modeling using free Slicer software. *Acta Neurochirurgica, 158*(11), 2195–2201. doi:10.100700701-016-2936-8 PMID:27543280

Han, P. P., Shetter, A. G., Smith, K. A., Fiedler, J. A., Rogers, C. L., Speiser, B., & Feiz-Erfan, I. (1999). Gamma knife radiosurgery for trigeminal neuralgia: Experience at the Barrow Neurological Institute. *Stereotactic and Functional Neurosurgery, 73*(1-4), 131–133. doi:10.1159/000029771 PMID:10853118

Hardy, D. G., & Rhoton, A. L. Jr. (1978). Microsurgical relationships of the superior cerebellar artery and the trigeminal nerve. *Journal of Neurosurgery, 49*(5), 669–678. doi:10.3171/jns.1978.49.5.0669 PMID:712389

Harness, D. M., & Chase, P. F. (1990). Lateralization of chronic facial pain: Fact or fiction. *Cranio, 8*(4), 339–341. doi:10.1080/08869634.1990.11678335 PMID:2098197

Harries, A. M., Dong, C. C. J., & Honey, C. R. (2012). Use of endotracheal tube electrodes in treating glossopharyngeal neuralgia: Technical note. *Stereotactic and Functional Neurosurgery, 90*(3), 141–144. doi:10.1159/000335714 PMID:22508038

Harries, A. M., & Mitchell, R. D. (2011). Percutaneous glycerol rhizotomy for trigeminal neuralgia: Safety and efficacy of repeat procedures. *British Journal of Neurosurgery, 25*(2), 268–272. doi:10.3109/02688697.2011.558946 PMID:21545328

Harris, W. (1912). Alcohol injection of the Gasserian ganglion for trigeminal neuralgia. *Lancet, 179*(4613), 218–221. doi:10.1016/S0140-6736(01)65362-5 PMID:19975621

Hartley, F. (1892). Intracranial Neurectomy of the Fifth Nerve. *Annals of Surgery, 17*, 511–526. doi:10.1097/00000658-189301000-00120 PMID:17859915

Hatem, J., Sindou, M., & Vial, C. (2001). Intraoperative monitoring of facial EMG responses during microvascular decompression for hemifacial spasm. Prognostic value for long-term outcome: A study in a 33-patient series. *British Journal of Neurosurgery, 15*(6), 496–499. doi:10.1080/02688690120105101 PMID:11814001

Headache Classification Committee of the International Headache S. (2013). The International Classification of Headache Disorders, 3rd edition (beta version). Cephalalgia, 33(9), 629-808. doi:10.1177/0333102413485658

Headache Classification Committee of the International Headache Society (IHS). (2013). The International Classification of Headache Disorders, 3rd edition (beta version). Cephalalgia, 33(9), 629–808. doi:10.1177/0333102413485658

Helbig, G. M., Callahan, J. D., & Cohen-Gadol, A. A. (2009). Variant intraneural vein-trigeminal nerve relationships: An observation during microvascular decompression surgery for trigeminal neuralgia. *Neurosurgery, 65*(5), 958–961, discussion 961. doi:10.1227/01.NEU.0000351757.29658.C0 PMID:19834410

Helis, C. A., Lucas, J. T. Jr, Bourland, J. D., Chan, M. D., Tatter, S. B., & Laxton, A. W. (2015). Repeat Radiosurgery for Trigeminal Neuralgia. *Neurosurgery, 77*(5), 755–761, discussion 761. doi:10.1227/NEU.0000000000000915 PMID:26214319

Hellsing, G. (1976). [Transcutaneous neural stimulation (TNS) in chronic pain in patients with temporomandibular joint disorders. A clinical report]. *Tandlakartidningen, 68*(13-14), 789–793. PMID:1077220

Henson, C. F., Goldman, H. W., Rosenwasser, R. H., Downes, M. B., Bednarz, G., Pequignot, E. C., ... Andrews, D. W. (2005). Glycerol rhizotomy versus gamma knife radiosurgery for the treatment of trigeminal neuralgia: An analysis of patients treated at one institution. *International Journal of Radiation Oncology, Biology, Physics, 63*(1), 82–90. doi:10.1016/j.ijrobp.2005.01.033 PMID:16111575

Hilton, D. A., Love, S., Gradidge, T., & Coakham, H. B. (1994). Pathological findings associated with trigeminal neuralgia caused by vascular compression. *Neurosurgery, 35*(2), 299–303, discussion 303. doi:10.1227/00006123-199408000-00017 PMID:7969838

Hiwatashi, A., Matsushima, T., Yoshiura, T., Tanaka, A., Noguchi, T., Togao, O., ... Honda, H. (2008). MRI of glossopharyngeal neuralgia caused by neurovascular compression. *AJR. American Journal of Roentgenology, 191*(2), 578–581. doi:10.2214/AJR.07.3025 PMID:18647935

Ho, A., Lo, A. T., Dieterich, S., Soltys, S. G., Gibbs, I. C., Chang, S. G., & Adler, J. R. (2012). Trigeminal neuralgia treatment dosimetry of the Cyberknife. *Medical Dosimetry: Official Journal of the American Association of Medical Dosimetrists*, *37*(1), 42–46. doi:10.1016/j.meddos.2010.12.012 PMID:21723113

Hodaie, M., & Coello, A. F. (2013). Advances in the management of trigeminal neuralgia. *Journal of Neurosurgical Sciences*, *57*(1), 13–21. PMID:23584217

Holsheimer, J. (2001). Electrical stimulation of the trigeminal tract in chronic, intractable facial neuralgia. *Archives of Physiology and Biochemistry*, *109*(4), 304–308. doi:10.1076/apab.109.4.304.4246 PMID:11935364

Hong, W., Zheng, X., Wu, Z., Li, X., Wang, X., Li, Y., ... Li, S. (2011). Clinical features and surgical treatment of trigeminal neuralgia caused solely by venous compression. *Acta Neurochirurgica*, *153*(5), 1037–1042. doi:10.100700701-011-0957-x PMID:21298451

Horsley, V. (1891). Remarks on the Various Surgical Procedures Devised for the Relief or Cure of Trigeminal Neuralgia (Tic Douloureux). *British Medical Journal*, *2*(1615), 1249–1252. doi:10.1136/bmj.2.1615.1249 PMID:20753459

Hsu, C., Chang, C., Peng, C., & Liang, C. (2014). Rapid Management of trigeminal neuralgia and comorbid major depressive disorder with duloxetine. *The Annals of Pharmacotherapy*, *48*(8), 1090–1092. doi:10.1177/1060028014532789 PMID:24788987

Huang, B. R., Chang, C. N., & Hsu, J. C. (2009). Intraoperative electrophysiological monitoring in microvascular decompression for hemifacial spasm. *Journal of Clinical Neuroscience*, *16*(2), 209–213. doi:10.1016/j.jocn.2008.04.016 PMID:19103492

Huang, B., Yao, M., Feng, Z., Guo, J., Zereshki, A., Leong, M., & Qian, X. (2014). CT-guided percutaneous infrazygomatic radiofrequency neurolysis through foramen rotundum to treat V2 trigeminal neuralgia. *Pain Medicine*, *15*(8), 1418–1428. doi:10.1111/pme.12440 PMID:24716880

Huang, C.-F., Chuang, J.-C., Tu, H.-T., & Chou, M.-C. (2006). Microsurgical outcomes after failed repeated Gamma Knife surgery for refractory trigeminal neuralgia. *Journal of Neurosurgery*, *105*(Suppl), 117–119. doi:10.3171up.2006.105.7.117 PMID:18503343

Hughes, B. (1950). Atypical trigeminal neuralgia. *British Dental Journal*, *89*(11), 243–249. PMID:14791847

Huo, X., Sun, X., Zhang, Z., Guo, W., Guan, N., & Luo, J. (2014). Dyna-CT-assisted percutaneous microballoon compression for trigeminal neuralgia. *Journal of Neurointerventional Surgery*, *6*(7), 521–526. doi:10.1136/neurintsurg-2013-010676 PMID:23904451

Hutchinson, B. (1822). *Cases of Neuralgia Spasmodica, Commonly Termed Tic Douloureux Successfully Treated.* London: Second.

Iannone, A., Baker, A. B., & Morrell, F. (1958). Dilantin in the treatment of trigeminal neuralgia. *Neurology*, *8*(2), 126–128. doi:10.1212/WNL.8.2.126 PMID:13504430

Ichikawa, T., Agari, T., Kurozumi, K., Maruo, T., Satoh, T., & Date, I. (2011). "Double-stick tape" technique for transposition of an offending vessel in microvascular decompression: technical case report. *Neurosurgery, 68*(2 Suppl), 377-382. doi:10.1227/NEU.0b013e318217141c

Ildan, F., Gocer, A. I., Bagdatoglu, H., Uzuneyupoglu, Z., Tuna, M., & Cetinalp, E. (1996). Isolated trigeminal neuralgia secondary to distal anterior inferior cerebellar artery aneurysm. *Neurosurgical Review, 19*(1), 43–46. doi:10.1007/BF00346609 PMID:8738365

Inoue, T., Shima, A., Hirai, H., Suzuki, F., & Matsuda, M. (2017). Nervus Intermedius Neuralgia Treated with Microvascular Decompression: A Case Report and Review of the Literature. *NMC Case Report Journal, 4*(3), 75–78. doi:10.2176/nmccrj.cr.2016-0261 PMID:28840083

Ischia, S., Luzzani, A., & Polati, E. (1990). Retrogasserian glycerol injection: A retrospective study of 112 patients. *The Clinical Journal of Pain, 6*(4), 291–296. doi:10.1097/00002508-199012000-00006 PMID:2135029

Isik, N., Pamir, M. N., Benli, K., Erbengi, A., Erbengi, T., & Ruacan, S. (2002). Experimental trigeminal glycerol injection in dogs: histopathological evaluation by light and electron microscopy. *Stereotact Funct Neurosurg, 79*(2), 94-106. doi: 7010570105

Ito, M., Yoshida, K., Kimura, H., Ozaki, N., & Kurita, K. (2007). Successful treatment of trigeminal neuralgia with milnacipran. *Clinical Neuropharmacology, 30*(3), 183–185. doi:10.1097/wnf.0b013e31803bb3da PMID:17545752

Jagia, M., Bithal, P. K., Dash, H. H., Prabhakar, H., Chaturvedi, A., & Chouhan, R. S. (2004). Effect of cerebrospinal fluid return on success rate of percutaneous retrogasserian glycerol rhizotomy. *Reg Anesth Pain Med, 29*(6), 592-595. doi: S1098733904005206

Jakobs, M., Unterberg, A., Treede, R. D., Schuh-Hofer, S., & Ahmadi, R. (2016). Subcutaneous trigeminal nerve field stimulation for refractory trigeminal pain: A cohort analysis. *Acta Neurochirurgica, 158*(9), 1767–1774. doi:10.100700701-016-2881-6 PMID:27372299

Jannetta, P. J. (2007). Arterial compression of the trigeminal nerve at the pons in patients with trigeminal neuralgia. 1967. *Journal of Neurosurgery, 107*, 216–219. doi:10.3171/JNS-07/07/0216

Jannetta, P. J. (1967). Arterial Compression of the Trigeminal Nerve at the Pons in Patients with Trigeminal Neuralgia. *Journal of Neurosurgery, 26*(1part2), 159–162. doi:10.3171/jns.1967.26.1part2.0159 PMID:6018932

Jannetta, P. J. (1974). Letter: Complications from microsurgical treatment of tic douloureux. *Journal of Neurosurgery, 40*(5), 675. PMID:4817815

Jannetta, P. J. (1985). Microsurgical management of trigeminal neuralgia. *Archives of Neurology, 42*(8), 800. doi:10.1001/archneur.1985.04210090068018 PMID:4026617

Jannetta, P. J., Fletcher, L. H., Grondziowski, P. M., Casey, K. F., & Sekula, R. F. (2010). Type 2 diabetes mellitus: A central nervous system etiology. *Surgical Neurology International, 1*(1), 31. doi:10.4103/2152-7806.66460 PMID:20847912

Jayasekera, B. A., Vergani, F., Gholkar, A., & Jenkins, A. J. (2014). Trigeminal neuralgia from an Arteriovenous malformation: An intra-operative diagnosis. *British Journal of Neurosurgery*, 1–2. PMID:25222749

Jefferson, A. (1963). Trigeminal Root and Ganglion Injections Using Phenol in Glycerine for the Relief of Trigeminal Neuralgia. *Journal of Neurology, Neurosurgery, and Psychiatry*, *26*(4), 345–352. doi:10.1136/jnnp.26.4.345 PMID:14043050

Jensen, M. P. (2003). The validity and reliability of pain measures in adults with cancer. *The Journal of Pain*, *4*(1), 2–21. doi:10.1054/jpai.2003.1 PMID:14622723

Jho, H. D., & Lunsford, L. D. (1997). Percutaneous retrogasserian glycerol rhizotomy. Current technique and results. *Neurosurgery Clinics of North America*, *8*(1), 63–74. PMID:9018706

Jia, D. Z., & Li, G. (2010). Bioresonance hypothesis: A new mechanism on the pathogenesis of trigeminal neuralgia. *Medical Hypotheses*, *74*(3), 505–507. doi:10.1016/j.mehy.2009.09.056 PMID:19900765

Jie, H., Xuanchen, Z., Deheng, L., Kun, G., Fengyang, X., Xiang, C., . . . Yiqing, L. (2013). The long-term outcome of nerve combing for trigeminal neuralgia. *Acta Neurochir (Wien)*, *155*(9), 1703-1708. doi:10.1007/s00701-013-1804-z

Johnson, M. D., & Burchiel, K. J. (2004). Peripheral stimulation for treatment of trigeminal postherpetic neuralgia and trigeminal posttraumatic neuropathic pain: a pilot study. *Neurosurgery*, *55*(1), 135-141.

Jorns, T., Johnston, A., & Zakrzewska, J. (2009). Pilot study to evaluate the efficacy and tolerability of levetiracetam in treatment of patients with trigeminal neuralgia. *European Journal of Neurology*, *16*(6), 740–744. doi:10.1111/j.1468-1331.2009.02585.x PMID:19475723

Jorns, T., & Zakrzewska, J. (2007). Evidence-based approach to the medical management of trigeminal neuralgia. *British Journal of Neurosurgery*, *21*(3), 253–261. doi:10.1080/02688690701219175 PMID:17612914

Jost, W. H., & Kohl, A. (2001). Botulinum toxin: Evidence-based medicine criteria in blepharospasm and hemifacial spasm. *Journal of Neurology*, *248*(S1), 21–24. doi:10.1007/PL00007813 PMID:11357234

Kaess, M. (1951). Etiology and treatment of idiopathic trigeminal neuralgia. *Munchener Medizinische Wochenschrift*, *93*(7), 330–335. PMID:14826732

Kanai, A., Saito, M., & Hoka, S. (2006). Subcutaneous sumatriptan for refractory trigeminal neuralgia. *Headache*, *46*(4), 577–582. doi:10.1111/j.1526-4610.2006.00405.x PMID:16643550

Kanai, A., Suzuki, A., Kobayashi, M., & Hoka, S. (2006). Intranasal lidocaine 8% spray for second-division trigeminal neuralgia. *British Journal of Anaesthesia*, *97*(4), 559–563. doi:10.1093/bja/ael180 PMID:16882684

Kanai, A., Suzuki, A., Osawa, S., & Hoka, S. (2006). Sumatriptan alleviates pain in patients with trigeminal neuralgia. *The Clinical Journal of Pain*, *22*(8), 677–680. doi:10.1097/01.ajp.0000210917.18536.0d PMID:16988562

Kanpolat, Y., Savas, A., Bekar, A., & Berk, C. (2001). Percutaneous controlled radiofrequency trigeminal rhizotomy for the treatment of idiopathic trigeminal neuralgia: 25-year experience with 1,600 patients. *Neurosurgery, 48*(3), 524-532.

Kanpolat, Y., Savas, A., Bekar, A., & Berk, C. (2001). Percutaneous controlled radiofrequency trigeminal rhizotomy for the treatment of idiopathic trigeminal neuralgia: 25-year experience with 1,600 patients. *Neurosurgery*, *48*(3), 524–532, discussion 532–534. doi:10.1097/00006123-200103000-00013 PMID:11270542

Karam, S. D., Tai, A., Snider, J. W., Bhatia, S., Bedrick, E. J., Rashid, A., ... Jean, W. (2014). Refractory trigeminal neuralgia treatment outcomes following CyberKnife radiosurgery. *Radiation Oncology (London, England)*, *9*(1), 257. doi:10.118613014-014-0257-8 PMID:25497053

Karatas, H., Erdener, S. E., Gursoy-Ozdemir, Y., Lule, S., Eren-Kocak, E., Sen, Z. D., & Dalkara, T. (2013). Spreading depression triggers headache by activating neuronal Panx1 channels. *Science*, *339*(6123), 1092–1095. doi:10.1126cience.1231897 PMID:23449592

Karibe, H., Shirane, R., Jokura, H., & Yoshimoto, T. (2004). Intrinsic arteriovenous malformation of the trigeminal nerve in a patient with trigeminal neuralgia: Case report. *Neurosurgery*, *55*(6), 1433. doi:10.1227/01.NEU.0000143147.57383.AA PMID:15574228

Karol, E. A., & Karol, M. N. (2009). A multiarray electrode mapping method for percutaneous thermocoagulation as treatment of trigeminal neuralgia. Technical note on a series of 178 consecutive procedures. *Surgical Neurology*, *71*(1), 11–17, discussion 17–18. doi:10.1016/j.surneu.2007.09.021 PMID:18328544

Katusic, S., Beard, C. M., Bergstralh, E., & Kurland, L. T. (1990). Incidence and clinical features of trigeminal neuralgia, Rochester, Minnesota, 1945-1984. *Annals of Neurology*, *27*(1), 89–95. doi:10.1002/ana.410270114 PMID:2301931

Katusic, S., Williams, D. B., Beard, C. M., Bergstralh, E. J., & Kurland, L. T. (1991). Epidemiology and clinical features of idiopathic trigeminal neuralgia and glossopharyngeal neuralgia: Similarities and differences, Rochester, Minnesota, 1945-1984. *Neuroepidemiology*, *10*(5-6), 276–281. doi:10.1159/000110284 PMID:1798430

Katusic, S., Williams, D. B., Beard, C. M., Bergstralh, E., & Kurland, L. T. (1991b). Incidence and clinical features of glossopharyngeal neuralgia, Rochester, Minnesota, 1945-1984. *Neuroepidemiology*, *10*(5-6), 266–275. doi:10.1159/000110283 PMID:1798429

Kellogg, R., Pendleton, C., Quinones-Hinojosa, A., & Cohen-Gadol, A. A. (2010). Surgical Treatment of Trigeminal Neuralgia: A History of Early Strides Toward Curing a "Cancerous Acrimony.". *Neurosurgery*, *67*(5), 1419–1425. doi:10.1227/NEU.0b013e3181f0ef13 PMID:20871443

Kerr, F. W. L., Miller, R. H., Bader, G., Coenen, H., Guarch, F. S., Lignac, G. O. E., ... Hager, W. (1966). The Pathology of Trigeminal Neuralgia. *Archives of Neurology*, *15*(3), 308. doi:10.1001/archneur.1966.00470150086014 PMID:5912011

Ketter, T., Wang, P., Chandler, R., Alarcon, A., Becker, O., Nowakowska, C., ... Schumacher, M. (2005). Dermatology precautions and slower titration yield low incidence of lamotrigine treatment-emergent rash. *The Journal of Clinical Psychiatry*, *66*(05), 642–645. doi:10.4088/JCP.v66n0516 PMID:15889953

Khan, M., Nishi, S. E., Hassan, S. N., Islam, M. A., & Gan, S. H. (2017). Trigeminal Neuralgia, Glossopharyngeal Neuralgia, and Myofascial Pain Dysfunction Syndrome: An Update. *Pain Research & Management*, *7438326*. doi:10.1155/2017/7438326 PMID:28827979

Khan, O. (1998). Gabapentin relieves trigeminal neuralgia in multiple sclerosis patients. *Neurology*, *51*(2), 611–614. doi:10.1212/WNL.51.2.611 PMID:9710050

Killian, J. M., & Fromm, G. H. (1968). Carbamazepine in the treatment of neuralgia. Use of side effects. *Archives of Neurology*, *19*(2), 129–136. doi:10.1001/archneur.1968.00480020015001 PMID:4877400

Kim, H. J., Park, Y. S., Ryu, J. S., Huh, R., Han, I., Shin, D. A., ... Chung, S. S. (2012). Intraoperative facial electromyography and brainstem auditory evoked potential findings in microvascular decompression for hemifacial spasm: Correlation with postoperative delayed facial palsy. *Stereotactic and Functional Neurosurgery*, *90*(4), 260–265. doi:10.1159/000338685 PMID:22777492

Kimura, T., Sako, K., Tohyama, Y., & Yonemasu, Y. (1999). Trigeminal neuralgia caused by compression from petrosal vein transfixing the nerve. *Acta Neurochirurgica*, *141*(4), 437–438. doi:10.1007007010050321 PMID:10352756

King, J. S., Jewett, D. L., & Sundberg, H. R. (1972). Differential blockade of cat dorsal root C fibers by various chloride solutions. *Journal of Neurosurgery*, *36*(5), 569–583. doi:10.3171/jns.1972.36.5.0569 PMID:5067506

Klein, J., Sandi-Gahun, S., Schackert, G., & Juratli, T. A. (2016). Peripheral nerve field stimulation for trigeminal neuralgia, trigeminal neuropathic pain, and persistent idiopathic facial pain. *Cephalalgia*, *36*(5), 445–453. doi:10.1177/0333102415597526 PMID:26209705

Ko, A. L., Lee, A., Raslan, A. M., Ozpinar, A., McCartney, S., & Burchiel, K. J. (2015a). Trigeminal neuralgia without neurovascular compression presents earlier than trigeminal neuralgia with neurovascular compression. *Journal of Neurosurgery*, *123*(6), 1519–1527. doi:10.3171/2014.11.JNS141741 PMID:26047411

Ko, A. L., Ozpinar, A., Lee, A., Raslan, A. M., McCartney, S., & Burchiel, K. J. (2015b). Long-term efficacy and safety of internal neurolysis for trigeminal neuralgia without neurovascular compression. *Journal of Neurosurgery*, *122*(5), 1048–1057. doi:10.3171/2014.12.JNS14469 PMID:25679283

Kolluri, S., & Heros, R. C. (1984). Microvascular decompression for trigeminal neuralgia. A five-year follow-up study. *Surgical Neurology*, *22*(3), 235–240. doi:10.1016/0090-3019(84)90005-3 PMID:6463831

Kondo, A. (2001). Microvascular decompression surgery for trigeminal neuralgia. *Stereotactic and Functional Neurosurgery*, *77*(1–4), 187–189. doi:10.1159/000064619 PMID:12378075

Kondziolka, D., & Lunsford, L. D. (2005). Percutaneous retrogasserian glycerol rhizotomy for trigeminal neuralgia: technique and expectations. *Neurosurg Focus, 18*(5), E7. doi: 180507

Kondziolka, D., Lacomis, D., Niranjan, A., Mori, Y., Maesawa, S., Fellows, W., & Lunsford, L. D. (2000). Histological effects of trigeminal nerve radiosurgery in a primate model: implications for trigeminal neuralgia radiosurgery. *Neurosurgery, 46*(4), 971-976-977.

Kondziolka, D., & Lunsford, L. D. (2005). Percutaneous retrogasserian glycerol rhizotomy for trigeminal neuralgia: Technique and expectations. *Neurosurgical Focus*, *18*(5), E7. doi:10.3171/foc.2005.18.5.8 PMID:15913283

Kondziolka, D., Lunsford, L. D., & Bissonette, D. J. (1994). Long-term results after glycerol rhizotomy for multiple sclerosis-related trigeminal neuralgia. *The Canadian Journal of Neurological Sciences*, *21*(2), 137–140. doi:10.1017/S0317167100049076 PMID:8087740

Kondziolka, D., Lunsford, L. D., Flickinger, J. C., Young, R. F., Vermeulen, S., Duma, C. M., ... Lindquist, C. (1996). Stereotactic radiosurgery for trigeminal neuralgia: A multiinstitutional study using the gamma unit. *Journal of Neurosurgery*, *84*(6), 940–945. doi:10.3171/jns.1996.84.6.0940 PMID:8847587

Kondziolka, D., Perez, B., Flickinger, J. C., Habeck, M., & Lunsford, L. D. (1998). Gamma Knife Radiosurgery for Trigeminal Neuralgia: Results and Expectations. *Archives of Neurology*, *55*(12), 1524–1529. doi:10.1001/archneur.55.12.1524 PMID:9865796

Koopman, J. S. H. A., Dieleman, J. P., Huygen, F. J., de Mos, M., Martin, C. G. M., & Sturkenboom, M. C. J. M. (2009). Incidence of facial pain in the general population. *Pain*, *147*(1-3), 122–127. doi:10.1016/j.pain.2009.08.023 PMID:19783099

Kosugi, S., Shiotani, M., Otsuka, Y., Suzuki, T., Katori, N., Hashiguchi, S., & Morisaki, H. (2015). Long-term outcomes of percutaneous radiofrequency thermocoagulation of gasserian ganglion for 2nd- and multiple-division trigeminal neuralgia. *Pain Practice: The Official Journal of World Institute of Pain, 15*(3), 223–228.

Kotecha, R., Kotecha, R., Modugula, S., Murphy, E. S., Jones, M., Kotecha, R., … Chao, S. T. (2016). Trigeminal Neuralgia Treated With Stereotactic Radiosurgery: The Effect of Dose Escalation on Pain Control and Treatment Outcomes. *International Journal of Radiation Oncology, Biology, Physics, 96*(1), 142–148. 10.1016/j.ijrobp.2016.04.013

Kotecha, R., Miller, J. A., Modugula, S., Barnett, G. H., Murphy, E. S., Reddy, C. A., ... Chao, S. T. (2017). Stereotactic Radiosurgery for Trigeminal Neuralgia Improves Patient-Reported Quality of Life and Reduces Depression. *International Journal of Radiation Oncology, Biology, Physics*, *98*(5), 1078–1086. doi:10.1016/j.ijrobp.2017.04.008 PMID:28721891

Kouzounias, K., Lind, G., Schechtmann, G., Winter, J., & Linderoth, B. (2010). Comparison of percutaneous balloon compression and glycerol rhizotomy for the treatment of trigeminal neuralgia. *Journal of Neurosurgery*, *113*(3), 486–492. doi:10.3171/2010.1.JNS091106 PMID:20187700

Krause, F. (1896). *Die Neuralgie des Trigeminus*. Leipzig: Vogel.

Kronfol, Z., & Remick, D. G. (2000). Cytokines and the brain: Implications for clinical psychiatry. *The American Journal of Psychiatry*, *157*(5), 683–694. doi:10.1176/appi.ajp.157.5.683 PMID:10784457

Kuchta, J., Møller, A. R., Wedekind, C., & Jannetta, P. J. (1998). Delayed hearing loss after microvascular decompression of the trigeminal nerve. *Acta Neurochirurgica*, *140*(1), 94–97. doi:10.1007007010050064 PMID:9522915

Kustermans, L., Van Buyten, J. P., Smet, I., Coucke, W., & Politis, C. (2017). Stimulation of the Gasserian ganglion in the treatment of refractory trigeminal neuropathy. *Journal of Cranio-Maxillo-Facial Surgery*, *45*(1), 39–46. doi:10.1016/j.jcms.2016.10.014 PMID:27919593

Laha, R. K., & Jannetta, P. J. (1977). Glossopharyngeal neuralgia. *Journal of Neurosurgery*, *47*(3), 316–320. doi:10.3171/jns.1977.47.3.0316 PMID:894337

Langley, G. B., & Sheppeard, H. (1985). The visual analogue scale: Its use in pain measurement. *Rheumatology International*, *5*(4), 145–148. doi:10.1007/BF00541514 PMID:4048757

Lang, S. S., Chen, H. I., & Lee, J. Y. (2012). Endoscopic microvascular decompression: A stepwise operative technique. *ORL; Journal for Oto-Rhino-Laryngology and Its Related Specialties*, *74*(6), 293–298. doi:10.1159/000342795 PMID:23235502

Larsen, A., Piepgras, D., Chyatte, D., & Rizzolo, D. (2011). Trigeminal neuralgia: Diagnosis and medical and surgical management. *JAAPA: Official Journal of the American Academy of Physician Assistants*, *24*(7), 20–25. doi:10.1097/01720610-201107000-00005 PMID:21748954

Latchaw, J. P. Jr, Hardy, R. W. Jr, Forsythe, S. B., & Cook, A. F. (1983). Trigeminal neuralgia treated by radiofrequency coagulation. *Journal of Neurosurgery*, *59*(3), 479–484. doi:10.3171/jns.1983.59.3.0479 PMID:6886761

Lazzara, B. M., Ortiz, O., Bordia, R., Witten, M. R., Haas, J. A., Katz, A. J., & Brown, J. A. (2013). Cyberknife radiosurgery in treating trigeminal neuralgia. *Journal of Neurointerventional Surgery*, *5*(1), 81–85. doi:10.1136/neurintsurg-2011-010125 PMID:22278932

Leal, P. R., Hermier, M., Froment, J. C., Souza, M. A., Cristino-Filho, G., & Sindou, M. (2010). Preoperative demonstration of the neurovascular compression characteristics with special emphasis on the degree of compression, using high-resolution magnetic resonance imaging: A prospective study, with comparison to surgical findings, in 100 consecutive patients who underwent microvascular decompression for trigeminal neuralgia. *Acta Neurochirurgica*, *152*(5), 817–825. doi:10.100700701-009-0588-7 PMID:20108106

Leal, P. R., Hermier, M., Souza, M. A., Cristino-Filho, G., Froment, J. C., & Sindou, M. (2011). Visualization of vascular compression of the trigeminal nerve with high-resolution 3T MRI: A prospective study comparing preoperative imaging analysis to surgical findings in 40 consecutive patients who underwent microvascular decompression for trigeminal neuralgia. *Neurosurgery*, *69*(1), 15–25, discussion 26. doi:10.1227/NEU.0b013e318212bafa PMID:21346659

Leandri, M., Lunardi, G., Inglese, M., Messmer-Uccelli, M., Mancardi, G. L., Gottlieb, A., & Solaro, C. (2000). Lamotrigine in trigeminal neuralgia secondary to multiple sclerosis. *Journal of Neurology*, *247*(7), 556–558. doi:10.1007004150070157 PMID:10993501

Lechin, F., van der Dijs, B., Lechin, M., Amat, J., Lechin, A., Cabrera, A., ... Jimenez, V. (1989). Pimozide therapy for trigeminal neuralgia. *Archives of Neurology*, *46*(9), 960–963. doi:10.1001/archneur.1989.00520450030015 PMID:2673161

Lee, A., McCartney, S., Burbidge, C., Raslan, A. M., & Burchiel, K. J. (2014). Trigeminal neuralgia occurs and recurs in the absence of neurovascular compression. *Journal of Neurosurgery*, *120*(5), 1048–1054. doi:10.3171/2014.1.JNS131410 PMID:24506241

Lee, C. C., Liao, C. H., Lin, C. F., Yang, T. F., Hsu, S. P., Yen, Y. S., & Shih, Y. H. (2014). Brainstem auditory evoked potential monitoring and neuro-endoscopy: Two tools to ensure hearing preservation and surgical success during microvascular decompression. *Journal of the Chinese Medical Association*, *77*(6), 308–316. doi:10.1016/j.jcma.2014.02.016 PMID:24768092

Lee, J. K., Choi, H. J., Ko, H. C., Choi, S. K., & Lim, Y. J. (2012). Long term outcomes of gamma knife radiosurgery for typical trigeminal neuralgia-minimum 5-year follow-up. *Journal of Korean Neurosurgical Society*, *51*(5), 276–280. doi:10.3340/jkns.2012.51.5.276 PMID:22792424

Lee, J. Y. K., Pierce, J. T., Sandhu, S. K., Petrov, D., & Yang, A. I. (2017). Endoscopic versus microscopic microvascular decompression for trigeminal neuralgia: Equivalent pain outcomes with possibly decreased postoperative headache after endoscopic surgery. *Journal of Neurosurgery*, *126*(5), 1676–1684. doi:10.3171/2016.5.JNS1621 PMID:27471895

Lee, L. T., Yeung, R. W., Wong, M. C., & McMillan, A. S. (2008). Diagnostic sub-types, psychological distress and psychosocial dysfunction in southern Chinese people with temporomandibular disorders. *Journal of Oral Rehabilitation*, *35*(3), 184–190. doi:10.1111/j.1365-2842.2007.01792.x PMID:18254795

Lee, S. H., Koh, J. S., & Lee, C. Y. (2011). Trigeminal neuralgia caused by an anomalous posterior inferior cerebellar artery from the primitive trigeminal artery: Case report. *Cerebellum (London, England)*, *10*(2), 199–203. doi:10.100712311-011-0249-2 PMID:21279490

Leksell, L. (1951). The stereotaxic method and radiosurgery of the brain. *Acta Chirurgica Scandinavica*, *102*(4), 316–319. PMID:14914373

Leksell, L. (1971). Sterotaxic radiosurgery in trigeminal neuralgia. *Acta Chirurgica Scandinavica*, *137*(4), 311–314. Retrieved from http://www.ncbi.nlm.nih.gov/pubmed/4948331 PMID:4948331

Lemos, L., Flores, S., Oliveira, P., & Almeida, A. (2008). Gabapentin supplemented with ropivacaine block of trigger points improves pain control and quality of life in trigeminal neuralgia patients when compared with gabapentin alone. *The Clinical Journal of Pain*, *24*(1), 64–75. doi:10.1097/AJP.0b013e318158011a PMID:18180639

Lettmaier, S. (2014). Radiosurgery in trigeminal neuralgia. *Physica Medica: PM: An International Journal Devoted to the Applications of Physics to Medicine and Biology: Official Journal of the Italian Association of Biomedical Physics*, *30*(5), 592–595. doi:10.1016/j.ejmp.2014.05.006 PMID:24889155

Leung, A., Donohue, M., Xu, R., Lee, R., Lefaucheur, J. P., Khedr, E. M., ... Chen, R. (2009). rTMS for suppressing neuropathic pain: A meta-analysis. *The Journal of Pain*, *10*(12), 1205–1216. doi:10.1016/j.jpain.2009.03.010 PMID:19464959

Levy, R., & Proudfit, H. (1977). The analgesic action of baclofen (beta-(4-chlorophenyl)-gamma-aminobutyric acid). *The Journal of Pharmacology and Experimental Therapeutics*, *202*, 437–445. PMID:886473

Leza, J. C., Garcia-Bueno, B., Bioque, M., Arango, C., Parellada, M., Do, K., ... Bernardo, M. (2015). Inflammation in schizophrenia: A question of balance. *Neuroscience and Biobehavioral Reviews*, *55*, 612–626. doi:10.1016/j.neubiorev.2015.05.014 PMID:26092265

Liang, X., Dong, X., Zhao, S., Ying, X., Du, Y., & Yu, W. (2017). A retrospective study of neurocombing for the treatment of trigeminal neuralgia without neurovascular compression. *Irish Journal of Medical Science*, *40*(1), 39–7. doi:10.100711845-016-1547-y PMID:28063126

Lichtor, T., & Mullan, J. F. (1990). A 10-year follow-up review of percutaneous microcompression of the trigeminal ganglion. *Journal of Neurosurgery*, *72*(1), 49–54. doi:10.3171/jns.1990.72.1.0049 PMID:2294184

Liebel, J. T., Menger, N., & Langohr, H. (2001). Oxcarbazepine in der Behandlung der Trigeminusneuralgie. *Nervenheilkunde: Zeitschrift für Interdisziplinaere Fortbildung*, *20*, 461–465.

Li, K., & Ma, L. (2004). Selective source blocking for Gamma Knife radiosurgery of trigeminal neuralgia based on analytical dose modelling. *Physics in Medicine and Biology*, *49*(15), 3455–3463. doi:10.1088/0031-9155/49/15/010 PMID:15379025

Lim, J. J., Ladd, B. M., Grande, A. W., & Haines, S. J. (2017). Letter: Prepackaged Instrument Kit for Percutaneous Balloon Compression Rhizotomy for the Treatment of Trigeminal Neuralgia: Improvised Solution for an Unexpected National Supply Shortage. *Operative Neurosurgery*, *13*(4), E19–E20. doi:10.1093/ons/opx061 PMID:28838119

Lim, M., Villavicencio, A. T., Burneikiene, S., Chang, S. D., Romanelli, P., McNeely, L., ... Adler, J. R. (2005). CyberKnife radiosurgery for idiopathic trigeminal neuralgia. *Neurosurgical Focus, 18*(5), E9. doi:10.3171/foc.2005.18.5.10 PMID:15913285

Lin, C. F., Chen, H. H., Hernesniemi, J., Lee, C. C., Liao, C. H., Chen, S. C., ... Hsu, S. P. (2012). An easy adjustable method of ectatic vertebrobasilar artery transposition for microvascular decompression. *Clinical Neurology and Neurosurgery, 114*(7), 951–956. doi:10.1016/j.clineuro.2012.02.021 PMID:22390889

Linderoth, B., & Lind, G. (2012). Retrogasserian Glycerol Rhizolysis in Trigeminal Neuralgia. In A. Quinones-Hinojosa (Ed.), Schmidek and Sweet: Operative Neurosurgical Techniques (6th ed.; Vol. 2, pp. 1393-1408). Philadelphia: Elsevier.

Linderoth, B., & Håkanson, S. (1989). Paroxysmal facial pain in disseminated sclerosis treated by retrogasserian glycerol injection. *Acta Neurologica Scandinavica, 80*(4), 341–346. doi:10.1111/j.1600-0404.1989.tb03890.x PMID:2816292

Lindquist, C., Kihlström, L., & Hellstrand, E. (1991). Functional neurosurgery--a future for the gamma knife? *Stereotactic and Functional Neurosurgery, 57*(1–2), 72–81. doi:10.1159/000099557 PMID:1725560

Lin, K.-H., Chen, Y.-T., Fuh, J.-L., & Wang, S.-J. (2015). Increased risk of trigeminal neuralgia in patients with migraine: A nationwide population-based study. *Cephalalgia: an International Journal of Headache, 36*(13), 1218–1227. doi:10.1177/0333102415623069 PMID:26692399

Lin, M. H.-C., Lee, M.-H., Wang, T.-C., Cheng, Y.-K., Su, C.-H., Chang, C.-M., & Yang, J.-T. (2011). Foramen ovale cannulation guided by intra-operative computed tomography with integrated neuronavigation for the treatment of trigeminal neuralgia. *Acta Neurochirurgica, 153*(8), 1593–1599. doi:10.100700701-011-1009-2 PMID:21503836

Linskey, M. E., Jho, H. D., & Jannetta, P. J. (1994). Microvascular decompression for trigeminal neuralgia caused by vertebrobasilar compression. *Journal of Neurosurgery, 81*(1), 1–9. doi:10.3171/jns.1994.81.1.0001 PMID:8207508

Linskey, M. E., Ratanatharathorn, V., & Penagaricano, J. (2008). A prospective cohort study of microvascular decompression and Gamma Knife surgery in patients with trigeminal neuralgia. *Journal of Neurosurgery, 109*(Suppl), 160–172. PMID:19123904

Liu, H., Li, H., Xu, M., Chung, K., & Zhang, S. (2010). A systematic review on acupuncture for trigeminal neuralgia. *The Journal of Alternative Therapies, 16*(6), 30–35. PMID:21280460

Lobato, R. D., Rivas, J. J., Sarabia, R., & Lamas, E. (1990). Percutaneous microcompression of the gasserian ganglion for trigeminal neuralgia. *Journal of Neurosurgery, 72*(4), 546–553. doi:10.3171/jns.1990.72.4.0546 PMID:2319312

Lopez, B. C., Hamlyn, P. J., & Zakrzewska, J. M. (2004). Systematic review of ablative neurosurgical techniques for the treatment of trigeminal neuralgia. *Neurosurgery, 54*(4), 973-982.

Lopez, B. C., Hamlyn, P. J., & Zakrzewska, J. M. (2004). Systematic review of ablative neurosurgical techniques for the treatment of trigeminal neuralgia. *Neurosurgery, 54*(4), 973-982; discussion 982-973.

Lopez, B. C., Hamlyn, P. J., & Zakrzewska, J. M. (2004). Stereotactic radiosurgery for primary trigeminal neuralgia: State of the evidence and recommendations for future reports. *Journal of Neurology, Neurosurgery, and Psychiatry, 75*(7), 1019–1024. doi:10.1136/jnnp.2003.018564 PMID:15201363

Lovell, B. (2015). Trigeminal herpes zoster: Early recognition and treatment are crucial. *BMJ Case Reports, 2015*(mar20 1), bcr2014208673. doi:10.1136/bcr-2014-208673 PMID:25795749

Lovely, T. J., & Jannetta, P. J. (1997). Microvascular decompression for trigeminal neuralgia. Surgical technique and long-term results. *Neurosurgery Clinics of North America, 8*(1), 11–29. PMID:9018702

Love, S., & Coakham, H. B. (2001). Trigeminal neuralgia: Pathology and pathogenesis. *Brain, 124*(Pt 12), 2347–2360. doi:10.1093/brain/124.12.2347 PMID:11701590

Lucas, J. T., Nida, A. M., Isom, S., Marshall, K., Bourland, J. D., Laxton, A. W., … Chan, M. D. (2014). Predictive Nomogram for the Durability of Pain Relief From Gamma Knife Radiation Surgery in the Treatment of Trigeminal Neuralgia. *International Journal of Radiation Oncology, Biology, Physics, 89*(1), 120–126. 10.1016/j.ijrobp.2014.01.023

Lunardi, G., Leandri, M., Albano, C., Cultrera, S., Fracassi, M., Rubino, V., & Favale, E. (1997). Clinical effectiveness of lamotrigine and plasma levels in essential and symptomatic trigeminal neuralgia. *Neurology, 48*(6), 1714–1717. doi:10.1212/WNL.48.6.1714 PMID:9191794

Lunn, M., Hughes, R., & Wiffen, P. (2014). Duloxetine for treating pain neuropathy, chronic pain or fibromyalgia. *Cochrane Database of Systematic Reviews, 3*(1). PMID:24385423

Lunsford, L. D. (1985). *Trigeminal neuralgia: treatment by glycerol rhizotomy*. New York: McGraw-Hill.

Lunsford, L. D., & Bennett, M. H. (1984). Percutaneous retrogasserian glycerol rhizotomy for tic douloureux: Part 1. Technique and results in 112 patients. *Neurosurgery, 14*(4), 424–430. doi:10.1227/00006123-198404000-00006 PMID:6728144

Lunsford, L. D., Bennett, M. H., & Martinez, A. J. (1985). Experimental trigeminal glycerol injection. Electrophysiologic and morphologic effects. *Archives of Neurology, 42*(2), 146–149. doi:10.1001/archneur.1985.04060020060016 PMID:3977642

Lv, M.-Y., Deng, S.-L., Long, X.-F., & Liu, Z.-L. (2017). Long-term outcome of microvascular decompression for hemifacial spasm. *British Journal of Neurosurgery, 31*(3), 322–326. doi:10.1080/02688697.2017.1297368 PMID:28288523

Maarbjerg, S., Di Stefano, G., Bendtsen, L., & Cruccu, G. (2017). Trigeminal neuralgia - diagnosis and treatment. *Cephalalgia: An International Journal of Headache*.

Maarbjerg, S., Di Stefano, G., Bendtsen, L., & Cruccu, G. (2017). Trigeminal neuralgia - diagnosis and treatment. *Cephalalgia, 37*(7), 648–657. doi:10.1177/0333102416687280 PMID:28076964

Maarbjerg, S., Gozalov, A., Olesen, J., & Bendtsen, L. (2014). Trigeminal neuralgia-a prospective systematic study of clinical characteristics in 158 patients. *Headache, 54*(10), 1574–1582. doi:10.1111/head.12441 PMID:25231219

MacDonald, B. K. (2000). The incidence and lifetime prevalence of neurological disorders in a prospective community-based study in the UK. *Brain, 123*(4), 665–676. doi:10.1093/brain/123.4.665 PMID:10733998

Macianskyte, D., Januzis, G., Kubilius, R., Adomaitiene, V., & Sciupokas, A. (2011). Associations between chronic pain and depressive symptoms in patients with trigeminal neuralgia. *Medicina (Kaunas, Lithuania), 47*(7), 386–392. PMID:22112988

Maesawa, S., Salame, C., Flickinger, J. C., Pirris, S., Kondziolka, D., & Lunsford, L. D. (2001). Clinical outcomes after stereotactic radiosurgery for idiopathic trigeminal neuralgia. *Journal of Neurosurgery, 94*(1), 14–20. doi:10.3171/jns.2001.94.1.0014 PMID:11147887

Mantella, R. C., Butters, M. A., Dew, M. A., Mulsant, B. H., Begley, A. E., Tracey, B., ... Lenze, E. J. (2007). Cognitive impairment in late-life generalized anxiety disorder. *The American Journal of Geriatric Psychiatry, 15*(8), 673–679. doi:10.1097/JGP.0b013e31803111f2 PMID:17426260

Marinković, S., Gibo, H., & Nikodijević, I. (1996). Trigeminocerebellar artery--anatomy and possible clinical significance. *Neurologia Medico-Chirurgica, 36*(4), 215–219. doi:10.2176/nmc.36.215 PMID:8741249

Martínez-Álvarez, R., Martínez-Moreno, N., Kusak, M. E., & Rey-Portolés, G. (2014). Glossopharyngeal neuralgia and radiosurgery. *Journal of Neurosurgery, 121*(Suppl), 222–225. doi:10.3171/2014.8.GKS141273 PMID:25434956

Martin, S., Teo, M., & Suttner, N. (2015). The effectiveness of percutaneous balloon compression in the treatment of trigeminal neuralgia in patients with multiple sclerosis. *Journal of Neurosurgery, 123*(6), 1507–1511. doi:10.3171/2014.11.JNS14736 PMID:26067615

Massager, N., Murata, N., Tamura, M., Devriendt, D., Levivier, M., & Régis, J. (2007). Influence of nerve radiation dose in the incidence of trigeminal dysfunction after trigeminal neuralgia radiosurgery. *Neurosurgery, 60*(4), 681–687, discussion 687–688. doi:10.1227/01.NEU.0000255393.77538.75 PMID:17415205

Massager, N., Nissim, O., Murata, N., Devriendt, D., Desmedt, F., Vanderlinden, B., ... Levivier, M. (2006). Effect of beam channel plugging on the outcome of gamma knife radiosurgery for trigeminal neuralgia. *International Journal of Radiation Oncology, Biology, Physics, 65*(4), 1200–1205. doi:10.1016/j.ijrobp.2006.01.043 PMID:16682146

Masuoka, J., Matsushima, T., Inoue, K., Nakahara, Y., Takase, Y., & Kawashima, M. (2015). Outcome of microvascular decompression for trigeminal neuralgia treated with the stitched sling retraction technique. *Neurosurgical Review*, *38*(2), 361–365, discussion 365. doi:10.100710143-015-0607-5 PMID:25663308

Masuoka, J., Matsushima, T., Kawashima, M., Nakahara, Y., Funaki, T., & Mineta, T. (2011). Stitched sling retraction technique for microvascular decompression: Procedures and techniques based on an anatomical viewpoint. *Neurosurgical Review*, *34*(3), 373–379, discussion 379–380. doi:10.100710143-011-0310-0 PMID:21347661

Matak, I., Bach-Rojecky, L., Fillipovic, B., & Lackovic, Z. (2011). Behavioral and immunohistochemical evidence for central antinocicpetive activity of botulinum toxin A. *Neuroscience*, *186*, 201–207. doi:10.1016/j.neuroscience.2011.04.026 PMID:21539899

Matsushima, T., Huynh-Le, P., & Miyazono, M. (2004). Trigeminal neuralgia caused by venous compression. *Neurosurgery*, *55*(2), 334–337, discussion 338–339. doi:10.1227/01.NEU.0000129552.87291.87 PMID:15271239

Matsushima, T., Yamaguchi, T., Inoue, T. K., Matsukado, K., & Fukui, M. (2000). Recurrent trigeminal neuralgia after microvascular decompression using an interposing technique. Teflon felt adhesion and the sling retraction technique. *Acta Neurochirurgica*, *142*(5), 557–561. doi:10.1007007010050469 PMID:10898363

Matthies, C., & Samii, M. (1997). Management of 1000 vestibular schwannomas (acoustic neuromas): clinical presentation. *Neurosurgery*, *40*(1), 1–9.

Ma, Z., & Li, M. (2009). "Nerve combing" for trigeminal neuralgia without vascular compression: Report of 10 cases. *The Clinical Journal of Pain*, *25*(1), 44–47. doi:10.1097/AJP.0b013e31817e138e PMID:19158545

McAllister-Williams, R. H., Bones, K., Goodwin, G. M., Harrison, J., Katona, C., Rasmussen, J., ... Young, A. H. (2017). Analysing UK clinicians' understanding of cognitive symptoms in major depression: A survey of primary care physicians and psychiatrists. *Journal of Affective Disorders*, *207*, 346–352. doi:10.1016/j.jad.2016.09.036 PMID:27743537

McCracken, L. M., MacKichan, F., & Eccleston, C. (2007). Contextual cognitive-behavioral therapy for severely disabled chronic pain sufferers: Effectiveness and clinically significant change. *European Journal of Pain (London, England)*, *11*(3), 314–322. doi:10.1016/j.ejpain.2006.05.004 PMID:16762571

McDonald, I. (2004). A History of Nerve Functions: From Animal Spirits to Molecular Mechanisms. *Brain*, *128*(1).

McLeod, N. M. H., & Patton, D. W. (2007). Peripheral alcohol injections in the management of trigeminal neuralgia. *Oral Surgery, Oral Medicine, Oral Pathology, Oral Radiology, and Endodontology*, *104*(1), 12–17. doi:10.1016/j.tripleo.2007.01.001 PMID:17428701

McWilliams, L. A., Cox, B. J., & Enns, M. W. (2003). Mood and anxiety disorders associated with chronic pain: An examination in a nationally representative sample. *Pain, 106*(1-2), 127–133. doi:10.1016/S0304-3959(03)00301-4 PMID:14581119

Mehrkens, J. H., & Steude, U. (2007). Chronic electrostimulation of the trigeminal ganglion in trigeminal neuropathy: Current state and future prospects. *Acta Neurochirurgica. Supplementum, 97*(Pt 2), 91–97. PMID:17691294

Melzack, R., Terrence, C., Fromm, G., & Amsel, R. (1986). Trigeminal neuralgia and atypical facial pain: Use of the McGill Pain Questionnaire for discrimination and diagnosis. *Pain, 27*(3), 297–302. doi:10.1016/0304-3959(86)90157-0 PMID:3808740

Meskal, I., Rutten, G. J., Beute, G. N., Salden, M. E., & Sitskoorn, M. M. (2014). Cognitive deficits in patients with trigeminal neuralgia: Opportunities to improve care and quality of life. *Acta Neurochirurgica, 156*(8), 1565–1566. doi:10.100700701-014-2100-2 PMID:24809528

Meyerson, B. A., & Hakanson, S. (1986). Suppression of pain in trigeminal neuropathy by electric stimulation of the gasserian ganglion. *Neurosurgery, 18*(1), 59–66. doi:10.1227/00006123-198601000-00010 PMID:2418383

Micheli, F., Scorticati, M. C., & Raina, G. (2002). Beneficial effects of botulinum toxin type a for patients with painful tic convulsive. *Clinical Neuropharmacology, 25*(5), 260–262. doi:10.1097/00002826-200209000-00006 PMID:12410057

Miller, J. P., Magill, S. T., Acar, F., & Burchiel, K. J. (2009). Predictors of long-term success after microvascular decompression for trigeminal neuralgia. *Journal of Neurosurgery, 110*(4), 620–626. doi:10.3171/2008.9.17660 PMID:19231931

Miller, L. E., & Miller, V. M. (2012). Safety and effectiveness of microvascular decompression for treatment of hemifacial spasm: A systematic review. *British Journal of Neurosurgery, 26*(4), 438–444. doi:10.3109/02688697.2011.641613 PMID:22168965

Minagar, A., & Sheremata, W. A. (2000). Glossopharyngeal neuralgia and MS. *Neurology, 54*(6), 1368–1370. doi:10.1212/WNL.54.6.1368 PMID:10746612

Mineka, Susan, & Kelly, Kelly A. (1989). The relationship between anxiety, lack of control and loss of control.

Mitsikostas, D. D., Pantes, G. V., Avramidis, T. G., Karageorgiou, K. E., Gartzonis, S. D., & Stathis, P. G. (2010). An observational trial to investigate the efficacy and tolerability of levetiracetam in trigeminal neuralgia. *Headache, 50*(8), 1371–1377. doi:10.1111/j.1526-4610.2010.01743.x PMID:21044281

Mittal, B., & Thomas, D. G. (1986). Controlled thermocoagulation in trigeminal neuralgia. *Journal of Neurology, Neurosurgery, and Psychiatry, 49*(8), 932–936. doi:10.1136/jnnp.49.8.932 PMID:3746327

Mohammad-Mohammadi, A., Recinos, P. F., Lee, J. H., Elson, P., & Barnett, G. H. (2013). Surgical outcomes of trigeminal neuralgia in patients with multiple sclerosis. *Neurosurgery*, *73*(6), 941–950, discussion 950. doi:10.1227/NEU.0000000000000128 PMID:23921703

Mohanty, A., Venkatrama, S. K., Rao, B. R., Chandramouli, B. A., Jayakumar, P. N., & Das, B. S. (1997). Experience with cerebellopontine angle epidermoids. *Neurosurgery, 40*(1), 24–9.

Møller, A. R. (1991). The cranial nerve vascular compression syndrome: II. A review of pathophysiology. *Acta Neurochirurgica*, *113*(1-2), 24–30. doi:10.1007/BF01402110 PMID:1799140

Møller, A. R., & Jannetta, P. J. (1987). Monitoring facial EMG responses during microvascular decompression operations for hemifacial spasm. *Journal of Neurosurgery*, *66*(5), 681–685. doi:10.3171/jns.1987.66.5.0681 PMID:3572493

Møller, A. R., & Møller, M. B. (1989). Does intraoperative monitoring of auditory evoked potentials reduce incidence of hearing loss as a complication of microvascular decompression of cranial nerves? *Neurosurgery*, *24*(2), 257–263. doi:10.1227/00006123-198902000-00017 PMID:2918977

Mongini, F., Ciccone, G., Ceccarelli, M., Baldi, I., & Ferrero, L. (2007). Muscle tenderness in different types of facial pain and its relation to anxiety and depression: A cross-sectional study on 649 patients. *Pain*, *131*(1-2), 106–111. doi:10.1016/j.pain.2006.12.017 PMID:17258397

Montano, N., Conforti, G., Di Bonaventura, R., Meglio, M., Fernandez, E., & Papacci, F. (2015). Advances in diagnosis and treatment of trigeminal neuralgia. *Therapeutics and Clinical Risk Management*, *11*, 289–299. doi:10.2147/TCRM.S37592 PMID:25750533

Morita, A., Fukushima, T., Miyazaki, S., Shimizu, T., & Atsuchi, M. (1989). Tic douloureux caused by primitive trigeminal artery or its variant. *Journal of Neurosurgery*, *70*(3), 415–419. doi:10.3171/jns.1989.70.3.0415 PMID:2915249

Morra, M., Elgebaly, A., Elmaraezy, A., Khalil, A., Altibi, A., Vu, T., ... Hirayama, K. (2016). Therapeutic efficacy and safety of Botulinum Toxin A Therapy in Trigeminal Neuralgia: A systematic review and metaanalysis of randomized controlled trials. *The Journal of Headache and Pain*, *17*(1), 63. doi:10.118610194-016-0651-8 PMID:27377706

Morrell, F., Bradley, W., & Ptashne, M. (1958). Effect of Diphenylhydantion on Peripheral Nerve. *Neurology*, *8*(2), 140–144. doi:10.1212/WNL.8.2.140 PMID:13504433

Mosberg, W. H., Jr. (1960). Trigeminal Neuralgia: Its History and Treatment. *The Journal of Nervous and Mental Disease*. Retrieved from http://journals.lww.com/jonmd/Citation/1960/07000/Trigeminal_Neuralgia__Its_History_and_Treatment.14.aspx

Motoyama, Y., Nakagawa, I., Takatani, T., Park, H. S., Kotani, Y., Tanaka, Y., ... Nakase, H. (2016). Microvascular decompression for glossopharyngeal neuralgia using intraoperative neurophysiological monitoring: Technical case report. *Surgical Neurology International*, *7*(3Suppl 2), S28–S35. doi:10.4103/2152-7806.173565 PMID:26862458

Mousavi, S. H., Niranjan, A., Huang, M. J., Laghari, F. J., Shin, S. S., Mindlin, J. L., ... Lunsford, L. D. (2015). Early radiosurgery provides superior pain relief for trigeminal neuralgia patients. *Neurology, 85*(24), 2159–2165. doi:10.1212/WNL.0000000000002216 PMID:26561286

Mousavi, S. H., Sekula, R. F., Gildengers, A., Gardner, P., & Lunsford, L. D. (2016). Concomitant depression and anxiety negatively affect pain outcomes in surgically managed young patients with trigeminal neuralgia: Long-term clinical outcome. *Surgical Neurology International*, *7*(1), 98. doi:10.4103/2152-7806.194145 PMID:28168085

Mullan, S., & Brown, J. A. (1996). Trigeminal neuralgia. *Neurosurgery Quarterly*, *6*(4), 267–288. doi:10.1097/00013414-199612000-00003

Mullan, S., & Lichtor, T. (1983). Percutaneous microcompression of the trigeminal ganglion for trigeminal neuralgia. *Journal ofNeurosurgery*, *59*(6), 1007–1012. doi:10.3171/jns.1983.59.6.1007 PMID:6631493

Murphy, J. B. (1896). Surgery of the Gasserian Ganglion with Demonstration and Report of Two Cases. In *Western Medical Review* (pp. 149–152). Western Medical Review Publishing Co.

Murphy, J. B. (1904). Osmic acid injections for relief of trifacial neuralgia. *Journal of the American Medical Association*, *43*(14), 947. doi:10.1001/jama.1904.92500140001f

Murphy, J. L., McKellar, J. D., Raffa, S. D., Clark, M. E., Kerns, R. D., & Karlin, B. E. (2014). *Cognitive behavioral therapy for chronic pain among veterans: therapist manual*. Washington, DC: US Department of Veterans Affairs.

Muzina, D. J., & Calabrese, J. R. (2005). Maintenance therapies in bipolar disorder: Focus on randomized controlled trials. *The Australian and New Zealand Journal of Psychiatry*, *39*(8), 652–661. doi:10.1080/j.1440-1614.2005.01649.x PMID:16050919

Nader, A., Bendok, B. R., Prine, J. J., & Kendall, M. C. (2015). Ultrasound-Guided Pulsed Radiofrequency Application via the Pterygopalatine Fossa: A Practical Approach to Treat Refractory Trigeminal Neuralgia. *Pain Physician*, *18*(3), E411–E415. PMID:26000688

Nader, A., Kendall, M. C., De Oliveria, G. S., Chen, J. Q., Vanderby, B., Rosenow, J. M., & Bendok, B. R. (2013). Ultrasound-guided trigeminal nerve block via the pterygopalatine fossa: An effective treatment for trigeminal neuralgia and atypical facial pain. *Pain Physician*, *16*(5), E537–E545. PMID:24077204

Nader, A., Schittek, H., & Kendall, M. C. (2013). Lateral pterygoid muscle and maxillary artery are key anatomical landmarks for ultrasound-guided trigeminal nerve block. *Anesthesiology*, *118*(4), 957. doi:10.1097/ALN.0b013e31826d3dfc PMID:23059449

Nair, P., Gharote, H., Singh, P., & Jain-Choudhary, P. (2014). Herpes zoster on the face in the elderly. *BMJ Case Reports*, *2014*(1). doi:10.1136/bcr-2013-200101 PMID:25331144

Nanda, A., Javalkar, V., Zhang, S., & Ahmed, O. (2015). Long term efficacy and patient satisfaction of microvascular decompression and gamma knife radiosurgery for trigeminal neuralgia. *Journal of Clinical Neuroscience*, *22*(5), 818–822. doi:10.1016/j.jocn.2014.11.028 PMID:25769254

Nicol, C. F. (1969). A four year double-blind study of tegretol in facial pain. *Headache*, *9*(1), 54–57. doi:10.1111/j.1526-4610.1969.hed0901054.x PMID:4896266

Nilsen, B., Le, K.-D., & Dietrichs, E. (2004). Prevalence of hemifacial spasm in Oslo, Norway. *Neurology*, *63*(8), 1532–1533. doi:10.1212/01.WNL.0000142080.85228.E8 PMID:15505186

Nishihara, K., Hanakita, J., Kinuta, Y., Kondo, A., Yamamoto, Y., & Nakatani, H. (1986). Importance of intraoperative monitoring of ABR and compound action potential of the eighth cranial nerve during microvascular decompression surgery. *No Shinkei Geka. Neurological Surgery*, *14*(4), 509–518. Retrieved from http://www.ncbi.nlm.nih.gov/pubmed/3713977 PMID:3713977

North, R. B., Kidd, D. H., Piantadosi, S., & Carson, B. S. (1990). Percutaneous retrogasserian glycerol rhizotomy. Predictors of success and failure in treatment of trigeminal neuralgia. *Journal of Neurosurgery*, *72*(6), 851–856. doi:10.3171/jns.1990.72.6.0851 PMID:2338568

Nugent, G. R. (1997). Radiofrequency treatment of trigeminal neuralgia using a cordotomy-type electrode. A method. *Neurosurgery Clinics of North America*, *8*(1), 41–52. PMID:9018704

Nugent, G. R., & Berry, B. (1974). Trigeminal neuralgia treated by differential percutaneous radiofrequency coagulation of the Gasserian ganglion. *Journal of Neurosurgery*, *40*(4), 517–523. doi:10.3171/jns.1974.40.4.0517 PMID:4592266

Nurmikko, T. J. (2009). Pathophysiology of MS-related trigeminal neuralgia. *Pain*, *143*(3), 165–166. doi:10.1016/j.pain.2009.03.019 PMID:19375226

Nurmikko, T. J., & Eldridge, P. R. (2001). Trigeminal neuralgia--pathophysiology, diagnosis and current treatment. *British Journal of Anaesthesia*, *87*(1), 117–132. doi:10.1093/bja/87.1.117 PMID:11460800

O'Neill, F., Nurmikko, T., & Sommer, C. (2017). Other facial neuralgias. *Cephalalgia: An International Journal of Headache*.

O'Reardon, J. P., Solvason, H. B., Janicak, P. G., Sampson, S., Isenberg, K. E., Nahas, Z., ... Sackeim, H. A. (2007). Efficacy and safety of transcranial magnetic stimulation in the acute treatment of major depression: A multisite randomized controlled trial. *Biological Psychiatry*, *62*(11), 1208–1216. doi:10.1016/j.biopsych.2007.01.018 PMID:17573044

Obermann, M. (2010). Treatment options in trigeminal neuralgia. *Therapeutic Advances in Neurological Disorders*, *3*(2), 107–115. doi:10.1177/1756285609359317 PMID:21179603

Obermann, M., Yoon, M.-S., Ese, D., Maschke, M., Kaube, H., Diener, H.-C., & Katsarava, Z. (2007). Impaired trigeminal nociceptive processing in patients with trigeminal neuralgia. *Neurology*, *69*(9), 835–841. doi:10.1212/01.wnl.0000269670.30045.6b PMID:17724285

Obermann, M., Yoon, M., Sensen, K., Maschke, M., Diener, H., & Katsarava, Z. (2008). Efficacy of pregabalin in the treatment of trigeminal neuralgia. *Cephalalgia*, *28*, 174–181. PMID:18039340

Obrador, S., & Boixados, J. R. (1955). Secondary trigeminal neuralgia due to basilar impression and platybasia. *Revista Clínica Española*, *58*(4), 232–234. PMID:13281048

O'Connor, A. B., Schwid, S. R., Herrmann, D. N., Markman, J. D., & Dworkin, R. H. (2008). Pain associated with multiple sclerosis: systematic review and proposed classification. *Pain, 137*(1), 96-111. doi: 10.1016/j.pain.2007.08.024

Oddsson, B. (1944). Electrocoagulation of the Gasserian ganglion by the Kirschner method. *Acta Psychiatrica Scandinavica, 19*(1–2), 293–299. doi:10.1111/j.1600-0447.1944.tb04571.x

Oesman, C., & Mooij, J. J. A. (2011). Long-term follow-up of microvascular decompression for trigeminal neuralgia. *Skull Base: Official Journal of North American Skull Base Society, 21*(5), 313–322. doi:10.1055/s-0031-1284213

Olesen, J., & Steiner, T. J. (2004). The International classification of headache disorders, 2nd edn (ICDH-II). *Journal of Neurology, Neurosurgery, and Psychiatry, 75*(6), 808–811. Retrieved from jnnp.bmj.com

Omeis, I., Smith, D., Kim, S., & Murali, R. (2008). Percutaneous balloon compression for the treatment of recurrent trigeminal neuralgia: Long-term outcome in 29 patients. *Stereotactic and Functional Neurosurgery, 86*(4), 259–265. doi:10.1159/000138770 PMID:18552523

Onofrio, B. M. (1975). Radiofrequency percutaneous Gasserian ganglion lesions. *Journal of Neurosurgery, 42*(2), 132–139. doi:10.3171/jns.1975.42.2.0132 PMID:1113146

Ordónez-Rubiano, E. G., García-Chingaté, C. C., Rodríguez-Vargas, S., Cifuentes-Lobelo, H. A., & Perilla-Cepeda, T. A. (2017). Microvascular Decompression for a Patient with a Glossopharyngeal Neuralgia: A Technical Note. *Cureus, 9*(7), e1494. doi:10.7759/cureus.1494 PMID:28948114

Ostwalt, F. (1906). On deep alcohol injections in the facial and other neuralgias and in histrionic spasm. *Lancet, 167*(4319), 1605–1607. doi:10.1016/S0140-6736(01)84034-4

Pal, H. K., Dinda, A. K., Roy, S., & Banerji, A. K. (1989). Acute effect of anhydrous glycerol on peripheral nerve: An experimental study. *British Journal of Neurosurgery, 3*(4), 463–469. doi:10.3109/02688698909002832 PMID:2803594

Pan, H.-C., Sheehan, J., Huang, C.-F., Sheu, M.-L., Yang, D.-Y., & Chiu, W.-T. (2010). Quality-of-life outcomes after Gamma Knife surgery for trigeminal neuralgia. *Journal of Neurosurgery, 113*(Suppl), 191–198. doi:10.3171/2010.8.GKS10879 PMID:21121802

Pan, S.-L., Yen, M.-F., Chiu, Y.-H., Chen, L.-S., & Chen, H.-H. (2011). Increased risk of trigeminal neuralgia after hypertension: A population-based study. *Neurology, 77*(17), 1605–1610. doi:10.1212/WNL.0b013e3182343354 PMID:21998318

Parekh, S., Shah, K., Kotdawalla, H., & Gandhi, I. (1989). Baclofen in carbamazepine resistant trigeminal neuralgia- a double blind clinical trial. *Cephalalgia, 9*(10_suppl), 392–393. doi:10.1177/0333102489009S10208

Park, C. K., Choi, H. J., Lee, S. H., & Rhee, B. A. (2014). Trigeminal neuralgia caused by persistent primitive trigeminal artery. *Journal of Korean Neurosurgical Society, 56*(3), 278–280. doi:10.3340/jkns.2014.56.3.278 PMID:25368776

Patel, J. P., & Frey, B. N. (2015). Disruption in the Blood-Brain Barrier: The Missing Link between Brain and Body Inflammation in Bipolar Disorder? *Neural Plasticity, 708306*. doi:10.1155/2015/708306 PMID:26075104

Pearce, J. M. S. (2003). Trigeminal neuralgia (Fothergill's disease) in the 17th and 18th centuries. *Journal of Neurology, Neurosurgery, and Psychiatry, 74*(12), 1688. doi:10.1136/jnnp.74.12.1688 PMID:14638891

Peiris, J. B., Perera, G. L. S., Devendra, S. V., & Lionel, N. D. W. (1980). Sodium valproate in trigeminal neuralgia. *The Medical Journal of Australia, 2*, 278. PMID:6776393

Peker, S., Kurtkaya, O., Uzün, I., & Pamir, M. N. (2006). Microanatomy of the central myelin-peripheral myelin transition zone of the trigeminal nerve. *Neurosurgery, 59*(2), 354-359. 10.1227/01.NEU.0000223501.27220.69

Perez, C., Navarro, A., Saldana, M. T., Martinez, S., & Rejas, J. (2009). Patient-reported outcomes in subjects with painful trigeminal neuralgia receiving pregabalin: Evidence from medical practice in primary care settings. *Cephalalgia, 29*(7), 781–790. doi:10.1111/j.1468-2982.2008.01792.x PMID:19522052

Perez, C., Saldana, M. T., Navarro, A., Martinez, S., & Rejas, J. (2009). Trigeminal neuralgia treated with pregabalin in family medicine settings: Its effect on pain alleviation and cost reduction. *Journal of Clinical Pharmacology, 49*(5), 582–590. doi:10.1177/0091270009333017 PMID:19299534

Peris-Celda, M., Graziano, F., Russo, V., Mericle, R. A., & Ulm, A. J. (2013). Foramen ovale puncture, lesioning accuracy, and avoiding complications: Microsurgical anatomy study with clinical implications. *Journal of Neurosurgery, 119*(5), 1176–1193. doi:10.3171/2013.1.JNS12743 PMID:23600929

Peters, G., & Nurmikko, T. J. (2002). Peripheral and gasserian ganglion-level procedures for the treatment of trigeminal neuralgia. *The Clinical Journal of Pain, 18*(1), 28–34. doi:10.1097/00002508-200201000-00005 PMID:11803300

Pinkus, R. L. (1984). Innovation in neurosurgery: Walter Dandy in his day. *Neurosurgery, 14*(5), 623–631. doi:10.1227/00006123-198405000-00022 PMID:6374495

Pollock, B. E. (2005). Percutaneous retrogasserian glycerol rhizotomy for patients with idiopathic trigeminal neuralgia: A prospective analysis of factors related to pain relief. *Journal of Neurosurgery, 102*(2), 223–228. doi:10.3171/jns.2005.102.2.0223 PMID:15739548

Pollock, B. E. (2012). Surgical management of medically refractory trigeminal neuralgia. *Current Neurology and Neuroscience Reports, 12*(2), 125–131. doi:10.100711910-011-0242-7 PMID:22183181

Pollock, B. E., & Boes, C. J. (2011). Stereotactic radiosurgery for glossopharyngeal neuralgia: Preliminary report of 5 cases. *Journal of Neurosurgery, 115*(5), 936–939. doi:10.3171/2011.5.JNS1133 PMID:21740122

Pollock, B. E., Phuong, L. K., Foote, R. L., Stafford, S. L., & Gorman, D. A. (2001). High-dose trigeminal neuralgia radiosurgery associated with increased risk of trigeminal nerve dysfunction. *Neurosurgery*, *49*(1), 58–64. PMID:11440460

Pollock, L. J., Potter, H. E., Patrick, H. T., Patrick, H. T., Härtel, F., Grinker, J., & Maes, U. (1916). Experimental studies of injection of the Gasserian ganglion. *Journal of the American Medical Association*, *LXVII*(19), 1357. doi:10.1001/jama.1916.02590190019007

Polo, G., Fischer, C., Sindou, M. P., & Marneffe, V. (2004). Brainstem auditory evoked potential monitoring during microvascular decompression for hemifacial spasm: Intraoperative brainstem auditory evoked potential changes and warning values to prevent hearing loss--prospective study in a consecutive series of 84 patients. *Neurosurgery*, *54*(1), 97–104, discussion 104–106. doi:10.1227/01.NEU.0000097268.90620.07 PMID:14683545

Pommier, B., Touzet, G., Lucas, C., Vermandel, M., Blond, S., & Reyns, N. (2017). Glossopharyngeal neuralgia treated by Gamma Knife radiosurgery: Safety and efficacy through long-term follow-up. *Journal of Neurosurgery*, 1–8. doi:10.3171/2017.3.JNS162542 PMID:28621622

Prasad, S., & Galetta, S. (2009). Trigeminal neuralgia: Historical notes and current concepts. *The Neurologist*, *15*(2), 87–94. doi:10.1097/NRL.0b013e3181775ac3 PMID:19276786

Premsagar, I. C., Moss, T., & Coakham, H. B. (1997). Teflon-induced granuloma following treatment of trigeminal neuralgia by microvascular decompression. Report of two cases. *Journal of Neurosurgery*, *87*(3), 454–457. doi:10.3171/jns.1997.87.3.0454 PMID:9285615

Putnam, T. J., Hampton, A. O., Harris, W., Härtel, F. F., Irger, I. M., Zander, P., ... Gama, C. (1936). A technic of injection into the Gasserian ganglion under roentgenographic control. *Archives of Neurology and Psychiatry*, *35*(1), 92. doi:10.1001/archneurpsyc.1936.02260010102007

Rachman, S. (1977). The conditioning theory of fear-acquisition: A critical examination. *Behaviour Research and Therapy*, *15*(5), 375–387. doi:10.1016/0005-7967(77)90041-9 PMID:612338

Radulović, N., Đorđević, N., Denić, M., Pinheiro, M. M. G., Fernandes, P. D., & Boylan, F. (2012). A novel toxic alkaloid from poison hemlock (Conium maculatum L., Apiaceae): Identification, synthesis and antinociceptive activity. *Food and Chemical Toxicology*, *50*(2), 274–279. doi:10.1016/j.fct.2011.10.060 PMID:22063758

Rahman, T., Campbell, A., O'Connell, C. R., & Nallapula, K. (2014). Carbamazepine in bipolar disorder with pain: Reviewing treatment guidelines. *The Primary Care Companion for CNS Disorders*, *16*(5). doi:10.4088/PCC.14r01672 PMID:25667814

Rand, R. W. (1981). The Gardner neurovascular decompression operation for trigeminal neuralgia. *Acta Neurochirurgica*, *58*(3–4), 161–166. doi:10.1007/BF01407123 PMID:7315548

Rand, R. W. (1997). Leksell Gamma Knife treatment of tic douloureux. *Neurosurgery Clinics of North America*, *8*(1), 75–78. Retrieved from http://www.ncbi.nlm.nih.gov/pubmed/9018707 PMID:9018707

Rappaport, Z. H., & Gomori, J. M. (1988). Recurrent trigeminal cistern glycerol injections for tic douloureux. *Acta Neurochirurgica*, *90*(1-2), 31–34. doi:10.1007/BF01541263 PMID:2449803

Rappaport, Z. H., Seltzer, Z., & Zagzag, D. (1986). The effect of glycerol on autotomy. An experimental model of neuralgia pain. *Pain*, *26*(1), 85–91. doi:10.1016/0304-3959(86)90175-2 PMID:3737232

Rasminsky, M. (1978). Ectopic generation of impulses and cross-talk in spinal nerve roots of "dystrophic" mice. *Annals of Neurology*, *3*(4), 351–357. doi:10.1002/ana.410030413 PMID:208454

Rasmussen, P. (1990a). Facial pain. II. A prospective survey of 1052 patients with a view of: Character of the attacks, onset, course, and character of pain. *Acta Neurochirurgica*, *107*(3-4), 121–128. doi:10.1007/BF01405790 PMID:2077848

Rasmussen, P. (1990b). Facial pain. I. A prospective survey of 1052 patients with a view of: Definition, delimitation, classification, general data, genetic factors, and previous diseases. *Acta Neurochirurgica*, *107*(3-4), 112–120. doi:10.1007/BF01405789 PMID:2077847

Rasmussen, P. (1991). Facial pain. IV. A prospective study of 1052 patients with a view of: Precipitating factors, associated symptoms, objective psychiatric and neurological symptoms. *Acta Neurochirurgica*, *108*(3-4), 100–109. doi:10.1007/BF01418516 PMID:2031469

Ray, J. P., & Price, J. L. (1992). The organization of the thalamocortical connections of the mediodorsal thalamic nucleus in the rat, related to the ventral forebrain-prefrontal cortex topography. *The Journal of Comparative Neurology*, *323*(2), 167–197. doi:10.1002/cne.903230204 PMID:1401255

Régis, J., Tuleasca, C., Resseguier, N., Carron, R., Donnet, A., Gaudart, J., & Levivier, M. (2016). Long-term safety and efficacy of Gamma Knife surgery in classical trigeminal neuralgia: A 497-patient historical cohort study. *Journal of Neurosurgery*, *124*(4), 1079–1087. doi:10.3171/2015.2.JNS142144 PMID:26339857

Rehm, L. P. (1977). A self-control model of depression. *Behavior Therapy*, *8*(5), 787–804. doi:10.1016/S0005-7894(77)80150-0

Rengachary, S. S., Watanabe, I. S., Singer, P., & Bopp, W. J. (1983). Effect of glycerol on peripheral nerve: An experimental study. *Neurosurgery*, *13*(6), 681–688. doi:10.1227/00006123-198312000-00012 PMID:6318149

Reus, G. Z., Titus, S. E., Abelaira, H. M., Freitas, S. M., Tuon, T., Quevedo, J., & Budni, J. (2016). Neurochemical correlation between major depressive disorder and neurodegenerative diseases. *Life Sciences*, *158*, 121–129. doi:10.1016/j.lfs.2016.06.027 PMID:27370938

Reuter, E., Krekeler, G., Krainick, J. U., Thoden, U., & Doerr, M. (1976). [Pain suppression in the trigeminal region by means of transcutaneous nerve stimulation]. *Deutsche Zahnarztliche Zeitschrift*, *31*(3), 274–276. PMID:1082811

Revuelta-Gutierrez, R., López-González, M. A., & Soto-Hernández, J. L. (2006). Surgical treatment of trigeminal neuralgia without vascular compression: 20 years of experience. *Surgical Neurology, 66*(1), 32–6. doi:10.1016/j.surneu.2005.10.018

Revuelta-Gutierrez, R., Martinez-Anda, J. J., Coll, J. B., Campos-Romo, A., & Perez-Peña, N. (2013). Efficacy and safety of root compression of trigeminal nerve for trigeminal neuralgia without evidence of vascular compression. *World Neurosurgery, 80*(3-4), 385–389. doi:10.1016/j.wneu.2012.07.030 PMID:22889619

Revuelta-Gutiérrez, R., Morales-Martínez, A. H., Mejías-Soto, C., Martínez-Anda, J. J., & Ortega-Porcayo, L. A. (2016). Microvascular decompression for glossopharyngeal neuralgia through a microasterional approach: A case series. *Surgical Neurology International, 7*(1), 51. doi:10.4103/2152-7806.181824 PMID:27213105

Rey-Dios, R., & Cohen-Gadol, A. A. (2013). Current neurosurgical management of glossopharyngeal neuralgia and technical nuances for microvascular decompression surgery. *Neurosurgical Focus, 34*(3), E8. doi:10.3171/2012.12.FOCUS12391 PMID:23451790

Rogers, C. L., Shetter, A. G., Fiedler, J. A., Smith, K. A., Han, P. P., & Speiser, B. L. (2000). Gamma knife radiosurgery for trigeminal neuralgia: The initial experience of The Barrow Neurological Institute. *International Journal of Radiation Oncology, Biology, Physics, 47*(4), 1013–1019. doi:10.1016/S0360-3016(00)00513-7 PMID:10863073

Rojas-Villabona, A., Kitchen, N., & Paddick, I. (2016). Investigation of dosimetric differences between the TMR 10 and convolution algorithm for Gamma Knife stereotactic radiosurgery. *Journal of Applied Clinical Medical Physics, 17*(6), 217–229. doi:10.1120/jacmp.v17i6.6347 PMID:27929495

Ro, L.-S., & Chang, K.-H. (2005). Neuropathic pain: Mechanisms and treatments. *Chang Gung Medical Journal, 28*(9), 597–605. PMID:16323550

Rose, F. C. (1993). European neurology from its beginnings until the 15th century: An overview. *Journal of the History of the Neurosciences, 2*(1), 21–44. doi:10.1080/09647049309525550 PMID:11618442

Rose, W. (1890). Removal of the Gasserian Ganglion for Severe Neuralgia. *Lancet, 136*(3505), 914–915. doi:10.1016/S0140-6736(01)78645-X

Rudy, T. E., Kerns, R. D., & Turk, D. C. (1988). Chronic pain and depression: Toward a cognitive-behavioral mediation model. *Pain, 35*(2), 129–140. doi:10.1016/0304-3959(88)90220-5 PMID:3237427

Rushworth, R. G., & Smith, S. F. (1982). Trigeminal neuralgia and hemifacial spasm: Treatment by microvascular decompression. *The Medical Journal of Australia, 1*(10), 424–426. Retrieved from http://www.ncbi.nlm.nih.gov/pubmed/7099070 PMID:7099070

Sabalys, G., Juodzbalys, G., & Wang, H. L. (2013). Aetiology and pathogenesis of trigeminal neuralgia: A comprehensive review. *Journal of Oral & Maxillofacial Research*, *3*(4), e2. doi:10.5037/jomr.2012.3402 PMID:24422020

Saers, S. J. F., Han, K. S., & de Ru, J. A. (2011). Microvascular decompression may be an effective treatment for nervus intermedius neuralgia. *The Journal of Laryngology and Otology*, *125*(5), 520–522. doi:10.1017/S0022215110002677 PMID:21223630

Saini, S. S. (1987). Reterogasserian anhydrous glycerol injection therapy in trigeminal neuralgia: Observations in 552 patients. *Journal of Neurology, Neurosurgery, and Psychiatry*, *50*(11), 1536–1538. doi:10.1136/jnnp.50.11.1536 PMID:3501000

Saito, K., Konishi, S., & Otsuka, M. (1975). Antagonism between Lioresal and substance P in rat spinal cord. *Brain Research*, *97*(1), 177–180. doi:10.1016/0006-8993(75)90928-2 PMID:1175037

Sakas, D. E., Panourias, I. G., Stranjalis, G., Stefanatou, M. P., Maratheftis, N., & Bontozoglou, N. (2007). Paroxysmal otalgia due to compression of the intermediate nerve: A distinct syndrome of neurovascular conflict confirmed by neuroimaging. Case report. *Journal of Neurosurgery*, *107*(6), 1228–1230. doi:10.3171/JNS-07/12/1228 PMID:18077963

Salagre, E., Sole, B., Tomioka, Y., Fernandes, B. S., Hidalgo-Mazzei, D., Garriga, M., ... Grande, I. (2017). Treatment of neurocognitive symptoms in unipolar depression: A systematic review and future perspectives. *Journal of Affective Disorders*, *221*, 205–221. doi:10.1016/j.jad.2017.06.034 PMID:28651185

Salama, H., Ben-Khayal, H., Mohamed, M. A. S., El-Mitwalli, A., Zaher, A. A., Ezzeldin, A., & ... . (2009). Outcome of medical and surgical management in intractable idiopathic trigeminal neuralgia. *Annals of Indian Academy of Neurology*, *12*(3), 173–178. doi:10.4103/0972-2327.56317 PMID:20174498

Salkovskis, P. M. (1991). The importance of behaviour in the maintenance of anxiety and panic: A cognitive account. *Behavioural and Cognitive Psychotherapy*, *19*(1), 6–19. doi:10.1017/S0141347300011472

Samadian, M., Bakhtevari, M. H., Nosari, M. A., Babadi, A. J., & Razaei, O. (2015). Trigeminal Neuralgia Caused by Venous Angioma: A Case Report and Review of the Literature. *World Neurosurgery*, *84*(3), 860–864. doi:10.1016/j.wneu.2015.04.063 PMID:25968963

Sandell, T., Ringstad, G. A., & Eide, P. K. (2014). Usefulness of the endoscope in microvascular decompression for trigeminal neuralgia and MRI-based prediction of the need for endoscopy. *Acta Neurochir (Wien), 156*(10), 1901-1909. doi:10.1007/s00701-014-2171-0

Sandell, T., & Eide, P. K. (2008). Effect of microvascular decompression in trigeminal neuralgia patients with or without constant pain. *Neurosurgery*, *63*(1), 93–99, discussion 99–100. doi:10.1227/01.NEU.0000335075.16858.EF PMID:18728573

Sato, O., Kanazawa, I., & Kokunai, T. (1979). Trigeminal neuralgia caused by compression of trigeminal nerve by pontine vein. *Surgical Neurology*, *11*(4), 285–286. PMID:441914

Schmidt, B. L., Gear, R. W., & Levine, J. D. (2003). Response of neuropathic trigeminal pain to the combination of low-dose nalbuphine plus naloxone in humans. *Neuroscience Letters, 343*(2), 144–146. doi:10.1016/S0304-3940(03)00356-2 PMID:12759184

Schwarz, W., & Fox, J. M. (1979). Effects of monochromatic X-radiation on the membrane of nodes of Ranvier under voltage and current clamp conditions. *Experientia, 35*(9), 1200–1201. doi:10.1007/BF01963288 PMID:314907

Seager, L. D., & Castelnuovo, G. (1947). Toxicity of stilbamidine; a study of the effects of chronic intoxication. *Archives of Pathology, 44*(3), 287–296. Retrieved from http://www.ncbi.nlm.nih.gov/pubmed/20267695 PMID:20267695

Sekula, R. F. Jr, Frederickson, A. M., Jannetta, P. J., Quigley, M. R., Aziz, K. M., & Arnone, G. D. (2011). Microvascular decompression for elderly patients with trigeminal neuralgia: A prospective study and systematic review with meta-analysis. *Journal of Neurosurgery, 114*(1), 172–179. doi:10.3171/2010.6.JNS10142 PMID:20653393

Sekula, R. F. Jr, Marchan, E. M., Fletcher, L. H., Casey, K. F., & Jannetta, P. J. (2008). Microvascular decompression for trigeminal neuralgia in elderly patients. *Journal of Neurosurgery, 108*(4), 689–691. doi:10.3171/JNS/2008/108/4/0689 PMID:18377247

Serpell, M. G. (2002). Neuropathic pain study group. Gabapentin in neuropathic pain syndromes: A randomized, double-blind, placebo-controlled trial. *Pain, 99*, 557–566. doi:10.1016/S0304-3959(02)00255-5 PMID:12406532

Shaikh, S., Yaacob, H., & Abd Rahman, R. B. (2011). Lamotrigine for trigeminal neuralgia: Efficacy and safety in comparison with carbamazepine. *Journal of the Chinese Medical Association, 74*(6), 243–249. doi:10.1016/j.jcma.2011.04.002 PMID:21621166

Sharim, J., Lo, W.-L., Kim, W., Chivukula, S., Tenn, S., Kaprealian, T., & Pouratian, N. (2017). Radiosurgical target distance from the root entry zone in the treatment of trigeminal neuralgia. *Practical Radiation Oncology, 7*(4), 221–227. doi:10.1016/j.prro.2016.12.006 PMID:28336479

Sharma, S. C., Ott, J. T., Williams, J. B., & Dickow, D. (2010). Clinical implications of adopting Monte Carlo treatment planning for CyberKnife. *Journal of Applied Clinical Medical Physics, 11*(1), 3142. doi:10.1120/jacmp.v11i1.3142 PMID:20160699

Shehata, H., El-Tamawy, M., Shalaby, N., & Ramzy, G. (2013). Botulinum toxin type A: Could it be an effective treatment option in intractable trigeminal neuralgia? *The Journal of Headache and Pain, 14*(1), 92. doi:10.1186/1129-2377-14-92 PMID:24251833

Sheinberg, M. A., & Sagher, O. (2002). Medical Management of Trigeminal Neuralgia. In K. J. Burchiel (Ed.), *Surgical Management of Pain*. Stuttgart: Georg Thieme Verlag; doi:10.1055/b-0034-45927

Shelden, C. H., Pudenz, R. H., Freshwater, D. B., & Crue, B. L. (1955). Compression Rather than Decompression for Trigeminal Neuralgia. *Journal of Neurosurgery, 12*(2), 123–126. doi:10.3171/jns.1955.12.2.0123 PMID:14368343

Sheng, B., Lv, F., Xiao, Z., Ouyang, Y., Lv, F., Deng, J., ... Liu, N. (2012). Anatomical relationship between cranial surface landmarks and venous sinus in posterior cranial fossa using CT angiography. *Surgical and Radiologic Anatomy*, *34*(8), 701–708. doi:10.100700276-011-0916-5 PMID:22160178

Siddon, R. L. (1985). Prism representation: A 3D ray-tracing algorithm for radiotherapy applications. *Physics in Medicine and Biology*, *30*(8), 817–824. doi:10.1088/0031-9155/30/8/005 PMID:4048266

Sidebottom, A., & Maxwell, S. (1995). The medical and surgical management of trigeminal neuralgia. *Journal of Clinical Pharmacy and Therapeutics*, *20*(1), 31–35. doi:10.1111/j.1365-2710.1995.tb00622.x PMID:7775611

Silver, M., Blum, D., Grainger, J., Hammer, A., & Quessy, S. (2007). Double-blind, placebo-controlled trial of lamotrigine in combination with other medications for neuropathic pain. *Journal of Pain and Symptom Management*, *34*(4), 446–454. doi:10.1016/j.jpainsymman.2006.12.015 PMID:17662571

Sindou, M., Howeidy, T., & Acevedo, G. (2002). Anatomical observations during microvascular decompression for idiopathic trigeminal neuralgia (with correlations between topography of pain and site of the neurovascular conflict). Prospective study in a series of 579 patients. *Acta Neurochirurgica*, *144*(1), 1–12. doi:10.1007/s007010200000

Sindou, M., Leston, J., Decullier, E., & Chapuis, F. (2007). *Microvascular decompression for primary trigeminal neuralgia: long-term effectiveness and prognostic factors in a series of 362 consecutive patients with clear-cut neurovascular conflicts who underwent pure decompression.* Academic Press.

Sindou, M. P., Chiha, M., & Mertens, P. (1994). Anatomical findings observed during microsurgical approaches of the cerebellopontine angle for vascular decompression in trigeminal neuralgia (350 cases). *Stereotactic and Functional Neurosurgery*, *63*(1-4), 203–207. doi:10.1159/000100316 PMID:7624636

Sindou, M., Fob, J.-L., Ciriano, D., & Fischer, C. (1992). Hearing Prognosis and Intraoperative Guidance of Brainstem Auditory Evoked Potential in Microvascular Decompression. *The Laryngoscope*, *102*(6), 678–682. doi:10.1288/00005537-199206000-00014 PMID:1602916

Sindou, M., Leston, J., Howeidy, T., Decullier, E., & Chapuis, F. (2006). Micro-vascular decompression for primary Trigeminal Neuralgia (typical or atypical). Long-term effectiveness on pain; prospective study with survival analysis in a consecutive series of 362 patients. *Acta Neurochirurgica*, *148*(12), 1235–1245, discussion 1245. doi:10.100700701-006-0809-2 PMID:16804643

Sindou, M., Mahmoudi, M., & Brînzeu, A. (2015). Hypertension of neurogenic origin: Effect of microvascular decompression of the CN IX-X root entry/exit zone and ventrolateral medulla on blood pressure in a prospective series of 48 patients with hemifacial spasm associated with essential hypertension. *Journal of Neurosurgery*, *123*(6), 1405–1413. doi:10.3171/2014.12.JNS141775 PMID:26230479

Sindrup, S. H., & Jensen, T. S. (2002). Pharmacotherapy of trigeminal neuralgia. *The Clinical Journal of Pain*, *18*(1), 22–27. doi:10.1097/00002508-200201000-00004 PMID:11803299

Singh, B., Srivastava, S. K., & Dang, R. (2001). Anatomic considerations in relation to the maxillary nerve block. *Regional Anesthesia and Pain Medicine*, *26*(6), 507–511. doi:10.1097/00115550-200111000-00004 PMID:11707787

Singh, R., Davis, J., & Sharma, S. (2016). Stereotactic Radiosurgery for Trigeminal Neuralgia: A Retrospective Multi-Institutional Examination of Treatment Outcomes. *Cureus*, *8*(4), e554. doi:10.7759/cureus.554 PMID:27182468

Sinoff, G., & Werner, P. (2003). Anxiety disorder and accompanying subjective memory loss in the elderly as a predictor of future cognitive decline. *International Journal of Geriatric Psychiatry*, *18*(10), 951–959. doi:10.1002/gps.1004 PMID:14533128

Sivakanthan, S., Van Gompel, J. J., Alikhani, P., van Loveren, H., Chen, R., & Agazzi, S. (2014). Surgical management of trigeminal neuralgia: use and cost-effectiveness from an analysis of the Medicare Claims Database. *Neurosurgery, 75*(3), 220-226. 10.1227/NEU.0000000000000430

Skirving, D. J., & Dan, N. G. (2001). A 20-year review of percutaneous balloon compression of the trigeminal ganglion. *Journal of Neurosurgery*, *94*(6), 913–917. doi:10.3171/jns.2001.94.6.0913 PMID:11409519

Slavin, K. V., Colpan, M. E., Munawar, N., Wess, C., & Nersesyan, H. (2006). Trigeminal and occipital peripheral nerve stimulation for craniofacial pain: A single-institution experience and review of the literature. *Neurosurgical Focus*, *21*(6), E5. doi:10.3171/foc.2006.21.6.8 PMID:17341049

Slavin, K. V., & Wess, C. (2005). Trigeminal Branch Stimulation for Intractable Neuropathic Pain: Technical Note. *Neuromodulation: Technology at the Neural Interface*, *8*(1), 7–13. doi:10.1111/j.1094-7159.2005.05215.x PMID:22151378

Slettebo, H., Hirschberg, H., & Lindegaard, K. F. (1993). Long-term results after percutaneous retrogasserian glycerol rhizotomy in patients with trigeminal neuralgia. *Acta Neurochirurgica*, *122*(3-4), 231–235. doi:10.1007/BF01405534 PMID:8372713

Smith, H. P., McWhorter, J. M., & Challa, V. R. (1981). Radiofrequency neurolysis in a clinical model. Neuropathological correlation. *Journal of Neurosurgery*, *55*(2), 246–253. doi:10.3171/jns.1981.55.2.0246 PMID:7252548

Smith, J. H., Robertson, C. E., Garza, I., & Cutrer, F. M. (2013). Triggerless neuralgic otalgia: A case series and systematic literature review. *Cephalalgia: an International Journal of Headache*, *33*(11), 914–923. doi:10.1177/0333102413477743 PMID:23444079

Smith, K. J., & McDonald, W. I. (1980). Spontaneous and mechanically evoked activity due to central demyelinating lesion. *Nature*, *286*(5769), 154–155. doi:10.1038/286154a0 PMID:7402307

Smith, K. J., & Mcdonald, W. I. (1999). The pathophysiology of multiple sclerosis: the mechanisms underlying the production of symptoms and the natural history of the disease. *Philosophical Transactions of the Royal Society of London. Series B, Biological Sciences*, *354*(1390), 1649–1673. doi:10.1098/rstb.1999.0510 PMID:10603618

Smith, Z. A., Gorgulho, A. A., Bezrukiy, N., McArthur, D., Agazaryan, N., Selch, M. T., & De Salles, A. A. F. (2011). Dedicated linear accelerator radiosurgery for trigeminal neuralgia: A single-center experience in 179 patients with varied dose prescriptions and treatment plans. *International Journal of Radiation Oncology, Biology, Physics*, *81*(1), 225–231. doi:10.1016/j.ijrobp.2010.05.058 PMID:21236592

Smyth, P., Greenough, G., & Stommel, E. (2003). Familial trigeminal neuralgia: Case reports and review of the literature. *Headache*, *43*(8), 910–915. doi:10.1046/j.1526-4610.2003.03172.x PMID:12940815

Sola, C., Raux, O., Savath, L., Macq, C., Capdevila, X., & Dadure, C. (2012). Ultrasound guidance characteristics and efficiency of suprazygomatic maxillary nerve blocks in infants: A descriptive prospective study. *Paediatric Anaesthesia*, *22*(9), 841–846. doi:10.1111/j.1460-9592.2012.03861.x PMID:22587691

Solaro, C., Messmer Uccelli, M., Uccelli, A., Leandri, M., & Mancardi, G. L. (2000). Low-dose gabapentin combined with either lamotrigine or carbamazepine can be useful therapies for trigeminal neuralgia in multiple sclerosis. *European Neurology*, *44*(1), 45–48. doi:10.1159/000008192 PMID:10894995

Solaro, C., Uccelli, M. M., Brichetto, G., Gaspperini, C., & Mancardi, G. (2001). Topiramate relieves idiopathic and symptomatic trigeminal neuralgia. *Journal of Pain and Symptom Management*, *21*(5), 367–368. doi:10.1016/S0885-3924(01)00275-5 PMID:11398791

Solmi, M., Veronese, N., Zaninotto, L., van der Loos, M. L., Gao, K., Schaffer, A., ... Correll, C. U. (2016). Lamotrigine compared to placebo and other agents with antidepressant activity in patients with unipolar and bipolar depression: A comprehensive meta-analysis of efficacy and safety outcomes in short-term trials. *CNS Spectrums*, *21*(5), 403–418. doi:10.1017/S1092852916000523 PMID:27686028

Son, B.-C., Kim, H.-S., Kim, I.-S., Yang, S.-H., & Lee, S.-W. (2011). Percutaneous radiofrequency thermocoagulation under fluoroscopic image-guidance for idiopathic trigeminal neuralgia. *Journal of Korean Neurosurgical Society*, *50*(5), 446–452. doi:10.3340/jkns.2011.50.5.446 PMID:22259692

Soriano-Baron, H., Vales-Hidalgo, O., Arvizu-Saldana, E., Moreno-Jimenez, S., & Revuelta-Gutierrez, R. (2015). Hemifacial spasm: 20-year surgical experience, lesson learned. *Surgical Neurology International*, *6*(1), 83. doi:10.4103/2152-7806.157443 PMID:26015871

Spina, A., Mortini, P., Alemanno, F., Houdayer, E., & Iannaccone, S. (2017). Trigeminal Neuralgia: Toward a Multimodal Approach. *World Neurosurgery*, *103*, 220–230. doi:10.1016/j.wneu.2017.03.126 PMID:28377244

Stajcic, Z. (1990). Evidence that the site of action of glycerol in relieving tic douloureux is its actual site of application. *Deutsche Zahnarztliche Zeitschrift*, *45*(1), 44–46. PMID:1701698

Steiger, H. J. (1991). Prognostic factors in the treatment of trigeminal neuralgia. Analysis of a differential therapeutic approach. *Acta Neurochirurgica*, *113*(1-2), 11–17. doi:10.1007/BF01402108 PMID:1799138

Steinberg, J., Sack, J., Wilson, B., Weingarten, D., Carter, B., Khalessi, A., ... Alksne, J. (2017). (In Press). Tentorial sling for microvascular decompression in patients with trigeminal neuralgia: A description of operative technique and clinical outcomes. *Journal of Neurosurgery*.

Stookey, B. (1928). Differential section of the trigeminal root in the surgical treatment of trigeminal neuralgia. *Annals of Surgery*, *87*(2), 172–178. doi:10.1097/00000658-192887020-00002 PMID:17865827

Stookey, B., & Ransohoff, J. (1959). *Trigeminal Neuralgia: Its History & Treatment*. Springfield, IL: Charles C Thomas.

Strandjord, R. (1973). Medicinal treatment planning in primary trigeminal neuralgia. *Tidsskrift for den Norske lageforening: tidsskrift for praktisk medicin, ny rakke, 93*(30), 2251-2252.

Strittmatter, M., Grauer, M., Isenberg, E., Hamann, G., Fischer, C., Hoffmann, K. H., ... Schimrigk, K. (1997). Cerebrospinal fluid neuropeptides and monoaminergic transmitters in patients with trigeminal neuralgia. *Headache*, *37*(4), 211–216. doi:10.1046/j.1526-4610.1997.3704211.x PMID:9150615

Stroud, M. W., Thorn, B. E., Jensen, M. P., & Boothby, J. L. (2000). The relation between pain beliefs, negative thoughts, and psychosocial functioning in chronic pain patients. *Pain*, *84*(2-3), 347–352. doi:10.1016/S0304-3959(99)00226-2 PMID:10666540

Sun, T., Saito, S., Nakai, O., & Ando, T. (1994). Long-term results of microvascular decompression for trigeminal neuralgia with reference to probability of recurrence. *Acta Neurochirurgica*, *126*(2–4), 144–148. doi:10.1007/BF01476425 PMID:8042547

Sweet, W. H. (1988). Percutaneous methods for the treatment of trigeminal neuralgia and other faciocephalic pain; comparison with microvascular decompression. *Seminars in Neurology*, *8*(4), 272–279. doi:10.1055-2008-1041389 PMID:3074421

Sweet, W. H., Cushing, H., Adson, A. W., Grant, F. C., Jefferson, G., Horrax, G., ... Orley, A. (1950). Trigeminal injection with radiographic control. *Journal of the American Medical Association*, *142*(6), 392. doi:10.1001/jama.1950.02910240010003 PMID:15402380

Sweet, W. H., Poletti, C. E., & Macon, J. B. (1981). Treatment of trigeminal neuralgia and other facial pains by retrogasserian injection of glycerol. *Neurosurgery*, *9*(6), 647–653. doi:10.1227/00006123-198112000-00006 PMID:6976524

Sweet, W. H., & Wepsic, J. G. (1974). Controlled thermocoagulation of trigeminal ganglion and rootlets for differential destruction of pain fibers. *Journal of Neurosurgery*, *40*(2), 143–156. doi:10.3171/jns.1974.40.2.0143 PMID:4587949

Taarnhøj, P. (1952). Decompression of the Trigeminal Root and the Posterior Part of the Ganglion as Treatment in Trigeminal Neuralgia. *Journal of Neurosurgery*, *9*(3), 288–290. doi:10.3171/jns.1952.9.3.0288 PMID:14939059

Taarnhøj, P. (1982). Decompression of the posterior trigeminal root in trigeminal neuralgia. *Journal of Neurosurgery*, *57*(1), 14–17. doi:10.3171/jns.1982.57.1.0014 PMID:7086492

Taha, J. M., & Tew, J. M. Jr. (1996). Comparison of surgical treatments for trigeminal neuralgia: Reevaluation of radiofrequency rhizotomy. *Neurosurgery*, *38*(5), 865–871. doi:10.1097/00006123-199605000-00001 PMID:8727810

Taha, J. M., Tew, J. M. Jr, & Buncher, C. R. (1995). A prospective 15-year follow up of 154 consecutive patients with trigeminal neuralgia treated by percutaneous stereotactic radiofrequency thermal rhizotomy. *Journal of Neurosurgery*, *83*(6), 989–993. doi:10.3171/jns.1995.83.6.0989 PMID:7490643

Taha, J. M., Tew, J. M. Jr, Keith, R. W., & Payner, T. D. (1994). Intraoperative monitoring of the vagus nerve during intracranial glossopharyngeal and upper vagal rhizotomy: Technical note. *Neurosurgery*, *35*(4), 775–777. doi:10.1227/00006123-199410000-00032 PMID:7808629

Taich, Z. J., Goetsch, S. J., Monaco, E., Carter, B. S., Ott, K., Alksne, J. F., & Chen, C. C. (2016). Stereotactic Radiosurgery Treatment of Trigeminal Neuralgia: Clinical Outcomes and Prognostic Factors. *World Neurosurgery*, *90*(Supplement C), 604–612.e11. doi:10.1016/j.wneu.2016.02.067 PMID:26915701

Talkovsky, A. M., Green, K. L., Osegueda, A., & Norton, P. J. (2017). Secondary depression in transdiagnostic group cognitive behavioral therapy among individuals diagnosed with anxiety disorders. *Journal of Anxiety Disorders*, *46*, 56–64. doi:10.1016/j.janxdis.2016.09.008 PMID:27707524

Tang, Y., Ma, L., Li, N., Guo, Y., Yang, L., Wu, B., ... Ni, J. X. (2016). Percutaneous trigeminal ganglion radiofrequency thermocoagulation alleviates anxiety and depression disorders in patients with classic trigeminal neuralgia: A cohort study. *Medicine; Analytical Reviews of General Medicine, Neurology, Psychiatry, Dermatology, and Pediatries*, *95*(49), e5379. doi:10.1097/MD.0000000000005379 PMID:27930513

Tan, N.-C., Chan, L.-L., & Tan, E.-K. (2002). Hemifacial spasm and involuntary facial movements. *QJM: Monthly Journal of the Association of Physicians*, *95*(8), 493–500. doi:10.1093/qjmed/95.8.493 PMID:12145388

Tartaro, S., Stroffolini, F., & Lepore, M. (1979). The importance of etiology for the successful treatment of secondary trigeminal neuralgia. Reviews of some clinical cases. *Journal of Medicine*, *10*(1-2), 121–128. PMID:290724

Tatli, M., Satici, O., Kanpolat, Y., & Sindou, M. (2008). Various surgical modalities for trigeminal neuralgia: Literature study of respective long-term outcomes. *Acta Neurochirurgica*, *150*(3), 243–255. doi:10.100700701-007-1488-3 PMID:18193149

Taub, E., Munz, M., & Tasker, R. R. (1997). Chronic electrical stimulation of the gasserian ganglion for the relief of pain in a series of 34 patients. *Journal of Neurosurgery*, *86*(2), 197–202. doi:10.3171/jns.1997.86.2.0197 PMID:9010419

Taylor, J., Brauer, S., & Espir, M. (1981). Long-term treatment of trigeminal neuralgia. *Postgraduate Medical Journal*, *57*(663), 16–28. doi:10.1136/pgmj.57.663.16 PMID:7279817

Teo, C., Nakaji, P., & Mobbs, R. J. (2006). Endoscope-assisted microvascular decompression for trigeminal neuralgia: technical case report. *Operative Neurosurgery, 59*(suppl_4).

Teo, Nakaji, & Mobbs. (2006). Endoscope-assisted microvascular decompression for trigeminal neuralgia: technical case report. *Neurosurgery, 59*(4 Suppl 2).

Teo, M. K., & Suttner, N. J. (2015). Effective management of lower divisional pain in trigeminal neuralgia using balloon traction. *British Journal of Neurosurgery*, *29*(3), 343–346. doi:10.3109/02688697.2014.990419 PMID:25496298

Terrence, C., & Fromm, G. (1981). Complications of Baclofen Withdrawal. *Journal of the American Medical Association*, *38*(9), 588–589. PMID:6791618

Tew, J. M., Jr., & Taha, J. M. (1995). Percutaneous rhizotomy in the treatment of intractable facial pain (trigeminal, glossopharyngeal, and vagal nerves). In Operative Neurosurgical Techniques (3rd ed.). Philadelphia: WB Saunders.

Theodros, D., Rory Goodwin, C., Bender, M. T., Zhou, X., Garzon-Muvdi, T., De la Garza-Ramos, R., ... Lim, M. (2016). Efficacy of primary microvascular decompression versus subsequent microvascular decompression for trigeminal neuralgia. *Journal of Neurosurgery*, 1–7. doi:10.3171/2016.5.JNS151692 PMID:27419826

Thirumala, P., Meigh, K., Dasyam, N., Shankar, P., Sarma, K. R., Sarma, D. R., ... Balzer, J. (2015). The incidence of high-frequency hearing loss after microvascular decompression for trigeminal neuralgia, glossopharyngeal neuralgia, or geniculate neuralgia. *Journal of Neurosurgery*, *123*(6), 1500–1506. doi:10.3171/2014.10.JNS141101 PMID:25932612

Tiller, J. W. (2013). Depression and anxiety. *The Medical Journal of Australia*, *199*(6Suppl), S28–S31. PMID:25370281

Toda, K. (2008). Operative treatment of trigeminal neuralgia: review of current techniques. *Oral Surg Oral Med Oral Pathol Oral Radiol Endod, 106*(6), 788-805.

Toda, H., Goto, M., & Iwasaki, K. (2015). Patterns and variations in microvascular decompression for trigeminal neuralgia. *Neurologia Medico-Chirurgica*, *55*(5), 432–441. doi:10.2176/nmc.ra.2014-0393 PMID:25925756

Tokita, K., Inoue, T., & Boughter, J. D. Jr. (2009). Afferent connections of the parabrachial nucleus in C57BL/6J mice. *Neuroscience*, *161*(2), 475–488. doi:10.1016/j.neuroscience.2009.03.046 PMID:19327389

Tolle, T., Dukes, E., & Sadosky, A. (2006). Patient burden of trigeminal neuralgia: Results from a cross-sectional survey of health state impairment and treatment patterns in six European countries. *Pain Practice*, *6*(3), 153–160. doi:10.1111/j.1533-2500.2006.00079.x PMID:17147591

Tomson, T., & Ekbom, K. (1981). Trigeminal neuralgia: Time course of pain in relation to carbamazepine dosing. *Cephalalgia*, *1*(2), 91–98. doi:10.1111/j.1468-2982.1981.tb00015.x PMID:7346177

Tremont-Lukats, I., Megeff, C., & Backonja, M. M. (2000). Anticonvulsants for neuropathic pain syndromes: Mechanisms of action and place in therapy. *Drugs*, *60*(5), 1029–1052. doi:10.2165/00003495-200060050-00005 PMID:11129121

Trojnik, T., & Ŝmigoc, T. (2012). Percutaneous trigeminal ganglion balloon compression rhizotomy: Experience in 27 patients. *TheScientificWorldJournal*, *328936*. doi:10.1100/2012/328936 PMID:22545013

Tronnier, V. M., Rasche, D., Hamer, J., Kienle, A. L., & Kunze, S. (2001). Treatment of idiopathic trigeminal neuralgia: Comparison of long-term outcome after radiofrequency rhizotomy and microvascular decompression. *Neurosurgery*, *48*(6), 1261–1267, discussion 1267–1268. PMID:11383728

Tsang, A., Von Korff, M., Lee, S., Alonso, J., Karam, E., Angermeyer, M. C., ... Watanabe, M. (2008). Common chronic pain conditions in developed and developing countries: Gender and age differences and comorbidity with depression-anxiety disorders. *The Journal of Pain*, *9*(10), 883–891. doi:10.1016/j.jpain.2008.05.005 PMID:18602869

Tubbs, R. S., Griessenauer, C. J., Hogan, E., Loukas, M., & Cohen-Gadol, A. A. (2014). Neural interconnections between portio minor and portio major at the porus trigeminus: Application to failed surgical treatment of trigeminal neuralgia. *Clinical Anatomy (New York, N.Y.)*, *27*(1), 94–96. doi:10.1002/ca.22299 PMID:23943366

Tuleasca, C., Carron, R., Resseguier, N., Donnet, A., Roussel, P., & Gaudart, J., … Régis, J. (2014). Repeat Gamma Knife surgery for recurrent trigeminal neuralgia: Long-term outcomes and systematic review. *Journal of Neurosurgery*, *121*(Suppl), 210–221. doi:10.3171/2014.8.GKS141487 PMID:25434955

Turk, D. C., Dworkin, R. H., Allen, R. R., Bellamy, N., Brandenburg, N., Carr, D. B., ... Witter, J. (2003). Core outcome domains for chronic pain clinical trials: IMMPACT recommendations. *Pain*, *106*(3), 337–345. doi:10.1016/j.pain.2003.08.001 PMID:14659516

Turk, D. C., & Rudy, T. E. (1986). Assessment of cognitive factors in chronic pain: A worthwhile enterprise? *Journal of Consulting and Clinical Psychology*, *54*(6), 760–768. doi:10.1037/0022-006X.54.6.760 PMID:3540044

Türp, J. C., & Gobetti, J. P. (1996). Trigeminal neuralgia versus atypical facial pain. A review of the literature and case report. *Oral Surgery, Oral Medicine, Oral Pathology, Oral Radiology, and Endodontics*, *81*(4), 424–432. doi:10.1016/S1079-2104(96)80018-7 PMID:8705588

Ucerler, H., & Govsa, F. (2006). Asterion as a surgical landmark for lateral cranial base approaches. *Journal of Cranio-Maxillo-Facial Surgery: Official Publication of the European Association for Cranio-Maxillo-Facial Surgery*, *34*(7), 415–420. doi:10.1016/j.jcms.2006.05.003 PMID:16963269

Van Buyten, J. P. (2015). Trigeminal Ganglion Stimulation. *Progress in Neurological Surgery*, *29*, 76–82. doi:10.1159/000434658 PMID:26394074

Van Buyten, J. P., Smet, I., & Van de Kelft, E. (2017). Electromagnetic Navigation Technology for More Precise Electrode Placement in the Foramen Ovale: A Technical Report. *Neuromodulation: Technology at the Neural Interface*, *12*(3), 244–249. doi:10.1111/j.1525-1403.2009.00222.x PMID:22151368

Varela-Lema, L., Lopez-Garcia, M., Maceira-Rozas, M., & Munoz-Garzon, V. (2015). Linear accelerator stereotactic radiosurgery for trigeminal neuralgia. *Pain Physician*, *18*(1), 15–27. PMID:25675056

Villavicencio, A. T., Lim, M., Burneikiene, S., Romanelli, P., Adler, J. R., McNeely, L., … Thramann, J. J. (2008). Cyberknife radiosurgery for trigeminal neuralgia treatment: a preliminary multicenter experience. *Neurosurgery, 62*(3), 647-655. 10.1227/01.neu.0000317313.46826.dc

Vilming, S., Lyberg, T., & Latase, X. (1986). Tizanidine in the management of trigeminal neuralgia. *Cephalalgia*, *6*(3), 181–182. doi:10.1046/j.1468-2982.1986.0603181.x PMID:3533272

Waltz, T. A., Dalessio, D. J., Copeland, B., & Abbott, G. (1989). Percutaneous injection of glycerol for the treatment of trigeminal neuralgia. *The Clinical Journal of Pain*, *5*(2), 195–198. doi:10.1097/00002508-198906000-00011 PMID:2520403

Wang, D. D., Raygor, K. P., Cage, T. A., Ward, M. M., Westcott, S., Barbaro, N. M., & Chang, E. F. (2017). Prospective comparison of long-term pain relief rates after first-time microvascular decompression and stereotactic radiosurgery for trigeminal neuralgia. *Journal of Neurosurgery*, 1–10. doi:10.3171/2016.9.JNS16149 PMID:28298026

Wang, J. Y., Bender, M. T., & Bettegowda, C. (2016). Percutaneous Procedures for the Treatment of Trigeminal Neuralgia. *Neurosurgery Clinics of North America*, *27*(3), 277–295. doi:10.1016/j.nec.2016.02.005 PMID:27324995

Wang, Q. P., & Bai, M. (2011). Topiramate versus carbamazepine for the treatment of classical trigeminal neuralgia: A meta-analysis. *CNS Drugs*, *25*(10), 847–857. doi:10.2165/11595590-000000000-00000 PMID:21936587

Wang, X., Thirumala, P. D., Shah, A., Gardner, P., Habeych, M., Crammond, D. J., ... Horowitz, M. (2013). Effect of previous botulinum neurotoxin treatment on microvascular decompression for hemifacial spasm. *Neurosurgical Focus*, *34*(3), E3. doi:10.3171/2012.11.FOCUS12373 PMID:23452316

Wang, Y., Cao, D. Y., Remeniuk, B., Krimmel, S., Seminowicz, D. A., & Zhang, M. (2017). Altered brain structure and function associated with sensory and affective components of classic trigeminal neuralgia. *Pain*, *158*(8), 1561–1570. doi:10.1097/j.pain.0000000000000951 PMID:28520647

Wang, Y., Li, D., Bao, F., Guo, C., Ma, S., & Zhang, M. (2016). Microstructural abnormalities of the trigeminal nerve correlate with pain severity and concomitant emotional dysfunctions in idiopathic trigeminal neuralgia: A randomized, prospective, double-blind study. *Magnetic Resonance Imaging*, *34*(5), 609–616. doi:10.1016/j.mri.2015.11.013 PMID:26747406

Watson, C. P. N. (2012). Trigeminal Neuralgia. *Pain Research & Management : The Journal of the Canadian Pain Society*, *17*(4), 297–298. doi:10.1155/2012/742324

Watson, C. P., Evans, R. J., Watt, V. R., & Birkett, N. (1988). Post-herpetic neuralgia: 208 cases. *Pain*, *35*(3), 289–297. doi:10.1016/0304-3959(88)90139-X PMID:2852344

Weber, K. (2017). Neuromodulation and Devices in Trigeminal Neuralgia. *Headache*, *57*(10), 1648–1653. doi:10.1111/head.13166 PMID:28905370

Weiss, A. L., Ehrhardt, K. P., & Tolba, R. (2017). Atypical Facial Pain: A Comprehensive, Evidence-Based Review. *Current Pain and Headache Reports*, *21*(2), 8. doi:10.100711916-017-0609-9 PMID:28251523

Wei, Y., Pu, C., Li, N., Cai, Y., Shang, H., & Zhao, W. (2016). Long-term therapeutic effect of microvascular decompression for trigeminal neuralgia: Kaplan-meier analysis in a consecutive series of 425 patients. *Turkish Neurosurgery*. doi:10.5137/1019-5149.JTN.18322-16.1 PMID:27593849

Wei, Y., Yang, W., Zhao, W., Pu, C., Li, N., Cai, Y., & Shang, H. (2017). Microvascular decompression for hemifacial spasm: Can intraoperative lateral spread response monitoring improve surgical efficacy? *Journal of Neurosurgery*, 1–6. doi:10.3171/2016.11.JNS162148 PMID:28498061

White, J. C., & Sweet, W. H. (1969). *Pain and the neurosurgeon: A forty-year experience*. Charles C. Thomas.

Wiffen, P. J., McQuay, H. J., Edwards, J. E., & Moore, R. A. (2005). Gabapentin for acute and chronic pain. *Cochrane Database of Systematic Reviews*, *20*(3), CD005452. doi:10.1002/14651858.CD005452 PMID:16034978

Wiffen, P. J., McQuay, H. J., & Moore, R. A. (2005). Carbamazepine for acute and chronic pain. *Cochrane Database of Systematic Reviews*, *3*(3), CD005451. doi:10.1002/14651858.CD005451 PMID:16034977

Wiffen, P., & Rees, J. (2007). Lamotrigine for acute and chronic pain. *Cochrane Database of Systematic Reviews*, *2*, CD006044. PMID:17443611

Wilkinson, H. A. (1999). Trigeminal nerve peripheral branch phenol/glycerol injections for tic douloureux. *Journal of Neurosurgery*, *90*(5), 828–832. doi:10.3171/jns.1999.90.5.0828 PMID:10223447

Wilkins, R. H. (1963). Neurosurgical Classic—XIV. *Journal of Neurosurgery*, *20*(12), 1090–1099. doi:10.3171/jns.1963.20.12.1090 PMID:14186111

Wilkins, R. H. (2002). Trigeminal Neuralgia: historical overview, with emphasis on surgical treatment. In K. J. Burchiel (Ed.), *Surgical Management of Pain* (pp. 288–301). New York: Thieme.

Williams, B. J., Schlesinger, D., & Sheehan, J. (2010). Glossopharyngeal neuralgia treated with gamma knife radiosurgery. *World Neurosurgery*, *73*(4), 413–417. doi:10.1016/j.wneu.2010.01.007 PMID:20849803

Wolf, A., & Kondziolka, D. (2016). Gamma Knife Surgery in Trigeminal Neuralgia. *Neurosurgery Clinics of North America*, *27*(3), 297–304. doi:10.1016/j.nec.2016.02.006 PMID:27324996

Woodhall, B., & Odom, G. L. (1956). Stilbamidine treatment of tic douloureux. *Transactions of the American Neurological Association*, 110–4. Retrieved from http://www.ncbi.nlm.nih.gov/pubmed/13312016

Wu, C., Lian, Y., Zheng, Y., Zhang, H., Chen, Y., Xie, N., & Wang, L. F. (2012). Botulinum toxin type A for the treatment of trigeminal neuralgia results from a randomized, double-blind, placebo-controlled trial. *Cephalalgia*, *32*(6), 443–450. doi:10.1177/0333102412441721 PMID:22492424

Wu, C., Xie, N., Lian, Y., Xu, H., Chen, C., Zheng, Y., ... Zhang, H. (2016). Central antinociceptive activity of peripherally applied botulinum toxin type A in lab rat model of trigeminal neuralgia. *SpringerPlus*, *5*(1), 431. doi:10.118640064-016-2071-2 PMID:27104119

Wu, C.-Y., Meng, F.-G., Xu, S.-J., Liu, Y.-G., & Wang, H.-W. (2004). Selective percutaneous radiofrequency thermocoagulation in the treatment of trigeminal neuralgia: Report on 1860 cases. *Chinese Medical Journal*, *117*(3), 467–470. doi:10.1142/S0192415X04002120 PMID:15043796

Wu, T. H., Hu, L. Y., Lu, T., Chen, P. M., Chen, H. J., Shen, C. C., & Wen, C. H. (2015). Risk of psychiatric disorders following trigeminal neuralgia: A nationwide population-based retrospective cohort study. *The Journal of Headache and Pain*, *16*(1), 64. doi:10.118610194-015-0548-y PMID:26174508

Xia, L., Zhong, J., Zhu, J., Wang, Y.-N., Dou, N.-N., Liu, M.-X., ... Li, S.-T. (2014). Effectiveness and Safety of Microvascular Decompression Surgery for Treatment of Trigeminal Neuralgia. *The Journal of Craniofacial Surgery*, *25*(4), 1413–1417. doi:10.1097/SCS.0000000000000984 PMID:24978453

Xiao, L., Cheng, J., Zuang, Y., Qu, W., Muir, J., Liang, H., & Zhang, D. (2013). Botulinum toxin type A reduces hyperalgesia and TRPV1 expression in rats with neuropathic pain. *Pain Medicine*, *14*(2), 276–286. doi:10.1111/pme.12017 PMID:23301515

Xu, A. Y., Bhatnagar, J., Bednarz, G., Niranjan, A., Kondziolka, D., Flickinger, J., ... Huq, M. S. (2015). Gamma Knife radiosurgery with CT image-based dose calculation. *Journal of Applied Clinical Medical Physics*, *16*(6), 119–129. doi:10.1120/jacmp.v16i6.5530 PMID:26699563

Xu-Hui, W., Chun, Z., Guang-Jian, S., Min-Hui, X., Guang-Xin, C., Yong-Wen, Z., & Lun-Shan, X. (2011). Long-term outcomes of percutaneous retrogasserian glycerol rhizotomy in 3370 patients with trigeminal neuralgia. *Turkish Neurosurgery*, *21*(1), 48–52. Retrieved from http://www.ncbi.nlm.nih.gov/pubmed/21294091 PMID:21294091

Xu, S.-J., Zhang, W.-H., Chen, T., Wu, C.-Y., & Zhou, M. (2006). Neuronavigator-guided percutaneous radiofrequency thermocoagulation in the treatment of intractable trigeminal neuralgia. *Chinese Medical Journal*, *119*(18), 1528–1535. PMID:16996006

Yaltho, T. C., & Jankovic, J. (2011). The many faces of hemifacial spasm: Differential diagnosis of unilateral facial spasms. *Movement Disorders: Official Journal of the Movement Disorder Society*, *26*(9), 1582–1592. doi:10.1002/mds.23692 PMID:21469208

Yamada, Y., Kondo, A., & Tanabe, H. (2006). Trigeminal neuralgia associated with an anomalous artery originating from the persistent primitive trigeminal artery. *Neurologia Medico-Chirurgica*, *46*(4), 194–197. doi:10.2176/nmc.46.194 PMID:16636511

Yang, D. B., Jiang, D. Y., Chen, H. C., & Wang, Z. M. (2015). Second microvascular decompression for trigeminal neuralgia in recurrent cases after microvascular decompression. *The Journal of Craniofacial Surgery*, *26*(2), 491–494. doi:10.1097/SCS.0000000000001523 PMID:25759921

Yang, J.-T., Lin, M., Lee, M.-H., Weng, H.-H., & Liao, H.-H. (2010). Percutaneous trigeminal nerve radiofrequency rhizotomy guided by computerized tomography with three-dimensional image reconstruction. *Chang Gung Medical Journal*, *33*(6), 679–683. PMID:21199613

Yang, M., Zhou, M., He, L., Chen, N., & Zakrzewska, J. (2011). Non-antiepileptic drugs for trigeminal neuralgia. *Cochrane Database of Systematic Reviews*, *1*, CD004029. PMID:21249658

Yap, A. U., Tan, K. B., Chua, E. K., & Tan, H. H. (2002). Depression and somatization in patients with temporomandibular disorders. *The Journal of Prosthetic Dentistry*, *88*(5), 479–484. doi:10.1067/mpr.2002.129375 PMID:12473996

Yeh, H. S., & Tew, J. M. (1984). Tic convulsif, the combination of geniculate neuralgia and hemifacial spasm relieved by vascular decompression. *Neurology*, *34*(5), 682–683. doi:10.1212/WNL.34.5.682 PMID:6538661

Yomo, S., Arkha, Y., Donnet, A., & Régis, J. (2009). Gamma Knife surgery for glossopharyngeal neuralgia. *Journal of Neurosurgery*, *110*(3), 559–563. doi:10.3171/2008.8.17641 PMID:19025360

Yoshino, N., Akimoto, H., Yamada, I., Nagaoka, T., Tetsumura, A., Kurabayashi, T., ... Sasaki, T. (2003). Trigeminal Neuralgia: Evaluation of Neuralgic Manifestation and Site of Neurovascular Compression with 3D CISS MR Imaging and MR Angiography. *Radiology*, *228*(2), 539–545. doi:10.1148/radiol.2282020439 PMID:12802002

Younes, W. M., Capelle, H.-H., & Krauss, J. K. (2010). Microvascular decompression of the anterior inferior cerebellar artery for intermediate nerve neuralgia. *Stereotactic and Functional Neurosurgery*, *88*(3), 193–195. doi:10.1159/000313873 PMID:20431332

Young, B., Shivazad, A., Kryscio, R. J., St Clair, W., & Bush, H. M. (2013). Long-term outcome of high-dose γ knife surgery in treatment of trigeminal neuralgia. *Journal of Neurosurgery*, *119*(5), 1166–1175. doi:10.3171/2013.1.JNS12875 PMID:23600932

Young, R. F. (1988). Glycerol rhizolysis for treatment of trigeminal neuralgia. *Journal of Neurosurgery*, *69*(1), 39–45. doi:10.3171/jns.1988.69.1.0039 PMID:2454304

Young, R. F., Vermulen, S., & Posewitz, A. (1998). Gamma knife radiosurgery for the treatment of trigeminal neuralgia. *Stereotactic and Functional Neurosurgery*, *70*(Suppl 1), 192–199. doi:10.1159/000056422 PMID:9782251

Zakrzewska, J. M., & Linskey, M. E. (2016). Trigeminal Neuralgia. (1532-0650 (Electronic)).

Zakrzewska, J. M. (2010). Medical management of trigeminal neuropathic pains. *Expert Opinion on Pharmacotherapy*, *11*(8), 1239–1254. doi:10.1517/14656561003767449 PMID:20426709

Zakrzewska, J. M. (2016). Chronic/Persistent Idiopathic Facial Pain. *Neurosurgery Clinics of North America*, *27*(3), 345–351. doi:10.1016/j.nec.2016.02.012 PMID:27325001

Zakrzewska, J. M., & Akram, H. (2011). Neurosurgical interventions for the treatment of classical trigeminal neuralgia [Review]. *Cochrane Database of Systematic Reviews*, (9). doi:10.1002/14651858.CD007312.pub2 PMID:21901707

Zakrzewska, J. M., Chaudhry, Z., Nurmikko, T. J., Patton, D. W., & Mullens, E. L. (1997). Lamotrigine in refractory trigeminal neuralgia: Results from a double-blind placebo controlled crossover trial. *Pain*, *73*(2), 223–230. doi:10.1016/S0304-3959(97)00104-8 PMID:9415509

Zakrzewska, J. M., Jassim, S., & Bulman, J. S. (1999). A prospective, longitudinal study on patients with trigeminal neuralgia who underwent radiofrequency thermocoagulation of the Gasserian ganglion. *Pain*, *79*(1), 51–58. doi:10.1016/S0304-3959(98)00145-6 PMID:9928776

Zakrzewska, J. M., & Linskey, M. E. (2014). Trigeminal neuralgia. *BMJ (Clinical Research Ed.)*, 348. PMID:24534115

Zakrzewska, J., & Patsalos, P. (1989). Oxcarbazepine: A new drug in the management of intractable trigeminal neuralgia. *Journal of Neurology, Neurosurgery, and Psychiatry*, *52*(4), 472–476. doi:10.1136/jnnp.52.4.472 PMID:2738589

Zakrzewska, J., & Patsalos, P. (2002). Long-term cohort study comparing medical (oxcarbazepine) and surgical management of intractable trigeminal neuralgia. *Pain*, *95*(3), 259–266. doi:10.1016/S0304-3959(01)00406-7 PMID:11839425

Zhang, H., Lian, Y., Ma, Y., Chen, Y., He, C., Xie, N., & Wu, C. (2014). Two doses of botulinum toxin type A for the treatment of trigeminal neuralgia: Observation of therapeutic effect from a randomized, double-blind, double-blind, placebo controlled trial. *The Journal of Headache and Pain, 15*(1), 65. doi:10.1186/1129-2377-15-65 PMID:25263254

Zhang, H., Qian, Y. L., Li, C., Liu, D., Wang, L., Wang, X. Y., ... Cao, J. L. (2017). Brain-Derived Neurotrophic Factor in the Mesolimbic Reward Circuitry Mediates Nociception in Chronic Neuropathic Pain. *Biological Psychiatry, 82*(8), 608–618. doi:10.1016/j.biopsych.2017.02.1180 PMID:28390647

Zhang, X., Xu, L., Zhao, H., Tang, Y. D., Zhu, J., Yuan, Y., ... Li, S. T. (2017). Long-term efficacy of nerve combing for the patients with trigeminal neuralgia who failed prior microvascular decompression. *World Neurosurgery, 108*, 711–715. doi:10.1016/j.wneu.2017.09.081

Zhao, C., Stillman, M., & Rozen, T. (2005). Traditional and evidence-based acupuncture in headache management: Theory, mechanism, and practice. *Headache, 45*(6), 716–730. doi:10.1111/j.1526-4610.2005.05139.x PMID:15953304

Zhao, H., Zhang, X., Tang, D., & Li, S. (2017). Nerve Combing for Trigeminal Neuralgia Without Vascular Compression. *The Journal of Craniofacial Surgery, 28*(1), e15–e16. doi:10.1097/SCS.0000000000003161 PMID:27875506

Zhao, Z.-F., Yang, L.-Z., Jiang, C.-L., Zheng, Y.-R., & Zhang, J.-W. (2010). Gamma Knife irradiation–induced histopathological changes in the trigeminal nerves of rhesus monkeys. *Journal of Neurosurgery, 113*(1), 39–44. doi:10.3171/2010.1.JNS091116 PMID:20170304

Zheng, X., Feng, B., Hong, W., Zhang, W., Yang, M., Tang, Y., ... Li, S. (2012). Management of intraneural vessels during microvascular decompression surgery for trigeminal neuralgia. *World Neurosurgery, 77*(5-6), 771–774. doi:10.1016/j.wneu.2011.08.031 PMID:22120295

Zhou, X., Liu, Y., Yue, Z., Luan, D., Zhang, H., & Han, J. (2016). Comparison of nerve combing and percutaneous radiofrequency thermocoagulation in the treatment for idiopathic trigeminal neuralgia. *Revista Brasileira de Otorrinolaringologia (English Ed.), 82*(5), 574–579. doi:10.1016/j.bjorl.2015.11.006 PMID:26832635

Zhu, S., Rong, Q., Chen, S., & Li, X. (2013). Pterygopalatine fossa segment neurectomy of maxillary nerve through maxillary sinus route in treating trigeminal neuralgia. *Journal of Cranio-Maxillo-Facial Surgery: Official Publication of the European Association for Cranio-Maxillo-Facial Surgery, 41*(7), 652–656. doi:10.1016/j.jcms.2013.01.002 PMID:23375531

Zorro, Lobato-Polo, Hideyuki, Flannery, Flickinger, & Lunsford. (2010). *Gamma Knife stereotactic radiosurgery for idiopathic trigeminal neuralgia*. Academic Press. doi:10.3171/2009.7.JNS09694

Zuniga, C., Piedimonte, F., Diaz, S., & Micheli, F. (2013). Acute Treatment of Trigeminal Neuralgia with Onabotulinum Toxin A. *Clinical Neuropharmacology, 36*(5), 146–150. doi:10.1097/WNF.0b013e31829cb60e PMID:24045604

About the Contributors

Steven D. Chang, MD is the Robert C. and Jeannette Powell Professor and Vice-Chair of the Department of Neurosurgery at the Stanford University School of Medicine. He is also the Director of the Stanford Cyberknife Program, the Stanford Neuromolecular Innovations Program, and the Stanford Neurogenetics Program. He is a world renown expert in tumor and cerebrovascular neurosurgery and a innovator in open, microscopic, endoscopic, and radiosurgical approaches to lesions of the brain and skull base. He is also a leader in the treatment of trigeminal neuralgia, with a large practice and clinical research effort dedicated specifically to patients with the disease and a specific emphasis on open microsurgical and non-invasive radiosurgical treatments.

Allen L. Ho, MD is a graduate of Harvard Medical School where he was a Howard Hughes Medical Research Fellow and is now a neurosurgery resident in the Department of Neurosurgery at the Stanford University School of Medicine. He is interested in expanding indications for neuromodulation, and technology-driven minimally-invasive and stereotactic approaches to cranial and spinal neurosurgery. He has won numerous national awards and grants for his research efforts and is specifically focused on how to improve treatment outcomes for patients with trigeminal neuralgia.

***

Huy M. Do, MD, is a Professor of Radiology and Neurosurgery at Stanford University School of Medicine, Medical Center, and Stroke Center. He is an interventional neuroradiologist with over 25 years of clinical practice. He is an expert in the treatment of neurovascular diseases (AVM, aneurysm, stroke, tumor) and pain related to the nervous system such as cranial facial pain syndromes and axial skeletal pain. He is on multiple editorial boards, and has published over 100 peer review papers.

Alexander Dru is currently a fourth-year medical student at the University of Arizona College of Medicine-Tucson.

Stephen Haines is professor of Neurosurgery, Otolaryngology and Pediatrics at the University of Minnesota. He is a graduate of the University of Vermont Larner College of Medicine and the Neurosurgical Residency Training Program at the University of Pittsburgh. His clinical interests are trigeminal neuralgia, skull base neurosurgery and pediatric neurosurgery. His research centers on the application of sophisticated clinical research methods to neurosurgical practice.

Alice L. Hung graduated college from Johns Hopkins University in 2013. She is currently a medical student at Johns Hopkins School of Medicine.

M. Yashar S. Kalani, MD, PhD, is Assistant Professor, Division of Neurological Surgery, Barrow Neurological Institute, Phoenix, Arizona, USA. Neurosurgical Resident Division of Neurological Surgery Barrow Neurological Institute St. Joseph's Hospital and Medical Center Phoenix, Arizona.

Michael R. Levitt, M.D., received his medical degree from Loyola University Stritch School of Medicine in Chicago, IL. He completed his neurological surgery residency at the University of Washington in Seattle, WA and at St. George's University of London in the United Kingdom. He is currently a fellow in endovascular neurosurgery at the Barrow Neurological Institute in Phoenix, AZ.

Celene Mulholland attended University of California, San Diego for her undergraduate studies in cognitive neuroscience. She subsequently completed a masters degree in public health at Rollins School of Public Health at Emory University and spent several years working at the Centers for Disease Control and Prevention. She was fortunate to return back to Los Angeles for medical school.

Peter Nakaji, MD, FACS, FAANS, Professor of Neurosurgery Director, Neurosurgery Residency Program Director, Minimally Invasive Neurosurgery Division of Neurological Surgery Barrow Neurological Institute Phoenix, Arizona.

James Pan is finishing up medical school at Stanford and is currently applying to residency programs in Neurosurgery.

J. Scott Pannell, M.D., is a board certified neurointerventional radiologist who specializes in endovascular neurosurgery and neuroradiology. Dr. Pannell specializes in the catheter-based treatment of ischemic stroke, cerebral aneurysms, arteriovenous malformations, carotid stenosis, vascular tumors, and interventional management of pain associated with disorders of the spine. His research interests include ischemic stroke, endothelial injury, and simulator based angiography training.

Bret Schneider specializes in brain neuromodulation technologies for interventional psychiatry, neurology and regenerative medicine including rTMS and radiomodulation. He earned a BA cum laude from Washington University in St. Louis, an MD degree from Rush University in Chicago, and graduated a clinical residency in Psychiatry at UCLA. He subsequently completed a post-doctoral fellowship in neurosurgical stereotactic radiosurgery and a post-doctoral fellowship in Advanced Psychiatry, both at Stanford University Bret is presently Chief Medical Officer for Zap Surgical Systems, where he is developing stereotactic radiosurgery as a tool for precise, non-invasive modulation of dysfunctional brain circuits, has a psychiatry private practice, and is Adjunct Professor of Psychiatry at the Stanford University School of Medicine.

Andrew Shetter, Barrow Neurological Institute, Division of Neurological Surgery Chairman, Section of Functional and Stereotactic Neurosurgery Co-Director, Gamma Knife Center.

Charlie Teo was born in Sydney, Australia and was educated at the Scots College. After graduating from the University of New South Wales medical school he embarked initially on a career in paediatric surgery and then neurosurgery, finally sub-specialising in paediatric neurosurgery. He was accepted at the Children's Medical Center, Dallas, Texas for a fellowship in paediatric neurosurgery and was strongly encouraged to stay in the United States. From Texas, Charlie moved to Little Rock, Arkansas, where he was rapidly promoted from Assistant Professor to Associate Professor of Neurosurgery at the University of Arkansas and developed an international reputation in the field of minimally invasive neurosurgery. Charlie has been an invited speaker and Visiting Professor to almost every continent and over 50 countries, including such prestigious centres in the USA, as Johns Hopkins, Vanderbilt, Emory, Stanford and Albert Einstein Universities and the Barrow Neurological Institute, as well as Marbourg University in Germany and the Karolinska Institute in Sweden. He was the International Scholar at UCSF in 2008. Since returning to Australia, Charlie has continued to develop pioneering procedures and is invited back to the USA at least 4 times a year to teach courses in these keyhole approaches. Indeed, a fellowship program started by him in 2000 is now filled with overseas neurosurgeons until the year 2017, all thirsty to learn his innovative techniques. In keeping with his passion for teaching and philanthropy, Charlie devotes 4 months of his time each year to educate neurosurgeons from developing countries such as Cuba, Peru, Indonesia and Vietnam, and to treat children with neurological conditions in those countries. Charlie primarily works at the Prince of Wales Private Hospital and has established an internationally acclaimed centre specialising in the treatment of adult and childhood brain tumours. The techniques and skills that he offers at the Centre have saved or extended the lives of many children from Australia and abroad with so called "inoperable" brain tumours. These patients have come to Sydney from all over the world. Charlie is currently the Director of the Centre for Minimally Invasive Neurosurgery, the author of the Australian Guidelines for the Management of Low Grade Gliomas, on the editorial board of several neurosurgical journals and a Founding Board Member of V.I.N.E. (volunteers for international neurosurgical education). He is the Founder of the Cure for Life Foundation which has successfully raised over 9 million dollars and is the largest charity devoted to the advancement and treatment of patients with brain tumours. Charlie has written over 100 publications, 30 book chapters and two books. He has been featured on Australian Story, "60 Minutes", "Good Medicine", "Last Chance Surgery" and "Today Tonight", highlighting patients with "inoperable" brain tumours that he has successfully removed. He is the subject of a best-selling book by Susan Wyndham "Life in his Hands". His dedication to neurosurgery and charitable efforts were rewarded in 2003 and 2009 when Charlie was NSW State finalist for the prestigious, Australian of the Year award and in 2005 he joined the ranks of such great Australians as Steve Waugh, Sir William Deane and Dame Joan Sutherland when awarded the Vocational Service Award by the Rotary Club. In 2007, he was given the Paul Harris Fellowship for his contribution to International Health and Welfare and in 2008 and 2014 the Humanitarian Service Award by Rotary International and the International Society of Brain Mapping and Therapeutics, respectively. In 2010 he was made a Member of the Order of Australia and in 2011 was asked to give the Australia Day Address to the Nation. In 2013 he became the first non-politician Australian to address the US Congress on the need for more funding for brain cancer research. He was most honoured to be the Invited Guest Speaker at the International Conference on Happiness and Its Causes and in 2009 shared the podium with His Holiness the Dalai Lama at the Mind and Its Potential Conference. Always the patient advocate, Charlie lives by the principle of treating all his patients as he would a member of his own family. Supported by his wife, Genevieve, and four daughters, Alex, Nikki, Katie and Sophie, Charlie has devoted his life to helping people with neurosurgical diseases.

Daivik Vyas is a medical student at the Stanford University School of Medicine.

Arvin Wali is a fourth-year medical student pursuing neurosurgical residency with a background in clinical and cost-effectiveness research.

Niushen Zhang is a board certified neurologist and clinical assistant professor in the Department of Neurology at Stanford University. She is the Headache Fellowship Program Director. She has a special interest in complementary and alternative medicine for the treatment of headache and facial pain. Dr. Zhang graduated from Yale University with a Bachelor of Science degree in Molecular, Cellular and Developmental Biology. She attended New York University School of Medicine and completed neurology residency and a fellowship in headache and facial pain at Stanford University.

Index

G

H

I

J

K

L

M

N

O

P

R

S

T

U

V

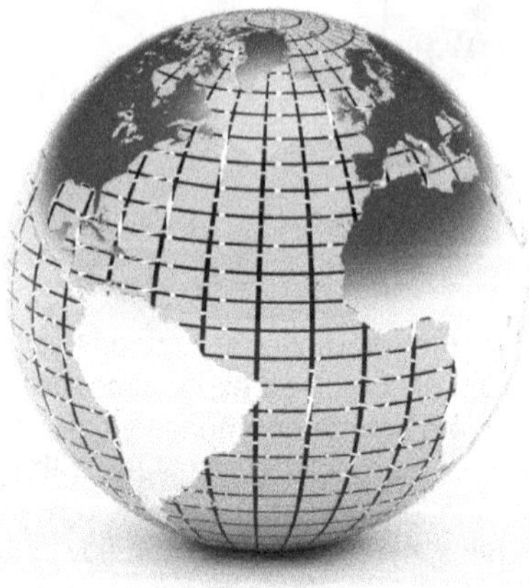

www.ingramcontent.com/pod-product-compliance
Lightning Source LLC
LaVergne TN
LVHW081249011026
849162LV00004BA/970